THE ULTIMATE MEDICAL TOURISM MANUAL

How to Save Thousands of Dollars on State-Of-The-Art Treatment Abroad

ಸೋ • ಧ

Bill Heid

The Ultimate Medical Tourism Manual: How to Save Thousands of Dollars on State-Of-The-Art Treatment Abroad
© 2011 Bill Heid

A product of Solutions From Science

Notice of Rights

Manufactured in the United States of America. All rights reserved. No part of this book may be reproduced in any form or by any electronic or mechanical means, including information storage or retrieval systems, without permission in writing by the copyright owner. For more products by Solutions From Science, please visit us on the web at www.solutionsfromscience.com

Notice of Liability

The information in this book is distributed on an "as is" basis, for informational purposes only, without warranty. While every precaution has been taken in the production of this book, neither the copyright owner nor Heritage Press Publications, LLC shall have any liability to any person or entity with respect to any liability, loss, or damage caused or alleged to be caused directly or indirectly by the instructions contained in this book.

Heritage Press Publications

Published by:
Heritage Press Publications, LLC
PO Box 561
Collinsville, MS 39325

ISBN 13: 978-1-937660-03-1
ISBN 10: 1-937660-03-6

Table of Contents

Acknowledgements	19
Foreword	21
Chapter 1: **The State of the U.S. Healthcare System**	25
Intro to Obamacare	27
Obamacare for Everyone!	27
There's No Assurance with This Insurance	28
Tighter Government Control Strangles Healthcare Freedom	29
Obamacare Is Socialized Medicine	30
The Eight U.S. Healthcare Myths Revealed	31
MYTH #1: The U.S. Healthcare Bill Is about Health	32
MYTH #2: Starting This Year, People with Pre-existing Conditions Will No Longer Be Denied Insurance	33
MYTH #3: The New Healthcare System Will Save Everyone Money	33
MYTH #4: Healthcare Reform Will Help Small Businesses	34
MYTH #5: Obamacare is Not Socialism at Work	35
MYTH #6: You Can Keep Your Current Insurance Plan	36
MYTH #7: The Quality of Medical Services Will Improve	37
MYTH #8: You Can Stay with Your Family Doctor	38

CONTENTS

How the New Healthcare Legislation Will Ruin America	39
Financial Costs	39
Ruining the Medical System	40
Unemployment	41
Taxes Will Cripple the Economy	43
Poverty Will Spread	43
The State of Control	44
The End of Market-Based Rationing	45
Who Does This New Healthcare System Really Benefit?	46
The U.S. Federal Government	46
Big Pharma	47
Wall Street	48
The Insurance Companies	48
Shutting Down the Health Industry	50
Goodbye Freedom – What Obamacare Means to Americans	50
The Freedom to Choose	50
Free Market System Collapses	51
No More Limits	51
Cover the Children	52
Your New Insurance Plan	52
Doctor Whisperers	52
Expanding Your Practice	53
Successful Career	53
Impact on the American Family	53
Your Constitutional Rights	54
The Road Ahead	54

Chapter 2: **Corruption, Greed and U.S. Politics**   58

   United We Stand, Dividing the Profits –
   How Healthcare Providers Get Away with Murder   58
      The Government Bankrupting America   59
      Death to Hospital Quality   62
      Death to American Patients   63
      Big Pharma, Big Sales   64
      Big Insurance, Limited Health   65

   Health Shock – The Hidden Legislation
   You Need to Know About   66
      Saving for Old Age   66
      Education Based on Race   67
      Again, More Taxes   68
      Obama's Private Army?   69
      Marriage Penalty   69
      Counting Calories   70
      Cosmetic Surgery Tax   71
      The Special Needs Tax   72
      Breastfeeding Rooms   72

   Why the U.S. Well of Health Will Run Dry   74
      Failure to Control Price Increases   75
      Failure to Give the People What They Want   76
      Failure to Keep Trained Medical
      Professionals Happy   76
      The Medical Brain Drain   77
      The Health Shortage   79

CONTENTS

Chapter 3: Finding a Solution to this Looming Problem — 82

Chronic Disease Treatment – Why Low Cost Isn't an Option — 83
- Coverage for All Means Coverage for None — 84
- Rationing Your Healthcare — 85
- Outright Denial of Treatment — 86
- Stunted Growth in Disease Treatment — 87
- Limited Access to Specialists and Medicine — 88
- Increase in Medical Malpractice — 89

The United States of Controlled Healthcare — 90
- Controlled Health of the Public — 90
- Public Health Measures — 91
- Mandatory Microchips — 93
- IRS and Control — 93
- Welcome to Big Brother — 94

The Effects of a Failing Healthcare System — 95
- The Short-term Effects of Obamacare — 95
- The Long-term Effects of Obamacare — 97

Why Medical Tourism Is Your Cost-effective Healthcare Alternative — 100
- Is It Really Cheaper to Get Medical Services Abroad? — 100
- Discovering the Real Cost of Medical Tourism — 102
- Saving Money the Smart Way — 103

Success Story: Medical Tourism Changing Lives — 104

Chapter 4: Introduction to Global Medical Tourism — 108

Why Choose to Travel Abroad for
Medical Services Now? — 109

The Four Types of Medical Travel — 111
- Elective Surgery — 111
- Emergency Surgery — 115
- Treatment for Chronic Disease — 119
- Alternative Medical Treatment — 123

Why Your Doctor Thinks It's a Bad Idea — 126
- Old-School Ideas of Medical Tourism — 127
- What about Legal Issues? — 128
- Higher Risk of Infection — 128

Beat the Cost Barriers with Medical Benefits Abroad — 129
- Your Medical Vacation — 129
- Increasing Quality of Care — 130
- Ease of Use — 130
- Working Out the Exact Cost — 131
- Licensed and JCI-approved — 132
- Competitive Care — 132
- The Two-Way Street — 132

Your First Steps to Improved Health
and Wellness Abroad — 133
- Determining Your Immediate Need — 133
- Destination Hospital — 134
- Doing It Alone — 135
- Going Through a Medical Travel Agent — 135

One Step Forward — 136

CONTENTS

Chapter 5: **Affordable Elective Surgery Abroad** — 138

Questions You Should Ask Your Doctor — 138
- Please tell me about your training and education — 138
- Would you send me your CV? — 139
- Is your hospital accredited? — 139
- Do you agree on the surgical procedures I need done, or are there other alternatives? — 140
- How safe is this elective procedure? — 140
- What is your personal success rate? — 140
- How is the surgery performed? — 141
- How long does it take? — 142
- What is the average recovery time for the surgery? — 142

Cosmetic Surgery — 143
- #1 Breast Augmentation — 144
- #2 Face and Neck Lift — 145
- #3 Liposuction — 146
- #4 Rhinoplasty — 147
- #5 Blepharoplasty — 148

Dental Surgery — 150
- #1 Dental Implants — 150
- #2 Jaw Bone Grafting — 151
- #3 Endodontic Surgery — 152
- #4 Extraction — 153
- #5 Dental Bridge — 154

Non-Surgical Dental Procedures — 156
- #1 Whitening your Teeth — 156
- #2 Dental Veneers — 157
- #3 Dental Fillings — 158

#4 Dentures	159
#5 Gum Treatment	160
Medical Procedures	**161**
#1 Orthopedic Surgery: Hip Replacement	162
#2 Cardiovascular Surgery: Pacemaker Implant	163
#3 Gynecological Surgery: Hysterectomy	164
#4 Diagnostic Surgery: Biopsy	164
Fertility Treatment	**165**
#1 In Vitro Fertilization	166
#2 Frozen Embryo Transfer	166
#3 Intracytoplasmic Sperm Injection	167
#4 Gamete Intrafallopian Transfer	168
#5 Ovary Transplant	169
Laser Eye Surgery	**169**
Testimonials from Elective Surgery Patients	**171**
Price Chart – Surgical Procedures Only	**174**

Chapter 6: **Affordable Emergency Surgery Abroad**   182

Questions You Should Ask Your Doctor in the Intensive Care Unit after Trauma Surgery	182
What is my current condition?	183
Please give me a full description of the surgeries I've had	183
What medications am I currently on?	183
What additional procedures or surgeries do I still need?	184

CONTENTS

What tests were performed, and what tests still need to be done? ... 184
How long will I have to stay in the hospital? ... 185
What are the risks involved if I travel? ... 185
How much will staying here cost? ... 185

Hiring an Air Ambulance or Other Medical Transport ... 186

General Surgery ... 186
    Emergency Gastrectomy ... 188
    Emergency Gall Bladder Removal ... 189
    Emergency Appendectomy ... 191
    Emergency Inguinal Hernia Repair ... 192
    Emergency Mastectomy ... 194
    Emergency Spleen Removal ... 195
    Lung Transplant ... 197
    Large Internal Hemorrhoid Surgery ... 199

Specialist Surgery ... 200
    Neurosurgery: Brain Tumor Surgery ... 201
    Orthopedic Surgery: Spinal Fusion ... 202
    Vascular Surgery:
    Abdominal Aortic Aneurysm Repair ... 204
    Cardiac Surgery: Aortic Valve Replacement ... 206
    Pediatric Surgery: Pyloromyotomy ... 208

Testimonials from Emergency Surgery Patients ... 210
    Name: Allen Miller, Washington ... 210
    Name: Sue Nagy, Illinois ... 210
    Name: Conchetta Procopio, Arizona ... 211

Price Chart – Surgical Procedures Only ... 212

Chapter 7: Affordable Chronic Disease Treatment Abroad — 216

Questions You Should Ask Your Doctor — 217
    Do you regularly provide treatment for my condition? — 217
    Do you have facilities for long-term care? — 218
    Is your surgical unit prepared for emergency surgeries arising from a chronic disease? — 218
    Does your hospital provide any alternative treatments in conjunction with mainstream modern medicine? — 219
    Do you offer counseling for patients and families dealing with my condition? — 219
    Are there any clinical trials I can participate in? — 219
    What can I expect when I arrive for my treatment? — 220
    What medical records and test results should I bring with me? — 220
    How much will my treatment cost? — 220

Cancer — 221
    Main Variants of Cancer — 221
    Treatment Options — 222
    Long-term Medical Care — 223

Type 2 Diabetes — 224
    Other Main Variants of Diabetes — 225
    Treatment Options — 225
    Long-term Medical Care — 227

CONTENTS

Heart Disease   227
    Main Variants of Heart Disease   228
    Treatment Options   229
    Long-term Medical Care   230

Kidney Disease   231
    Main Variants of Kidney Disease   231
    Treatment Options   232
    Long-term Medical Care   233

Chronic Respiratory Illness   234
    Main Variants of Chronic Respiratory Illness   234
    Treatment Options   235
    Long-term Medical Care   236

Obesity   236
    Main Diseases Linked to Obesity   237
    Treatment Options   238
    Long-term Medical Care   239

Stem Cell Treatment   240
    Main Diseases That Can Be Treated with Stem Cells: 240
    Cancer Stem Cell Transplantation   241
    Stem Cell Treatment You Can't Get in the U.S.   241
    Long-term Medical Care   241

Mental Illness   242
    Main Variants of Mental Illness   243
    Treatment Options   243
    Long-term Medical Care   244

Addiction	245
Main Variants of Addiction	246
Treatment Options	246
Long-term Medical Care	247
Chronic Disease Care	247
Prevent Illness	248
Get Regular Diagnostic Testing	248
Follow Your Doctor's Plan	248
Testimonials from Chronic Disease Patients	249
Name: Rand Loftness, WA	249
Name: Dr. O, Oklahoma	249
Price Chart	251

Chapter 8: **Affordable Alternative Medicine Abroad**   256

Questions You Should Ask Your Doctor	257
Which alternative treatments do you specialize in?	257
Tell me about the process. How does it work?	258
What benefits can I expect from this treatment?	258
Will I be given herbal medicine, and if so,	
what are the side effects?	259
What kind of facilities do you have?	259
How are you uniquely qualified	
to do these treatments?	260
Have you treated anyone with my specific	
condition before?	260
Alternative Cancer Treatments	261
Immunotherapy	261
Nutritional Therapies	262

CONTENTS

Adjunctive Therapies	263
Biological Therapies	263
Revici Therapy	264
Antineoplastons	264
Homeopathy	**264**
Classical Medicine	265
Constitutional Medicine	265
Allergodes, Nosodes and Sarcodes	266
Complex Medicine	266
Homeopathy Abroad	267
Chelation Therapy	**267**
Naturopathic Medicine	**269**
Physical Medicine	269
Psychological Medicine	269
Light Surgery	270
Nutrition	270
Homeopathic Medicine	270
Botanical Medicine	270
Naturopathic Obstetrics	271
Ayurvedic Medicine	**272**
The Vata Type	272
The Pitta Type	273
The Kapha Type	273
Acupuncture	**273**
Chinese Acupuncture	274
Japanese Acupuncture	274
Korean Acupuncture	275
Five-Element Acupuncture	275

Auricular Acupuncture	275
Trigger Point Acupuncture	275
Hyperbaric Oxygen Therapy	276
Oxygen Concentrators	277
Compressed Oxygen Cylinders	277
Liquid Oxygen Systems	277
Multiplace Chamber	278
Biofeedback Therapy	278
Electromyography (EMG)	279
Thermal Biofeedback	279
Electroencephalography (EEG)	279
Finger Pulse Measurements	280
Respiration Biofeedback	280
Spa Retreats	281
Health Spa	281
Resort Spa	282
Day Spa	282
Mineral Springs Spa	283
Medical Spa	283
Testimonial from an Alternative Medicine Patient	284
Price Chart	285

Chapter 9: **Everything You Need to Know Before You Go** 288

Become a Successful Medical Traveler	289
Breaking through the Culture Clash	289
Medical Tourism Safety	290
JCI-approved Hospitals and Other Accreditations	291

CONTENTS

Finance at the Ready	292
Informing Your Local Doctor	294
Planning Your Medical Expedition Abroad	**294**
Step 1: Behold, Fast Information!	295
Step 2: Making a Quick Getaway	298
Step 3: The Finer Points of Travel	299
Step 4: Your Safety Net	301
Step 5: Preparing Yourself	303
When You Arrive	**305**
Meeting Your Doctor	305
Discussing Treatment Options	305
Handing Over Medical Records	306
Poking Around the Hospital	307
Pre-Operative Checks	307
Make Copies of Your Test Results	307
Getting the Most Out of Your Stay	**308**
Vacation Time Planning	308
Tours	309
Things to Pack	309
Your Guide to Recovery	**311**
Hospital Stay	311
Private Nurses	312
The Dos and Don'ts after Surgery or Treatment	313
Medications	313
Post-Op Checks	314
New Medical Records	314
Continuity of Care	**314**
Returning Home	315

Contacting Your Local Doctor 315
What to Do if the Worst Happens 316
Spreading the Word 316

Medical Tourism Solves the U.S. Healthcare Crisis ... 317

Chapter 10: **Destination Profiling: Countries, Facilities and Treatments** 320

Where Do I Go for My Specific Medical Concern? ... 320
   Spotlight on Panama: Orthopedics 321
   Spotlight on Dubai: Dental Care 321
   Spotlight on South Africa: Cosmetic Surgery ... 321
   Spotlight on Singapore: Neurosurgery 321
   Spotlight on Saudi Arabia: Diabetes 322
   Spotlight on New Zealand: Pediatrics 322
   Spotlight on India: Cardiology 322
   Spotlight on Mexico: Emergency Surgery 322
   Spotlight on Thailand: Alternative Medicine ... 323
   Spotlight on Philippines: Weight Loss Surgery ... 323
   Spotlight on South Korea: Spinal Disorders 323
   Spotlight on Europe: Stem Cell Treatment 323
   Spotlight on Malaysia: Reproductive Health ... 323
   Spotlight on Costa Rica: Oncology 324
   Spotlight on Belize: Eye Surgery 324

The Top Four Destinations for Fast,
Excellent Medical Care 324
   Top Destination #1: Panama 324
   Top Destination #2: Belize 328
   Top Destination #3: Mexico 331
   Top Destination #4: Costa Rica 333

Other Worthy Destinations for
Global Medical Travel   336
    Dubai   336
    South Africa   340
    Singapore   342
    Saudi Arabia   344
    New Zealand   346
    India   348
    Thailand   350
    Philippines   352
    South Korea   354
    Europe   356
    Malaysia   359

Medical Glossary   362

Resources for the Medical Traveler   380

Endnotes   385

References   405

Index   451

Acknowledgements

This book is the result of months of research and collaboration with medical professionals and medical tourism agencies. A big thank you to Hospital Punta Pacifica's CEO Richard Larison and its Marketing & Communications Director, Asbell Burillo, who provided much useful information about their country and hospital. Your contribution and friendly collaboration were greatly appreciated! Another mention must go to Lorraine Melvill, of Surgeon and Safari (South Africa), for her wonderful conversation and contributions to this book; and to Life Smile Healthcare at HealthToursIndia.com, for their many touching testimonials and their assistance throughout the writing process. To all of the other medical tourism companies, doctors and patients who contributed: Thank you for your willingness to participate. This book could not have been created without the time, knowledge and involvement of these wonderful contributors.

Foreword

Medical tourism was once an experience for the brave, courageous and determined souls of the Western world. These days, with the cost of American healthcare growing and the new changes in legislation coming into effect, the medical traveler has morphed into a savvy medical pioneer, seeking alternatives to remain healthy, happy and financially secure. For many people, medical travel has become an increasingly popular choice. This book was created to inform you that there are alternatives available to you for quality medical care and professionalism outside of the United States.

The Republic of Panama, for example, is a rising star in international medical care. The solid steps taken by the country towards democracy in the last two decades have fostered a steady period of growth, attracting foreign investment capital throughout the 1990s and 2000s. Panama's economic stability and increasing role in international commerce are two of the factors that motivated a group of highly-trained local physicians to establish Hospital Punta Pacifica, the first medical facility in Latin America affiliated with Johns Hopkins Medicine International. With the hospital's inception in 1999, the creators of Hospital Punta Pacifica aspired to establish a medical center that would offer first-class services for all Panamanians, and that would expand its services to international patients through medical tourism. Today, they continue to cater to medical travelers who desire the best medical services possible at significantly reduced prices.

Started as a single-person operation in the office of Asbell Burillo, the hospital's Marketing & Communications Director, Punta Pacifica's Medical Tourism department has grown into a program capable of receiving e-mails and phone calls from around the world 24/7, and handling all medical cases of the country's growing cruise ship industry. Although the sector as a whole is still growing, Punta Pacifica's service structure is well developed. In Panama, most private medical facilities maintain a traditional approach to business, something we were able to use to our advantage. Panama features all the elements needed for a rapid development of the medical tourism sector. We have everything that a patient from North America or Europe looks for in terms of comfort and quality: a cosmopolitan, first-world capital city full of excellent restaurants and hotels; and a large Spanish/English bilingual population. The concept of medical tourism in the region is not new. However, this presents no threat to the hospital's medical tourism program as other countries offering medical tourism packages tend to focus on "low-end treatments." Our program offers high-end procedures such as neurosurgery, plastic surgery, orthopedics, in vitro fertilization, bariatric medicine and other specialties – all at a fraction of the cost of similar procedures up north.

The present state of the world's economy, the increasing costs of medical services in the United States, and the rising number of uninsured families are also contributing to boost Punta Pacifica's program. Many people in the U.S. and Canada are looking for options. Our services, for example, have been extremely beneficial for numerous Hispanic residents who often struggle with insurance costs. The hospital staff has launched an aggressive marketing campaign that involves establishing contact with international brokers, attending various trade fairs overseas, and joining forces with the ATP, Panama's Tourism Authority. The program is rapidly helping to raise the standards of the country's tourism industry, the members of which are improving their services tremendously in order to offer our patients an enjoyable stay and recovery period.

Dr. Julio Arias, a specialist in hand and microsurgery, is a passionate member of Punta Pacifica's medical tourism staff. Arias, who trained at the universities of Panamá, Arkansas and Yale, stated that "being capable of treating patients from all over the world who have not been able to get answers elsewhere is a gratifying experience for me.... Panama is state-of-the-art in this field, and other countries are aware of that." The country's role as an international business center has been one of the main factors behind the development of Punta Pacifica's Plastic Surgery department. Our patients, many of whom are businesspeople visiting Panama, come from everywhere: the U.S., Canada, South America, and even as far away as Australia and New Zealand. Punta Pacifica is equipped to offer a wide range of aesthetic and reconstructive treatments with the latest technology. A good percentage of Punta Pacifica's foreign patients are baby boomers seeking orthopedic treatment for age and sports-related problems and injuries. Many of them are referred to Dr. Salomon Dayan, one of the most prominent Panamanian physicians in the field of orthopedic surgery. A graduate of the University of Panama and prestigious New York City institutions, Dr. Dayan, whose clinic is part of the Punta Pacifica complex, says that his greatest pleasure in working at the hospital is to help people transform their lives. "I recently had the honor of treating a gentleman who came to me in a wheelchair with both of his hips completely damaged. Due to the success of his first surgery, he decided to have the second one with us. He is now able to walk perfectly, and visits Panama regularly with his family for pleasure."

One of the program's happy faces is that of Brenda Hill, an expat from San Francisco, California who lived for 18 months in the mountain town of Boquete before moving to Panama City in September of 2009. A retiree getting used to her new environs, Hill immediately started searching the web for high-quality healthcare facilities. "I found a number of articles published in local newspapers, and decided to try Punta Pacifica. The services are nothing less than excellent. I was welcomed at the hospital by bilingual professionals who explained each

FOREWORD

plan and package available in full detail and in perfect English.... It was truly a positive experience." With hospitals like Punta Pacifica just hours away, Americans are guaranteed quality medical care, even when there is none to be had in the States.

This definitive medical text will explain to you, the American patient, what is actually going on in your country, how it will impact your life, and how medical tourism can stand by your side through it all. After months of intensive research, investigation and compilation, it's all here for you to discover. Follow Bill Heid through this life-saving medical text, and add your name to the list of people who have read the most outspoken and important medical book ever released in America.

Regards,
Richard Larison, CEO
Hospital Punta Pacifica

CHAPTER 1

THE STATE OF THE U.S. HEALTHCARE SYSTEM

The State of the U.S. Healthcare System

☙ • ❧

America offers the most expensive healthcare services in the world – did you know that? Hospital bills and prescription medication are more costly here than anywhere else on the globe. Couple this with the fact that 47 million Americans don't have health insurance because premiums are so high, and you're looking at a lot of people who will never get the medical attention they deserve. Now, imagine if everyone had medical insurance! Sounds great – but what do you think would happen if prices weren't lowered at the same time so that people could afford their new insurance? What would happen if the government taxed the hell out of your personal income so they could provide medical care for everybody else? What would happen if you couldn't get medical attention because you were still uninsured?

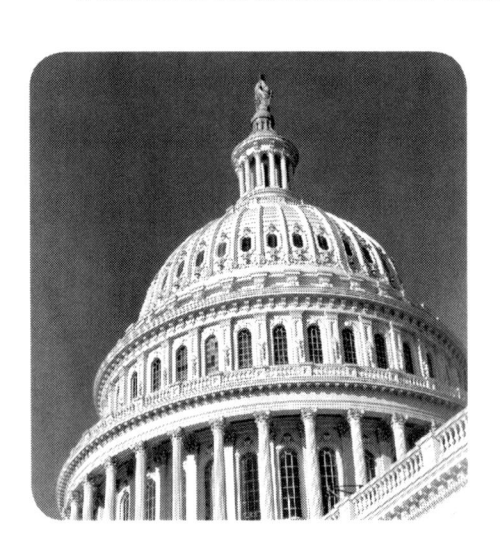

Welcome to the state of the new U.S. healthcare system. In this book, we explore our reformed healthcare legislation and expose it for what it really is: another step toward supreme government control of America. There's nothing we can do about it now except find better healthcare alternatives abroad. That is what this book is all about. Our goal is to help you understand Obamacare, and how it will affect your life and the lives of your loved ones. If the worst should happen, we want you to be informed and prepared. You need to know how, why and where you can get world-class medical services abroad without going bankrupt. This is your complete guide to surviving the U.S. healthcare system.

Intro to Obamacare

For the past several years, we have been told that our healthcare system is crumbling, and that without reform, the nation's medical services are going to take a nosedive. When President Barack Obama moved into the White House, Americans were sure that his healthcare reform plan would cure the ills that had been plaguing the system since before Clinton was president. We were sure Obama would guide us toward a solution – but we were wrong. Today we face the biggest threat that we as nation have ever gone up against: the new U.S. healthcare legislation[1] recently passed by Congress. The most troubling thing about it is that we are being told that it's for the good of America – that this bill will save us. Somehow, even without the support of the American people and half of Congress itself, the House of Representatives pushed the bill through.[2] Now we all have to live with the consequences of Obamacare. We've been told that the new bill is a giant leap in the right direction by the government-controlled media,[3] and thus many average Americans have accepted it as a welcome change. We need to strip away the media façade and discover for ourselves exactly what is going on here, and how we can survive this move toward universal medical care. While the media fills our heads with President Obama's promises, we need to look closer and separate the dreams from the reality of the situation.

Obamacare for Everyone!

On March 30th, 2010, President Obama signed a bill called the "Patient Protection and Affordable Care Act" that changed the healthcare system

THE STATE OF THE U.S. HEALTHCARE SYSTEM

in America forever. As aptly named as the "Patriot Act" passed under the Bush administration in 2001, the healthcare bill won't "protect patients" nor provide "affordable" healthcare for anyone, despite its claims of being for the people. The federal government now controls healthcare in America[4] and you're the one who's going to pay for it – literally. With a delightful set of new taxes and rationed healthcare,[5] standards are going to plummet and costs are going to soar. Need a clearer picture? You are going to suffer. Universal healthcare is a great idea – but that's where it ends. Shortages are guaranteed. People will die. That's the reality of Obamacare. When everybody gets standardized healthcare, nobody wins.[6] It's a deeply flawed system and we've hardly even tasted it yet. Soon, families all over America will need to find medical alternatives if they are going to survive this socialized madness.

One of the fantastic highlights of our new Obamacare system provides for forced medical aid membership, whether you want it or not. If you don't have it, then you don't get any medical services and, even better than that, the government will tax you for not consenting to their socialized system. Ramifications for the economic stability of America are even worse – as if Obama's Stimulus Plan didn't put us into enough debt,[7] even more debt will be generated by his new healthcare plan. All of a sudden, you aren't getting the medical help you need because the government dictates what you deserve and when you deserve it. It's the end of medical capitalism in America.

There's No Assurance with This Insurance

The biggest implication of the Obamacare system lies in its core policy – in the realm of medical insurance. When a government decides to fund public medical insurance for the masses, bad things happen. First of all, our government-controlled insurance will be cheaper than private insurance company rates. Over time, these privately-owned businesses will be forced to close[8] because they can't compete with standardized government insurance rates. Before we know it, everyone will be forced to adhere to the government medical body, which will control everything from medical procedures to medication for chronic illnesses. In other words, if they don't think you need an operation, you can't have one. That's the beauty of a socialist medical system: it takes away your right to choose.[9]

The same thing will happen in other private sectors. Privately-owned hospitals will be forced to follow the new bill to the letter and, as a result, many doctors will pack up and leave for greener pastures.[10] Proposed pay cuts for doctors who decide to stay isn't much of an incentive. This of course leaves America in a very tight spot. If all the good doctors leave, what kind of healthcare do we have to look forward to?

Tighter Government Control Strangles Healthcare Freedom

Obamacare creates a new rule of law for doctors, nurses and hospitals to abide by. This is quite unfortunate, because if it were up to President Obama – which it is – there would be fewer specialists in America and a whole lot more general practitioners.[11] According to the theories which created the new healthcare reform, Americans waste a lot of money on unnecessary hospital and doctors' visits. This absurd idea has far-reaching implications. What Obama really wants is to limit healthcare as a whole, reaching down to the poor by taxing the middle class like crazy.[12] Obama believes that

> According to the theories which created the new healthcare reform, **Americans waste a lot of money on unnecessary hospital and doctors' visits**

in order for this new system to work, people who can afford medical treatment must have less of it so that those who can't afford it at all can have some. When something as personal as healthcare is consumed by the federal government, everything becomes clinical, processed and suited to the masses instead of the individual. A middle class cancer patient, for example, will be limited in treatment of the disease so that a hundred others who don't have jobs can go see the doctor about a headache. This is an extreme example, but one that will repeatedly manifest itself in our new system as the years pass. How will anyone be able to get the treatment they need with these laws in place? Our medical standards will plummet as our doctors, surgeons and nurses become government employees, with the sole purpose of giving everyone equal medical care.

Obamacare Is Socialized Medicine

Make no mistake: "universal medical care" means that socialized medicine is alive and well here in America.[13] Our health as a nation is now in the hands of the corrupt bureaucrats who have let the country down on so many occasions. The government will have access to your medical records – which means that they can track certain groups of people. This has become evident with the new "Childhood Obesity Task Force Report" announced by Michelle Obama in May 2010.[14] The federal government will now be tracking children's weight and immunization records. On the surface, this may seem like a perfectly innocent tactic to help kids maintain the right body mass index. On closer inspection, though, it's more likely that the government is scanning for indicators of future health issues that children would be prone to should their weight remain out of control. The tracking system also gives the government a clear view of which children have had their vaccinations and which haven't. It's only a matter of time before immunization becomes compulsory as well.[15]

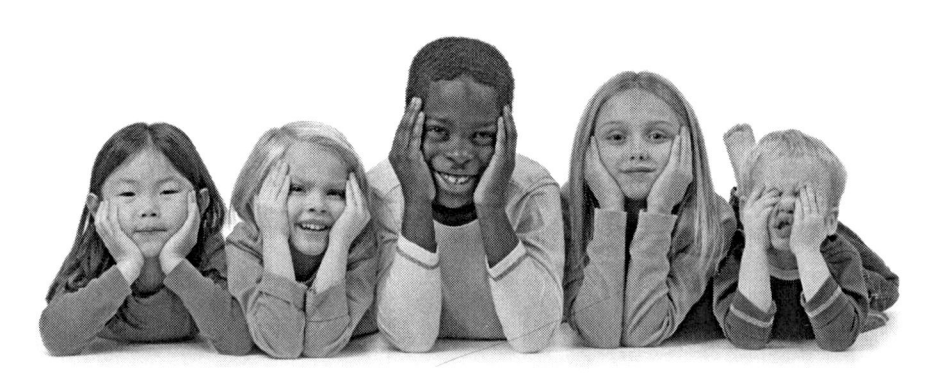

It would behoove you to realize now that Obamacare is not here to help you. The government will use Obamacare to expand its power, to exercise more efficient population control, and to pay back private investors who have government contracts in the medical industry. You can choose to see this new healthcare reform for what it is and take actions to find better medical care for your family. There are alternatives – and as long as we have alternatives, there is hope.

The Eight U.S. Healthcare Myths Revealed

Misinformation seems to be the order of the day with the "Patient Protection and Affordable Care Act." President Obama has made a number of claims about how it will help people; but so far, it has only caused a complete upheaval of our entire medical system and sent a quiver of rage through established medical centers and hospitals.[16] Trust politicians, with the help of the mainstream media, to skew the story to such a point that no one can tell truth from lies anymore. The media claims that the many "rumors" that have spread come from conspiracy theorists on the Internet. What they fail to point out is that many of these "rumors" are plausible, and are based on facts and information received from verifiable news sources, members of Congress, and town meetings.[17] The Obama administration, like many before it, uses vague language to outline what is clearly socialized medicine[18] without ever calling it that so they have plausible deniability. To clear up a few grand myths about our new healthcare system, we have to go a little deeper into the behind-the-scenes workings of our government. Here we thresh the truth from the lies, and put a spotlight on the misinformation the government wants you to believe.

MYTH #1
The U.S. Healthcare Bill Is about Health

This is perhaps the most shocking claim that the Obama administration has made about the new U.S. healthcare legislation. If you take away all the false promises and evaluate how this system would work in reality, both fiscally and socially, the sector that will suffer the most is healthcare.[19] When the government assumes control of medical services in America, the only people who benefit are those in power and those who provide medicine for the government's health plan.[20] If this bill really was about health, it would work to keep doctors, nurses and hospitals happy. But, it doesn't keep them happy. Instead, it forces the industry to adopt a government-controlled method of practice that treats people like cattle and stunts hospital growth.[21]

Real Life Examples!
Doctor-owned hospitals are not allowed to expand their services anymore, thanks to section 6001 of the new healthcare legislation. Before the bill was passed, McBride Orthopedic Hospital planned to open a new intensive care unit and operating rooms.[22] Now, those additional features of the hospital will never see the light of day. Instead, like every other doctor-owned hospital in America, McBride has to implement new practices and prepare annual transparency reports to satisfy government requirements. Who does this kind of policy hurt? You, the patient.

MYTH #2
Starting This Year, People with Pre-existing Conditions Will No Longer Be Denied Insurance

It's a nice idea to think that kids who have been denied insurance in the past because of illness will now be able to get it. In fact, this very promise is what delivered the support Obama desperately needed to pass the bill. Our president openly stated at a Virginia healthcare rally that this new policy would be immediately implemented, playing on people's hopes for better healthcare for their sick children.[23] It was only a matter of days after the bill was pushed through before the real truth came out: pre-existing conditions in children won't be covered until 2014. Until then, I'm afraid your child will still be at the mercy of unscrupulous insurance companies who view your son or daughter as a liability.

MYTH #3
The New Healthcare System Will Save Everyone Money

Our new money-saving healthcare system is not as sound as you may think. The federal government insists that it will bring about positive change and save the U.S. a lot of money in the long run.[24] Basically, Obama has tried to convince the public that extending healthcare to another 50 million people will help America cut costs. You'd expect there to be some truth to that statement since it was one of the core reasons they implemented such a radical new system. And yet, even with the many new taxes buried in the legislation it's simply not true that money will be saved, as many financial analysts have repeatedly claimed since the bill was passed. Unfortunately,

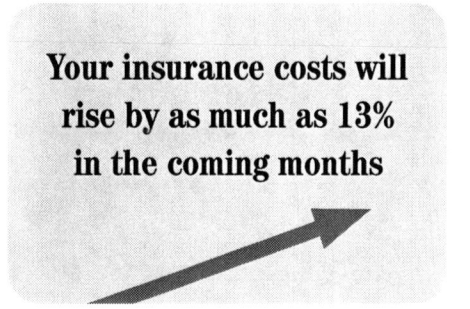

Your insurance costs will rise by as much as 13% in the coming months

even the Congressional Budget Office admits that, in the long run, this legislation will destabilize the budget and increase spending in the healthcare sector.[25] Don't get any fanciful ideas about healthcare being cheaper for the individual either. According to the CBO, your insurance costs will rise by as much as 13% in the coming months. So what is the point of this new system? If it isn't going to cut costs for the government and it isn't going to help families save money on insurance premiums, what exactly is the underlying purpose? The main function of the new law is to seize regulatory control of the healthcare system.[26]

MYTH #4
Healthcare Reform Will Help Small Businesses

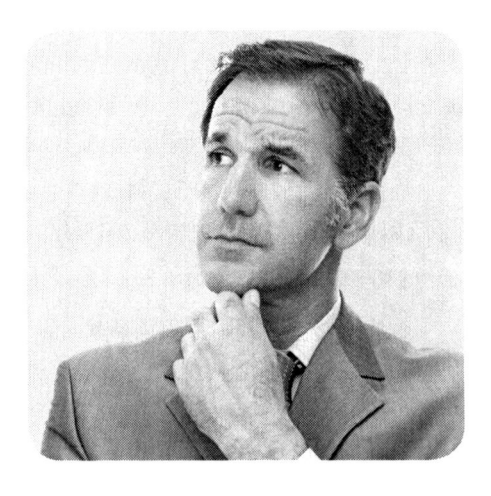

Small businesses have always been "supported" by the federal government, which is why the health bill provides tax breaks along with the new mandatory employee insurance structure. Small businesses with 50 employees or more are now required by law to pay for their employees' medical insurance. It doesn't sound too unreasonable – until you consider the implications. Healthcare costs are still high, so this move will have the average small business forking over thousands of dollars for this previously optional benefit. This means that in order for these small businesses to survive, they will have to reduce their overall costs either by firing some of their workforce or by lowering their standard salary payments.[27] If these businesses don't comply with the new law by purchasing government-controlled insurance, there is a nice provision in the bill that fines them $750 per employee. There is another hidden gem in the bill that targets small construction companies, forcing them to pay for insurance even if they only employ five full-time employees. This is a blatant move by the government to restrict and regulate the growth of these businesses.

The federal government will also have you believe that the rich will pay for the poor's insurance premiums. Did you know that "the rich" means middle income earners, many of whom own small businesses? These business owners will have additional taxes to pay on top of their employees' insurance premiums – a combination which will limit the growth of their businesses. Money will go to the government instead of back into the trade market. The economy will take a severe hit when these small businesses feel the full wrath of Obamacare.[28]

MYTH #5
Obamacare is Not Socialism at Work

With all of the political rhetoric at work trying to convince Americans that this new health bill is not a move toward socialized medicine, let's look up the real definition of the phrase and see how it truly relates to our new healthcare system.

The Merriam-Webster Dictionary defines "socialized medicine" as: "medical and hospital services for the members of a class or population administered by an organized group (as a state agency) and paid for from funds obtained usually by assessments, philanthropy, or taxation." We already know that the government has seized control of the medical services in America, regulating all private hospitals, doctors and nurses.

Bureaucrats take on roles that should be held by qualified medical professionals

The entire medical industry is now under their watchful eye, and these institutions and private individuals have to adopt the new system or face hefty fines. The whole sector falls under the government umbrella as bureaucrats take on roles that should be held by qualified medical professionals.[29] Plus, the bulk of this system is being paid for by a collection of new taxes to be imposed on businesses and on the private individual.[30] So, while the government never mentions socialized medicine, Obamacare certainly reeks of it. Our healthcare reform bill seized the opportunity to advance one of the core ideals of a socialist society: that the rich need to pay for the inadequacies of the poor because owning more than others is socially unjust.

MYTH #6
You Can Keep Your Current Insurance Plan

In the fantasy world of the Obama Administration, no Americans who are already on medical insurance plans will have to switch plans as a result of the new legislation. This is an untenable statement that the government has professed throughout the implementation of the healthcare bill. Once again, the Administration fails to recognize reality: millions of U.S. citizens will be forced to change their plans, whether they want to or not.[31] This is because the law states that if you don't have medical insurance, you have to sign up for the government-controlled option that they now conveniently offer; and if you ever change plans, you will have to change to the government option. President Obama's government insurance plan will progressively outbid private companies, drawing more people in due to its lower rates and premiums. Millions of Americans will ultimately have no choice but to opt for the more affordable option. The Lewin Group, a successful team of actuaries, predicts that up to 118 million Americans will have to switch to government insurance in the coming years.[32]

MYTH #7
The Quality of Medical Services Will Improve

This myth is perhaps the most shocking and transparent of all. Everyone knows that when government takes over a portion of the private sector, the quality rapidly drops. Most government-run programs are crippled with backlogs and poor service.[33] It's difficult to believe that our healthcare sector will be any different. Imagine the government dictating how, when and where you get medical care. What will eventually happen is that the government will view cutting costs as their main imperative rather than providing quality services to Americans. This will lead to the government cutting off research that leads to life-saving technological breakthroughs, denying medical procedures to people who need them, and spreading (what is left of) the budget so thin that the entire system becomes inefficient.[34] This is the true cost of government-controlled healthcare: instead of everyone getting great healthcare, everyone will get standardized, low-quality care.

The healthcare bill also tries to turn your doctor against you in order to keep costs low. There is a provision in the legislation that fines your doctor if he refers you to a specialist when you're sick.[35] Because of the potentially severe financial impact of these penalties on medical practices, many patients will go without proper medical care. The government wants fewer people going to surgeons or having expensive procedures done, and the result will be medical practitioners downright refusing to treat people who are very sick in order to avoid fines.

MYTH #8
You Can Stay with Your Family Doctor

> It's only a matter of time before all the good doctors are gone from your life

If you're on Medicare, Obama's medical insurance plan, then no, you probably won't get to keep seeing your family doctor. You see, only doctors who choose to accept patients who are on the Medicare plan will be able to see you. Consider the fact that thousands of doctors all over America have outright rejected Medicare, and you have a problem. If you're on government medical insurance, then you will be assigned a local doctor that accepts this form of payment. Recently, the Houston Chronicle published an article about the alarming rate at which doctors in Texas are opting out of the Medicare plan.[36] This is because the reimbursement that they usually get from insurance has been cut, which means they lose money if they decide to treat a patient on Medicare. With the new healthcare bill forcing people onto Medicare, it's only a matter of time before all the good doctors are gone from your life. After months of reaffirming the fact that people will be able to keep their doctors, President Obama finally admitted that this is not the case: "If you want to keep the health insurance you got, you can keep it, then **you're not going to have anybody getting in between you and your doctor** in your decision making. *And I think that some of the provisions that got snuck in might have violated that pledge.*" He had to concede that what he had been saying the entire time about keeping your doctor is just not going to happen.

•

These eight horrifying myths[37] about Obama's healthcare reform plan are still circulating, giving people false hope about a system that is going to fail. If you are ever denied coverage for a medical procedure that you must have in order to live a healthy life, don't give up hope! There are solutions in this book that will help you.

How the New Healthcare Legislation Will Ruin America

So far you've read about Obamacare, and how many lies the government has told in order to create support for their new system. But what is the actual impact this legislation will have on America as a whole? How will things change? Is this really the end of freedom of choice? Let's take a look at the healthcare reform bill – and how it will ruin America for all of us.

Financial Costs

Despite the constant clamor coming from Congress about how this new legislation will rectify America's healthcare crisis, figures don't lie. What makes the deceit even worse is that the projected numbers arrived on the doorstep of Health Secretary Kathleen Sebelius a week before the bill was pushed through the House of Representatives.[38] The Obama Administration knew that the system would cause massive increases in government spending – but they chose to ignore the report and lie to everyone instead. This was the projection: according to the Department of Health and Human Services, the cost of the government-implemented system will rise by a staggering $389 million in the coming years.

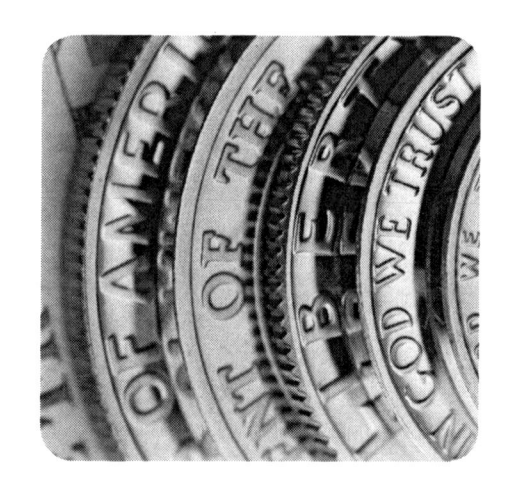

Accompanying this report were figures outlining the impact on the American family, which showed that there would still be millions without insurance and therefore millions excluded from most medical services. So exactly how is this new system going to "save money and protect the uninsured"? The simple answer is that it won't. Financial strain will come from all directions as the healthcare bill saddles small businesses, hospitals, doctors, families, and even the government with price hikes. The federal budget deficit is set to increase by one trillion dollars over the next ten years, with millions of Americans losing their health insurance coverage due to increasing costs. Couple these figures with the $500 billion cuts in Medicare, and we're looking at a system that forces hospitals to close because they just aren't making enough money. With figures like this flying around after the passing of the bill, we have to wonder how it was ever passed at all.

Ruining the Medical System

We have already examined many of the myths about how much better the new legislation will make the medical system. What we haven't gone through yet is exactly how Obamacare will ruin our medical infrastructure. First of all, the private medical industry in America is going to take the biggest hit. Because of the provisions in the bill limiting how many specialist referrals each doctor can make, specialists will lose money and even go out of business. The doctor-to-specialist system that has helped millions of Americans will be hamstrung, and everyone will suffer.[39] With government control of private insurance companies come many ramifications. For example, Obamacare indirectly promotes *not* getting insurance at all.[40] This is because insurers are now

> **Obamacare indirectly promotes not getting insurance at all**

required by law to accept anyone for overall coverage, with or without pre-existing medical conditions. What is preventing the average American family from coasting through life without insurance until they get sick, and then buying coverage? If the penalties for not having insurance are cheaper than the expensive premiums for a basic policy, many people will simply choose not to have any.[41] The insurance companies will have a small stream of revenue coming in from chronically ill people who are forced to stay on their insurance plans, but this won't be enough to sustain them. This will cause many, if not all. private insurance companies to close. The only option left will be Medicare or Medicaid, both government-controlled – and both garbage. The government conveniently gets rid of the private sector, thus eliminating the competition and establishing full control of the medical industry. Suddenly, the government can set prices for doctor's visits, operations, procedures and surgeries, and there is no industry competition to bring costs down. Prices will rise while private hospitals and small practices feel the pain of miniscule Medicare payments. They will be reimbursed less and consistently lose money until these doctors, like the private insurers, are forced to close shop and either stop practicing or start working for a government-owned hospital.[42] This will impact medical education, encouraging many young people to learn something other than medicine. To cut costs, the government will abandon technology, new innovations and progress in the medical field. Standards will fall rapidly, and the entire healthcare system in America will be ruined.

Unemployment

One of the worst consequences of the new healthcare reform bill is that it will force people out of business. People will lose their jobs as their employers have to downscale because of new taxes and mandated employee insurance. Unemployment will rise in America, and the small business sector will be forever damaged.[43] The law also fosters unemployment in low income earning groups. Because of certain provisions in the legislation, if a company hires an employee from a low income family, it will be charged taxes of up to $3,000. It makes more fiscal sense for that employer to hire someone from a middle-income family with a working spouse. The bill also forces businesses to hire people on a part-time basis, thereby excluding them from the compulsory employee insurance that they should otherwise be getting. Right off the bat, the insurance, medical and small business sectors will suffer, and millions of people will find themselves unemployed. Even big business will take a hit with the new law forcing them to hand over millions in insurance coverage for their employees.[44] An unpleasant side effect of this process will be the massive price increases imposed by all businesses affected by the bill. In order to cover costs, a business will have to raise its prices just to break even every quarter, or it risks losing the business altogether.[45]

Real Life Examples!

Maria's Italian Kitchen is a successful chain of restaurants owned by entrepreneur Madelyn Alfano. In an interview with a CNBC news correspondent, Madelyn discussed how the new healthcare legislation will affect her business.[46] She expressed the concern that paying healthcare coverage for all 400 of her employees would put her out of business. "From what I gather, it would cost over $120,000 a month or $1.4 million a year.... We don't make that much money." Like many other business owners all over America, Madelyn is upset about the enormous healthcare cost that the government expects Maria's Italian Kitchen to incur. Her only options under these laws are to cut her employees' salaries... or close down. This is the reality that Obamacare has unleashed upon small businesses in America.

Taxes Will Cripple the Economy

One of the main reasons that the government decided to implement this new bill was to bring about a new and exciting range of taxes (which, of course, senior government officials are exempt from paying themselves).[47] Naturally, these taxes will only take effect after the next election, so that voters won't be carrying pitchforks and torches to burn them all at the stake. There are 18 new taxes created by the healthcare bill. Health insurance will be subject to a 40% excise tax, with individuals and businesses forced to pay penalties if they refuse to cooperate with the new system. Overall taxes will increase to $36 billion from the previously modest $12 billion that the government demands from us now. There's even a 10% tax on tanning services![48] Charles Krauthammer, a world famous conservative commentator, predicts that a National Sales Tax is also lurking around the corner. This sales tax would force prices through the roof as businesses scramble to cover this added overhead cost on their products and services without losing their profit margin. Annual fees, penalties and taxes are the government's way of "helping" us – by taking away all of our hard-earned money. Our economy is going to suffer, and those hardest hit will be the poor – the very people Obama claimed to want to help.[49]

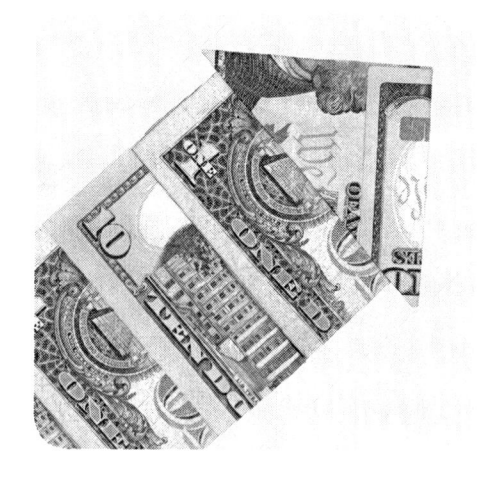

Poverty Will Spread

Currently in America, there are millions of people living below the bread line. Some of these poor work as much as they can and own small houses in bad areas. How would you feel about a bill that promised you medical insurance, but actually ended up being the reason that you lost the little money you have because of taxes and penalties? A full-time waiter, for example, would be fined if he or she didn't sign up for Medicare. That penalty of $750 could be the difference between living at home and living on the street. The jobs that help the poor will now be even scarcer because employers will be required by law to provide medical insurance for all full-time employees. Instead of doing this, most businesses will simply keep them as temp workers or fire them altogether, causing mass unemployment for Americans who really need the work. The lucky ones who do manage to keep their jobs will be paying more for products and services as the dollar weakens and interest rates skyrocket. Their income will be taxed even more – and worse, the chances of ever receiving quality medical care at a hospital will be virtually zero.[50]

The State of Control

Imagine if you've just lost your job, like millions of Americans will, and you can't afford to have medical insurance or pay the fine. According to Congress, you'll be fined $1,900 or you'll have to go to jail for up to a year. It's a scary reality that is bound to come true for many law-abiding Americans. With all of these new taxes, layoffs, price hikes and penalties, more than one family will be ripped apart by this new system. How in the world can you afford the $1,900 fine if you couldn't pay the fine of $750? "Do what we tell you, or you're going to jail."[51] It's just another injustice that will tear through America as this bill comes into effect. Such severe consequences will surely ruin the fabric of America, until

> **According to Congress**
> **You'll be fined $1900, or you'll have to go to jail for up to 1 year**

nothing is left but a police state where you do what you're told or else.[52] But of course, all prisons will be on the government-controlled healthcare system, so you can enjoy free healthcare for the year you are in jail.

The End of Market-Based Rationing

The days of competitive market-based medical care are over. Our old system was far from perfect, but at least if you really needed an operation and you had the money, you could get it. These days, with Obama's blanket coverage and "everyone receives equal benefits" plan, medical capitalism is dead. If they say no, the answer is no. Now we can look forward to waiting periods, lightning-fast doctor's visits, and limited medical care.[53] This means that if you're on Medicare, and you need an operation but they don't think it's necessary... good luck to you! The answer's still no. This will force the average American to fork over even more money, in addition to the expensive insurance premium being paid, to get that operation. And you'd better get it while private medical centers are still in existence. Soon, all hospitals will be government-run. Best case scenario: you'll be scheduled for an operation in three years because of ridiculous waiting periods. If you're not insured and you get into a car accident, you're left to foot the entire bill. Don't forget to pay your fines; those aren't waived because you were almost killed. Filing for bankruptcy is also an option, which is what you'll have to do anyway once you get the gigantic hospital bill. This is the reality that we all have to look forward to – and only time will tell how bad this government-created disaster will get.

So what's the point of all these new laws? And why has the government spent so much time and energy making sure that they come into existence?

> **If you need an operation but they don't think it's necessary— the answers is NO**

Who Does This New Healthcare System Really Benefit?

With all of these new, destructive laws coming into play, it's time to ask the difficult question: Who does this new healthcare system really benefit? Surely there must be some solid reasons why Obama so hastily forced the bill through. Right?

The U.S. Federal Government

The most obvious and most sinister beneficiary of this healthcare bill is, of course, the federal government itself. President Obama and his cabinet want more power, and therefore need to accumulate more control in sectors like the medical services industry. We mere mortals are now stuck with awful medical insurance options while the senior staff enjoys exemption from the harmful effects of this new healthcare regime. On page 158 of the bill, a provision states that those on congressional committees and in senior staff positions don't have to comply with the new health laws. They can have whatever medical insurance they choose – which means that President Obama remains completely untouched by the new healthcare reform, and gets to broaden his scope of power at the same time. It's the old "have your cake and eat it" politics that have caused so many debacles in the past.

The U.S. government is becoming more and more powerful under the Obama administration.[54] As new laws are passed, the government takeover of the private sector is apparent even through the lies and misinformation that the government releases. The big players in business have a vested interest in Obama, and he in them – something that is evident from his move toward universal healthcare. There is an ongoing debate about whether the U.S. government is really trying to help the people, or whether it's trying to eliminate free enterprise. With Obamacare, free enterprise certainly does suffer as hospitals, doctors and patients foot the bill for this new reform. Government is freeing itself from its previous limitations so it can expand its reach and exert true control over the economy – channeling money into big business, and ignoring the needs of the average American. Money, power and control seem to be the driving forces behind our federal government.[55]

Big Pharma

Big Pharma is one of the biggest lobbying groups on Capitol Hill, with a whopping $26.2 million being spent last year alone. It comes as no shock then that this financial giant benefits almost as much as the government does with the new healthcare bill. You could say that the new reform act goes above and beyond, protecting the interests of Big Pharma and squashing any threats that would lose it money over the next few years. Big Pharma chief Billy Tauzin was seen flitting in and out of the White House eleven times in the months leading up to the bill proposal.[56] As usual, Big Pharma has come out on top, with all of their interests protected and codified into law in the pages of Obama's healthcare reform legislation.

The health reform bill clearly states that the importation of drugs is prohibited; in other words, cheaper drugs from other countries are not allowed into the U.S. This harms the average American family, forcing them to buy branded Big Pharma drugs that are much more expensive and further cutting into their already limited budgets. During his election campaign, before the lobbyists hit him with cash incentives, Obama supported low-cost imported medicine. Clearly, like so many other promises, it was just talk. Now, drugs have to be bought from U.S. manufacturers at whatever price they demand. This protectionism that Big Pharma enjoys means bigger profits and a secured consumer demand for their medicine, and Obama keeps his biggest lobby happy.

This wasn't the only provision passed for Big Pharma. The legislation also preserved Medicare's overpayment for drugs, meaning that generics in the U.S. will still be expensive, grossly affecting people's choices and limiting options for seniors. Biotech drugs are now also exclusively provided by Big Pharma, with billions in subsidies bought through Medicaid. With Democrats topping the charts as the politicians who pocket the most cash from lobbyists, this comes as no surprise. The bill was centered on getting more people on Medicare and Medicaid so that the drug companies could eventually reap the benefits. This, of course, dooms Americans to accept overpriced medication for the next ten years.[57]

Wall Street

How could Wall Street possibly profit from the new healthcare reform bill? Congressman Dennis Kucinich said at one time that the new healthcare reform was designed to benefit Wall Street. There has been much discussion about the involvement of bankers in American politics, and their plans to seize control of the U.S. by bankrupting everyone. If this is the case, then they have one hell of an ally in the form of the Obama administration. Let's not forget that the banks own a lot of politicians, and have been steadily pushing their way into politics for some time. At the core of everything is money, and we've already explored how much more it will cost America and each of its citizens to implement this new health reform. When all is said and done, the real winners are the money lenders.[58] It seems that as long as campaign contributions are more important than the American people, bankers will always have a say in American politics.

The Insurance Companies

Startling as it may sound, many insurance companies will benefit from this new healthcare system.[59] Large companies will earn hundreds of millions as a result of this new mandatory insurance coverage for all Americans. While many private insurance companies will close, the profits of some others will rise because costs won't decrease as Obama had previously promised. This means that even though you are paying the same or higher insurance rates, you'll be getting fewer benefits for your money. This saves insurance companies a lot of money. The new law that limits specialist referrals also reduces the chances of big insurance companies having to pay for expensive operations and procedures. It seems that despite the "lobbying against the bill" façade that these insurance companies put up, many of them still stand to make a heap of cash.

All in all, Obama's healthcare bill was clearly passed for the benefit of private interests like Wall Street bankers, Big Pharma and large insurance firms. By making it seem as though some of the lobbyists were against the bill, the administration managed to mask this blatant collusion from the general public. Worst of all is that this entire new healthcare system will destroy what little we have left of our Constitution.[60] Obama is bent on ushering in a socialist system that benefits the few and brings more hardship to the many. With so much money flowing into the government from these private interests, what chance do we ever have of getting quality medical services that will reduce the cost of care? Evan Newmark of the Wall Street Journal writes: "Obamacare is a bad deal made to look good through funny accounting." All of these private interests had one bottom line – profit. The health bill was never about helping people, reducing costs or designing a more efficient system. It was all about the hidden agendas of lobbyists on Capitol Hill, and their extensive political influence.

> **Even though you are paying more or the same insurance rates, you'll be getting less medical services for it**

Shutting Down the Health Industry

There were supposed to be provisions in the health reform bill that would essentially fill the gaps in budget spending. Instead, Obama ignored the segments of the medical industry that would suffer, leaving them to close down and make more room for the large, dominant companies. While he could have negotiated prices with the drug companies like the Veteran's Administration does, lowering costs on prescription medication, Obama instead outlawed cheaper drugs from other countries. Nothing about Obama's actions has been noble or for the benefit of the American people.[61] We are in a country that rewards the corrupt and stomps on everyone else. We are now facing a threat to our freedom that will only prove more powerful with time.

Goodbye Freedom – What Obamacare Means to Americans

Though most Americans opposed the bill, it passed, and Obamacare became the law of the land. President Obama and all of his private interests are moving against the liberty of the American people. This is a play to restrict our freedoms as a nation. All across America, cries of protest are falling on deaf ears.[62] Individual states are fighting against the bill – but it's too little, too late. The federal government is already rolling toward controlling the medical industry, creating huge debt, and destabilizing everything that America has built as a nation of free people. If you still aren't convinced, take a closer look at what the bill will force you to do.

The Freedom to Choose

Government-mandated insurance packages will all be alike, taking away your freedom to choose which coverage best suits you and your family.[63] This effectively removes your right to spend more money on a comprehensive health plan, or less if you can't afford it. The promise of better healthcare is gone – the promise of cheaper healthcare is gone. Even if you are young and are in great health, it doesn't matter. You will be forced to get the same package at the same rate as a 40-year-old with a range of chronic conditions.

Free Market System Collapses

Obamacare is ushering in a socialist medical system; but more than that – it is ushering out our free market system that encourages growth and development. No one has been more vocal about this simple but important point than Ron Paul.[64] On his website, RonPaul.com, he states that people don't realize that if they are for Obamacare, then they are not only against quality healthcare but also against the free market system that has made our nation great. A free market allows the government to regulate the economy, but it does not force ownership on people. With Obamacare, the government has so much control over our health care system that they have effectively removed that fundamental freedom of choice. Now the government alone has the power to dictate prices, services and products within our medical system. It's only a matter of time before Obama's administration pushes for an end to our entire free market system. Ron Paul explains that America will collapse under this new bill, and that the Constitution has become nothing more than an old bit of paper, disregarded by those currently in power. With a domino effect so imminent, it's no wonder America is up in arms about this government play for control.

No More Limits

You can't customize your insurance anymore. This means that you will be paying extra for a nice variety of options you've never had and will never use – because it's all part of the package. Section 2711 of the legislation even prohibits the sale of policies with lifetime limits on rates – policies that young, healthy people often find affordable and useful.[65]

Cover the Children

The new law allows kids to stay on their parents' plans until the age of 26.[66] This means that as a small business, every single one of your employees has the option to make you pay for coverage for their kids, regardless of whether or not the children are working. Though this may sound great to parents, remember: the law probably means that your overall salary will be lowered to make up for these insured kids, and the medical services provided will be terrible.

Your New Insurance Plan

There are so many useless extras that you will never need or use in a government-controlled insurance plan. But, they exist and you will pay for them. Ever been a drug addict? It doesn't matter to the government. You'll still have to pay for coverage for substance abuse treatment services and rehabilitation fees. Ever been to a psychiatrist? Whether you have or haven't, you've still got to include mental healthcare in your plan. All men must have pediatric coverage, regardless of whether or not they have kids; women must have maternity coverage, even if they are physically unable to have kids. Look forward to a large selection of useless features on your insurance plan, with nothing covering what you actually need.

Doctor Whisperers

If you are a doctor and you own your own practice, you can look forward to the government telling you how to run your business, who to treat, how to carry out procedures and what medicines to prescribe. This is because the government now dictates what goes on in the medical industry. Goodbye, doctor-to-individual-patient treatment in your practice.[67]

Expanding Your Practice

As a successful doctor, you can no longer open your own hospital. You have to work for the government now, using Medicare as your insurance reimbursement strategy. If you have already started building your own hospital, you have to stop: the government won't let you open it.

Successful Career

If you ever reach the point in your life when you are earning more than $250,000 a year, say hello to a whole new lineup of taxes. All of your alternative income will also be taxed, and any of your existing policies, trusts or plans will be taxed – again.[68]

Impact on the American Family

The Patient Protection and Affordable Care Act was touted as a family-friendly bill. But is it really? With a limited number of plans within the new government-controlled system, the legislation doesn't benefit families at all. In fact, they are forced to pay higher rates for less choice. These plans will also contain a number of ethically-gray areas that families may have a problem with – such as abortion. If your family doesn't believe in abortion, tough. You still have to pay for the coverage.[69]

And as if this wasn't bad enough, there is now a marriage penalty. If you decide to get married, you could be subject to enormous penalties for it. This

> **If your family doesn't believe in abortion its tough, you still have to pay for it**

tax will have far-reaching consequences as many American couples will refuse to marry, or will get divorced to end the drain on their finances. However you look at it, this bill is a destructive force against the American family.

Your Constitutional Rights

In the past, our Constitution has prevented the government from overstepping its bounds; but, over the past ten years, that document seems to be counting for less and less.[70] This statement rings true in the context of the healthcare reform bill. Never before has our government been empowered to force people to buy something they don't need or want. The increasingly intrusive Commerce Clause has made mincemeat of our former rights. The government has inched forward, and now we are suffering at the hands of the most blatant disregard for our rights since the Bush Executive Orders. Obamacare includes constitutional violations like the new Student Loan Program, which offers student loans via the government instead of private companies. This will cause even more job losses and put your children's futures in the hands of a corrupt government selection program.[71] As unconstitutional provisions like this become more common, we will begin to see the move toward a government-controlled America where state law is under the direct control of the President and his cabinet.

The Road Ahead

With this healthcare reform, the federal government shows a complete disregard for our constitutional rights. They take away our right to choose, telling us what we can and cannot have. By limiting us, they save on costs while we deal with the consequences of standardized medicine. Senator Orrin Hatch of Utah is firmly against the health bill, which he states is not "constitutionally justifiable." Speaking on CNSNews, Hatch goes on to say that if the government can force people to buy insurance, then they can do anything.[72] This is a disturbing sentiment coming from a man whose career includes more than 33 years as a United States Senator.

If someone can't afford to buy medical insurance, or doesn't have it provided by an employer, then that person is giving money to the government for nothing. This mandatory health coverage is just the government's way of ensuring that everyone pays, regardless of whether they want to or not. The shocking truth is that costs will increase instead of decrease, standards will fall, and within a matter of years the U.S. healthcare system will come crashing down. This is due in large part to the many bureaucracies, commissions and boards that will be in control of the entire medical industry in America. Your life and the lives of your loved ones are at risk with this new system.[73] Don't make the mistake of believing that the government system will work, or you might discover the truth the hard way. The U.S. Healthcare System is in shambles. As a nation, we can no longer depend on our government to do the right thing and defend the rights of its people. As we delve deeper into the realm of greed, corruption and politics, we will uncover how damaging this system will actually be, for us and for the American economy.

> **Your life and the lives of your loved ones are at risk with this new system**

CHAPTER 2

CORRUPTION, GREED AND U.S. POLITICS

Corruption, Greed and U.S. Politics

The federal government is no longer a single entity, and no longer creates policy that is in the best interests of the American people. With the U.S. healthcare reform bill comes the sudden realization of how much clout the lobbyists actually hold over our senior government officials. The secret back-room deals are becoming more obvious as the government desperately tries to keep the public at arm's length from the truth. Unfortunately, the armies of industry lobbyists that assault Capitol Hill on a daily basis have become more powerful than our own legislative process. As money is pumped into the greedy hands of the politicians, laws are bought – not made according to the needs of the country. With a system built on corruption, greed and politics, what chance does America have for a brighter future? We are now living under a government that compromises the urgent needs of the people to enrich third-party operators.

United We Stand, Dividing the Profits – How Healthcare Providers Get Away with Murder

It's amazing how a law can come into focus when you see through the lies and misinformation that surround it. As a united force, the health insurance industry and the pharmaceutical industry ensured that the new health bill was tailor-made to line their pockets. Did you know that in the final weeks of debate on the legislation, both of these industries experienced increases in their stock value despite the government's prediction that these companies would lose a ton of money under the new system?[74] This raises red flags for anyone who has a basic understanding of how stock trading works. If a company is set to lose money in the coming financial year, stock values decrease. The system is based on future predictions of the profit that a company will make. So, how in the world did pharmaceutical and health insurance stocks go up while Obama was proclaiming so adamantly that these sectors would lose money?

The truth is that they won't lose money at all. How can they when they all but wrote the bill themselves? The top insurance companies experienced growth of nearly 79% in the year preceding the bill, while the top pharmaceutical companies enjoyed a tidy 24% rise in their stock value.[75] Stock prices don't rise if huge losses are around the corner. If Obama's version had been true, we would have seen a big dip in the market values of these companies. The deal has worked out in the insurance industry's favor as more people will be forced onto expensive health insurance plans. Meanwhile, pharmaceutical companies will benefit from the new influx of prescriptions to be filled for the millions of new insurance holders. It's a win-win for these corrupt bedfellows, who laugh in the face of average Americans and their naïve belief that the system is set up to help them. We citizens are left to foot the bill for this corrupt new system while the ultra-powerful lobbyists enjoy their new summer homes in Monaco. The agenda has been set, with the Government – Big Pharma – Big Insurance triad steamrolling over the rights of the American people.

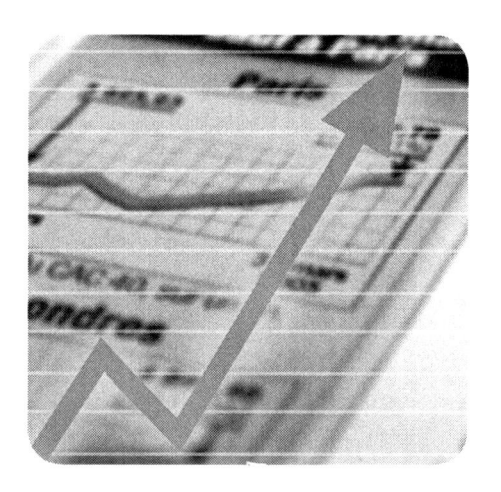

The Government Bankrupting America

Money is the source of all of America's current problems. With the worst recession in economic history supposedly "behind us," President

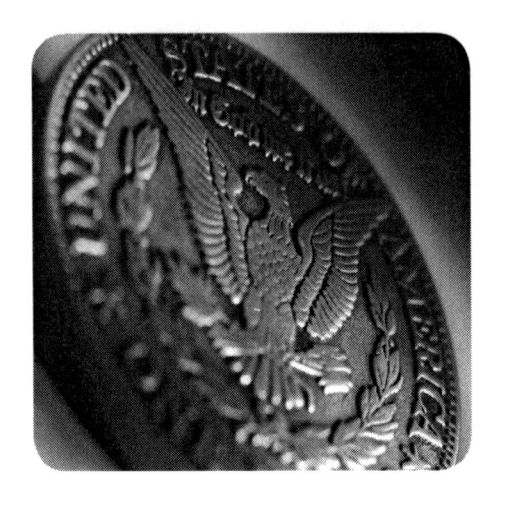

Obama is working to make sure that the culture of bankruptcy reaches your children, and your children's children. Every step the government takes is a step toward greater debt for the country, and poverty for millions of Americans. Now that Obama is openly in bed with big corporations, there is little left to save us from his damaging policies as they pass into law, one by one. The U.S. healthcare reform bill is his greatest triumph, crossing lines and expanding government further than any president has accomplished in almost 100 years. His reckless spending and open disregard for public opinion is sinking America into a deep hole, one that we cannot escape from.

If you think healthcare was expensive in the past, just wait until these new laws take effect. With this new blanket insurance coverage, we will all have to suffer the costs of additional extras and inflated prices. Ron Paul describes it as an "economic fantasy" – one that forces Americans to comply, regardless of the stringent and damaging effect on their quality of life. We are supposed to live in a free country, in which people have the right to choose for themselves. With this new law fully enacted, what hope does the average American have of reaching a point of financial stability?

So why exactly are Obama and his government working so hard to bankrupt America? The answer lies in his political ideology. After he was elected, rumors began to circulate about President Obama being a socialist. Since then, even his most ardent followers have come to question his choices and intentions. Obama openly ignores the declining state of the U.S. economy, and moves forward with laws, programs and policies that will put America into even greater debt. Why would he do that unless he was aiming for the system to fail altogether? By pushing America into debt, Obama makes way for his new socialist form of government, replacing the old capitalist system that "failed." His actions speak far louder than his words on this matter. There is scarcely an informed American who would still argue that Obama's actions are in the best interest of the people. He works to blight the free market economy in order to replace it with a collection of government-controlled bodies. The new healthcare legislation is a crucial step in his plan for the future of America. It is impossible to believe that he doesn't realize that he is driving our economy into the ground. Obama is an intelligent man who is trying to force America into a nationalized system – without us even realizing it![76] The downward spiral of his agenda includes bankrupting the middle class to pay for sustaining the poor; killing small business, so that there is no direct competition for his government-run system; and, worst of all, sacrificing the lives of thousands in order to make his vision come true. That is what this new healthcare system will do. People will die because of the terrible healthcare they receive in government-run hospitals and medical centers. We can all look forward to worsening health conditions and increased debt, thanks to the vision of our President. Suddenly, his statement that America will go bankrupt without healthcare reform seems ironic. It's because of Obamacare that America will go bankrupt.

> **Obama is an intelligent man who is trying to force America into a nationalized system without us even realizing it!**

Death to Hospital Quality

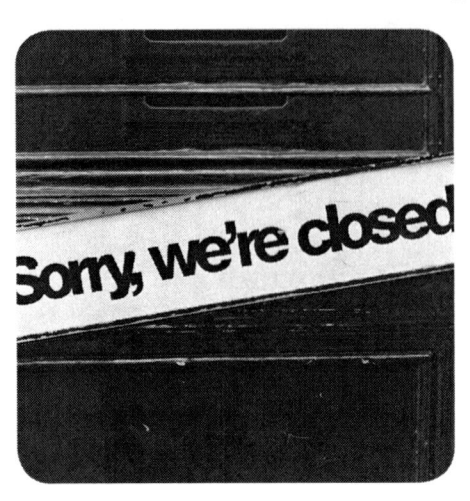

Obamacare has torn through the medical industry, destroying 60 doctor-owned hospitals already – all for "the good of the people." This has been nothing but a blatant ploy to remove these privately-owned facilities as competitors to the government-run options. With 60 hospitals already closed due to the new health laws, and 200 more projected to go to wrack and ruin in the coming years, who is benefiting from this loss? It certainly isn't the patients.[77] By closing these hospitals and limiting where the American people can get medical care, Obama's laws will lead to millions of deaths around the country. But don't worry: you'll still be able to get care from the American Hospital Association's membership of low-quality, expensive hospitals. It comes as no surprise that this association is one of the biggest lobbying groups on Capitol Hill.[78] It's just another in the long list of corrupt companies and organizations that were on board with the new healthcare bill.

The legislation effectively stunts the growth of quality medical care and kills the future expansion of the industry. This puts thousands of qualified professionals out of work, and forces thousands more to accept massive pay cuts in order to work for government-controlled hospitals. If Obama succeeds in eliminating competition in the medical industry, standards will plummet and quality healthcare will go into permanent decline.

Death to American Patients

Obamacare is Obama's final solution for sick people who he sees as putting financial strain on our economy. The new legislation will lead to nationwide neglect of those Americans who are in serious need of effective healthcare. Instead of helping them get better, provisions in the bill leave them to die – with limited care, expensive insurance and overpriced medicine. Even if all you need is to find a specialist for your condition, you're out of luck – because your doctor can't give you a name without suffering severe penalties. Most of the time, if you're in terrible shape they won't even treat you, because the insurance reimbursements won't cover the cost of your medical care. You'll bounce from one government-run hospital to the next, until your time runs out. You could try appealing to the government medical board, but they judge your case on how much it will cost them, not how much you need the treatment. This is what happens when the decisions lie with third parties, and not the doctors or patients themselves. The bureaucrats who dictate how, when and where you get your medical care will waste time, and won't make the necessary decisions fast enough, causing thousands of senseless deaths.

In Britain, the socialist model of medicine has been in place for some years now. During the course of a full-scale probe into a particular hospital to assess how well this system has been functioning, British Secretary of Health Andy Burnham discovered an alarmingly high death rate. This was due to the hospital's need to cut costs so that they could meet government targets. The result? Widespread neglect. This

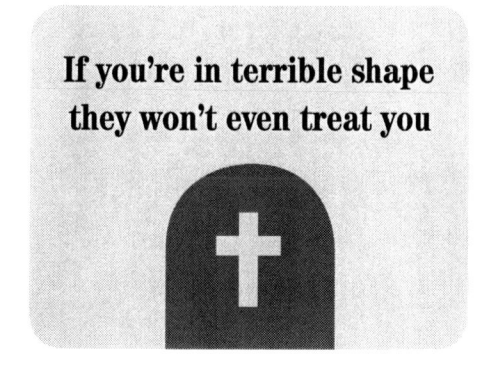

If you're in terrible shape they won't even treat you

is what we have to look forward to in America – patients left in soiled sheets, patients being given the wrong medication by untrained nurses, patients dying of starvation or of contagious infections contracted in the hospital... all caused by fear of the punishing axe of a cost-paranoid government.

Big Pharma, Big Sales

Big Pharma stands firmly with the government on the new U.S. healthcare legislation. This is because they transformed what everyone was sure would be a price curb into a price hike. They were able to accomplish this magical feat through systematic and frequent depositing of money into the bank accounts of the right officials. When millions of Americans are forced to accept the new government-controlled health insurance, no one will profit more than Big Pharma. Many people can't afford medication because they are uninsured; but now, with this delightful mandatory insurance going around, Big Pharma is going to make big profits. As the second co-writer of the health bill, they have everything to gain and nothing to lose. While government cuts will initially cost them money, whatever they lose will be won back – in spades.[79] With almost all of America able to "afford" medicine, Big Pharma is looking at quite a successful sales year. In one of their many legislative victories, they managed to slip into the bill a provision that will keep generic medication off the market for up to 12 years, keeping brand-name medicines safe from competitors. Big Pharma stands to make billions off the new laws, which were passed without any of the potential restrictions that many of the nation's senators called for during the debate. Doctors who want only to cure their patients will be forced to

> **Big Pharma stands to make billions off the new laws**

prescribe medicine instead. We are already struggling as a nation to deal with the effects of prescribed medication and the many problems it causes. With this new legislation, more Americans will fall victim to dependency, addiction and even death from pharmaceutical "solutions." Giving Big Pharma more power in the healthcare industry is a mistake that we will all regret. Expensive medications will bankrupt American families, and no cheaper alternatives will arrive on the market in time. However, America won't feel the full impact for some years to come.

Big Insurance, Limited Health

The government-run insurance companies that will benefit from the health care bill will cause endless problems for the medical services industry. Working together with government bureaucrats, these companies will do everything in their power to make sure that you don't force them to spend money. This means longer waiting periods for insurance approval, limited coverage for expensive procedures, and round-the-clock policing of what you may and may not spend on your medical care. While there are many "hits" that the insurance industry will take – such as the reduction of payments, and having to accept people with pre-existing conditions – the long-term benefits will more than make up for any lost revenue. In fact, the system was designed to put smaller insurance companies out of business, allowing the big ones to thrive with millions of extra clients forced to sign on. This is just another example of the blatant support the Obama administration lends to big business, in an attempt to quash free trade in the private sector. What chance does a small business have when laws are passed to prevent it from ever growing? As usual, you will be the one to suffer – as prices are regulated, treatment is limited and costs are barely covered.

There is nothing secret about the alliance that government has formed with Big Pharma, Big Insurance and Big Hospital Groups. These lobbyists have won and will get away with murder. They, rather than American families, are protected by the new legislation. With millions of people facing bankruptcy, failing medical services and illness, Obamacare is set to kill thousands, if not hundreds of thousands, in the future. And they won't be held accountable for their actions. You must make the decision to find better medical services for you and your family, before the U.S. system comes crashing down. The truth is that we have been excluded from decisions that could one day save our lives. Instead, these decisions are in the hands of the greedy, the corrupt and the immoral, who are only interested in making money.

Health Shock – The Hidden Legislation You Need to Know About

The gigantic 2000+ page healthcare act has so many provisions and inclusions in it that we will probably still be discovering new things about it in the coming years. But, what we already know is that the government tried to sneak a few pretty radical things into this bill… and succeeded.[80] When dealing with such a massive game-changer like this health bill, it's important to try to understand as much of it as possible. Here are some hidden details that have recently come to light about the healthcare bill, and what they mean for you.

Saving for Old Age

A nice little provision snuck into the healthcare reform bill gives your employer license to take as much as $240 off your paycheck at the end of every month. This is unrelated to the many other taxes that Obama is now forcing you to pay – and is something that you need to be aware of. The average monthly deduction from your paycheck, which is determined by age, will be $146 according to the Congressional Budget Office or $240 according to the Centers for Medicare and Medicaid Services. It is specifically designed to help you save for your twilight years. In other words, this program forces you to save, since there's a chance you'll need help when you're older. It also happens to relieve the financial strain on Medicaid. The government claims that this provision will keep seniors at home instead of in nursing homes. Eventually, you should be able to draw $75 a day for in-home care in your old age. Though this may sound like a great option, the government has no business pushing extra costs on people who are already struggling, and they certainly have no right to dictate how much you should be putting away every month.

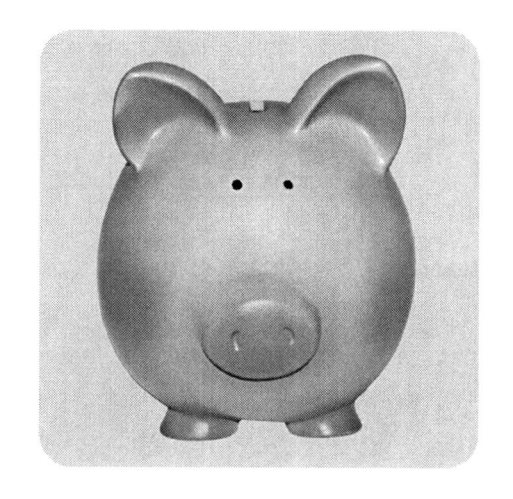

Education Based on Race

America is supposed to be the land of the free. You're free to hire whoever you want, free to get education if you want it. Unfortunately, under a provision on page 879 of the health bill, freedom of education is no longer a guarantee. This section clearly states that, in order for a medical institution or school to be eligible for government-controlled grants, the school has to make damn sure that they have a "demonstrated record" of enrolling underrepresented minority groups. This means that if they don't choose African Americans or Hispanic Americans over other students, then they won't get to benefit from any government-funded contracts. Since when did the government start singling

> **Since when did the government start singling out people based on race?**

people out based on race? Is this a form of reverse discrimination against the Jewish, Caucasian, Chinese and privileged classes? Any non-merit-based system causes problems. A person should get into a good school based on performance records, not based on the fact that he or she is poor. The government is trying to strong-arm medical education facilities into teaching certain people; and, as a result, students who would have made excellent doctors will never get taught, while those who struggled in the past will find their way into the medical services field.

Again, More Taxes

Among the many new taxes and juicy penalties that the government is using to take more than their pound of flesh, one damaging tax provision was passed into law while everyone was looking the other way. According to Section 9006 of the healthcare legislation, taxes will now be levied on all sales and purchases of goods and services.[81] This is a massive inconvenience for businesses as it gives them a whole lot of extra paperwork to do, both during the year and at year end. An IRS 1099 form now has to be sent to the businesses you buy goods from; and, if it is a continuous monthly order, the 1099 has to be sent to that business at the end of the year to help the government track exactly what you are spending. This has little resemblance to the original 1099, the purpose of which was to track your personal income. The 1099 form now covers personal and corporate sales – leaving small businesses to drown in a sea of paperwork. If your business simply buys a new computer online, you have to fill out a 1099 form. This allows the government to closely watch your spending habits, and make sure that they are getting their fair share of it – especially if your known income is less than what you are spending. Essentially, it's the government's way of tracking any additional income that you don't report. This enormous new regulation will see thousands of hours wasted on filling out forms, and it further damages small businesses by consuming what little time they have to grow.

Obama's Private Army?

Sections 5210 and 203 of the healthcare reform bill state that President Obama may create a "reserve force" army and a "regular corps" army in the public health sector – realizing his desire to have a national force, funded by the government, right here in the United States.[82] This move toward Obama's own personal army is startling; even more disturbing is the fact that these public servants may be called to active duty whether they want to or not. But first, why the hell is there a section in our healthcare reform bill about a 6,000-strong national army?[83] Even if they really are for helping in times of healthcare crises and natural disasters, and to advance studies in medicine – why are they also allowed to police the population during terrorist attacks? This new provision in our reform bill lets Obama give military training to doctors and equip them with guns. It also gives Obama the opportunity to finally put together his "civilian army" he was so adamant about in 2008. We should all be outraged that such a dangerous provision was pushed through Congress and is now law. Who knows what rule of law these physician armies will abide by, and what they will be allowed to do in the name of healthcare emergency situations. We will need to watch our President and his new army very closely.

> **We will need to watch our President and his new army very closely**

Marriage Penalty

This provision was touched on earlier, but is so ridiculous that it's worth exploring. Paying for health insurance is going to be a costly business for an individual, but not nearly as costly as a joint payment for a married couple. The new healthcare reform act dictates that if an individual is earning $30,000 a year, that person's insurance payments would be around $1,320 – expensive, but manageable. If two people earning that same amount married, their new combined insurance premium would skyrocket to $12,000 per year! This provision has severe consequences for the sanctity of marriage in America. It discourages young couples from taking the leap – and if they do dare to get married, it subjects them to enormous financial hardship right off the bat. Millions of Americans will exceed the combined income that triggers this tax leap – and this was all done in the name of easing the financial strain on the poor. This bill shows a complete disregard for the concept of equality in collecting taxes from middle class citizens so that lower income people can afford healthcare. This tax forces married couples to fork over their hard-earned cash to pay for certain benefits – but not just for themselves. Now, middle-class couples are footing the bill for the exact same set of benefits for the poor.

Counting Calories

If you're a successful franchise or restaurant owner, the new legislation is going to force you to invest in determining the exact calorie count for every meal you prepare, and to print the results next to each meal on your menu.[84] A clause in the healthcare reform bill forces owners to add the nutritional content of their food to all promotional content in their restaurants. The law applies to owners who run more than 20 restaurant outlets, and also extends to vending machine operators. This will hit the food service industry hard as people are discouraged from eating high-calorie foods and become more wary of what they choose to eat. The hard costs involved will also set these restaurant owners back thousands of dollars as they are forced to reprint menus that include this new information. While there is nothing wrong with displaying the caloric content to the public, this requirement is yet another financial blow to businesses across America.

Cosmetic Surgery Tax

What do you know – another tax. This one targets women who choose to have elective cosmetic surgery.[85] The bill states that, if you choose to have particular kinds of surgery, you may be subject to a tax of up to 7% depending on the supplies and implants required for your procedure. This tax specifically targets middle class women and assumes that most cosmetic surgery is a waste of money. This is simply not true. While many cosmetic surgery procedures are performed purely to enhance looks and self-esteem, many people have a real need for these surgeries to correct scarring, deformation and skin problems. This provision was included for the sole purpose of raking in more money for the insurance redistribution plan. Most women who undergo plastic surgery procedures are fit and healthy, so in essence, these healthy women are paying for medical coverage for unhealthy people – something that more than one cosmetic surgeon has complained about. This is just another source of revenue for Obamacare – one that will inflate prices, and may lead to patients seeking less expensive surgery elsewhere, thus hurting the industry.

As if the tax on cosmetic surgery wasn't preposterous enough, the government also included a 10% tax on tanning salon services. This is an example of the government reaching deep into the healthcare sector for money. It has been labeled a "sin tax," because tanning is all about looking good rather than about health. Tanning salons all over America have been forced to raise their prices, which could threaten these small businesses and result in many salons closing.[86] The tax has also outraged regular tanning salon customers, some of whom were already suffering under Obama's tax-happy bill.

The Special Needs Tax

> **Currently there are over 35 million people in America who rely on flex accounts to cover their large medical bills**

If you or a loved one has special needs, prepare to lose many of your tax benefits under the new Obamacare bill. This is also true for people with chronic illnesses, who will now be liable for their medication if they exceed the new $2,500 cap. This is as a result of the new flexible spending cap that Obama and his administration have imposed on those most in need of the extra help of a flex account. Your account will now be capped at $2,500. Anything beyond that – you'll have to pay in cash. Parents of kids with special needs use flexible spending accounts to save for future medical expenses. These accounts cover costs that aren't provided for by their insurance companies. This new cap brings financial hardship to those Americans with chronic conditions, or who are disabled or have special needs. Naturally, the fact that flex accounts aren't taxed disturbed the government; so, they took measures to limit it, making all additional money spent for medical necessities subject to taxes. Currently, there are over 35 million people in America who rely on flex accounts to cover their large medical bills. Now, like so many others, many of them will be left wanting for much needed medications, services and care when their accounts run dry.

Breastfeeding Rooms

Mothers who are breastfeeding during work hours can now look forward to regular breaks throughout the day, and special mandatory rooms that they can use to express milk for their child. The new law adds a provision to the Fair Labor and Standards Act that forces businesses with more than 50 employees to build or allocate a special room for this purpose. Unfortunately, this is just another provision that is going to make employers spend thousands of dollars for no particular reason. In the past, mothers have been fine with using a clean bathroom facility for pumping milk – but that's not good enough, says the government. Instead, employers must invest money to make conditions more private for these women. This appears to be another pointless tactic to get businesses to needlessly spend money, further stretching their tight budgets.

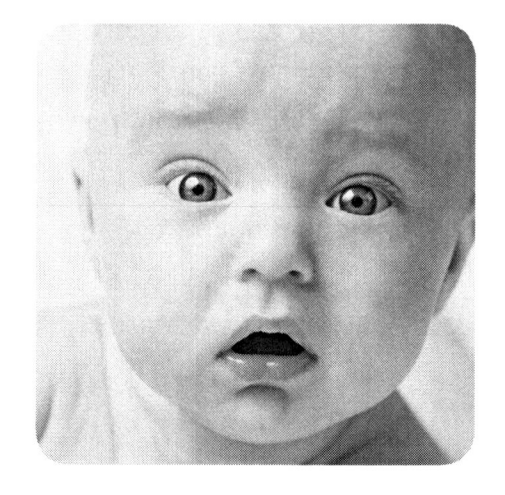

Obamacare places a lot of emphasis on taxes, with the middle class taking on huge burdens in their private lives, married lives, businesses and recreational activities.[87] Imagine for a moment that you are a businesswoman who is engaged, owns her own chain of restaurants and frequents tanning salons. The government will tax you for getting married, force you to invest money on reprinting nutritional information on your menus, push you to decrease all of your employees' salaries (because you are liable for their insurance premiums) and tax you for getting a nice tan. With all of these additional costs, how will you and your business survive? How many of your staff will leave in search of better salaries? What kind of a budget will you have to live on? The initial outlay for complying with these taxes will be bigger than most small businesses can handle. So far, this bill is proving to be far more expensive for the average American than Obama has ever admitted. His "affordable healthcare for all" slogan is wearing thin. The government has heaped huge taxes on the middle class to fund their insane healthcare bill. The only people who are winning are the few poor who have a steady job – and even they will experience the inflated prices caused by Obamacare. The "rich" are being crippled, stunted and controlled, while Obama blankets the country with his socialist healthcare system. Hundreds of thousands of people will lose their jobs and descend into poverty. People who are very sick will have to pay extra for medical care they can't afford, or be forced to accept the limited help they can find within this new system. After all is said and done, it's the American people who are going to suffer the most for this healthcare catastrophe.

Why the U.S. Well of Health Will Run Dry

America is now entering a new era in the medical services field. With the healthcare reform bill thinly disguised as a solution to our spiraling health costs, the U.S. will feel the full impact of a socialized medical system over the next ten years.[88] Instead of confronting the failures of Obamacare that the government knew would eventually come to light, they distracted the American people with threats of doom, and with partisan fighting between Democrats and Republicans. Obama seems to think that as long as his intentions are viewed as honorable, he can get away with anything, even the complete dismantling of our Constitution. With the integrity of that document lying in pieces on the floor of the Congressional building, Obama did what any power-hungry, profit-mongering Democrat would do: he pretended as though it didn't happen.[89] All the American people can say is thank God for YouTube. It puts Obama's endless storytelling and fabrication out in the open. This Obamacare system will cause a slow descent into economic bankruptcy for America, the loss

> **Obama seems to think that as long as his intentions are viewed as honorable, he can get away with anything**

of our world-class medical service industry and countless other social implications for the average American family. In this section, we explore why the new legislation will crash and burn, and what the ramifications will be for American citizens. While it remains to be seen what the full impact of this new system will be, there is enough information to conclude that it's not going to be good for anyone – except, of course, for the chosen parties who drafted the legislation. Let's take a look at the problems facing America thanks to Obamacare.

Failure to Control Price Increases

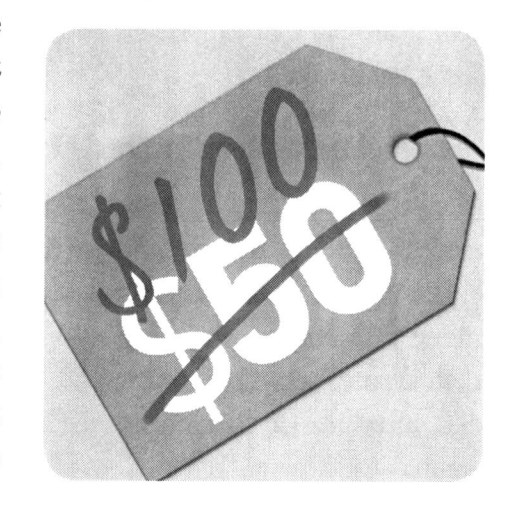

With the new laws already in place, the entire country is coming to the realization that prices in the medical service industry are still out of control. The bill has failed miserably to control soaring medical costs and provide cheaper insurance to everyone. In fact, it has only exacerbated the situation.[90] While Obama's idealistic claims gained him many allies in his fight to pass the new bill, his execution has come up short – delivering a cash-crunching blow to the middle class, stealing millions in extra tax levies, and handing the American people over to Big Pharma on a silver platter. To make things even worse, the bill forces cost cuts where they can do the most damage. The government takes your money to make up for its severe lack of planning, greedily inhaling your bank account in order to pay for this mess of a system. Over the next four years, prices will inflate, your medical benefits will be cut and your freedom as a patient entitled to quality medical care will be cut off. It's very hard to imagine that Obama and his team, who drew up this legislation, had no idea that this would be the result. What happened to those shiny promises that Obama made before the bill was passed? Now that it's in the books and people are combing through it, the truth is being revealed.

Failure to Give the People What They Want

All Americans wanted was less expensive, better quality healthcare. They didn't want insurance reform, taxes, mandatory plans, low quality healthcare and bureaucratic bilge – but that's what Obama gave them. Instead of spending two trillion dollars on insurance, pharmaceuticals and government-controlled hospitals, he could have spent a third of that on expanding the free market system and creating positive change. But that wasn't his agenda.[91] Obama's agenda was to create more wealth for the big corporations who own Congress and the White House. Now we have to deal with a whole new collection of problems, in addition to the escalating bankruptcy stimulated by the medical industry. Millions of people must now change their plans, despite Obama's reassurances that this wouldn't happen. In short, Obamacare amounted to the worst healthcare bill that Americans could have imagined – because it wasn't about health at all.

Failure to Keep Trained Medical Professionals Happy

Doctors, specialists, surgeons and nurses are the backbone of the medical services industry. Without their support and dedication, the entire system would crumble – which is basically what is happening. Along with blanket insurance coverage comes the horrible realization that Obamacare does nothing to ensure that there will be enough doctors to take on so many extra patients.[92] Acting for the big insurance companies, Obama decided to force Medicare on people instead, knowing that doctors would have to treat patients on this insurance plan. Unfortunately for doctors, massive cuts were made in an attempt to balance out the blanket coverage; so, doctors will lose money when treating Medicare patients. This removes your doctor's incentive to provide you with top quality care, and replaces it with a weak moral obligation to do so. And with blanket coverage, your doctor will also be spread thin and close to burn-out because of the sheer number of patients seen on a daily basis. Combine these trends and you're looking at low-quality, rushed care that is profit-centered and not based on your individual needs. Imagine being a highly-regarded doctor with 15 years of experience and qualifications – and the government tells you that you have to take a pay cut. The new law will not only increase your patient load, but it will limit your resources, prevent your practice from expanding and force you to comply with government-mandated cost-cutting strategies. No wonder doctors all over America are angry – they are getting a raw deal!

The Medical Brain Drain

For all of the reasons mentioned, the Obamacare system is bound to fail. The inevitable consequence of putting such powerful pressures on doctors will be a medical brain drain. Some doctors will choose to close their practices and find a new career, and others will choose to leave America in search of greener pastures. This will aggravate the shortage, and lead to even worse healthcare conditions for

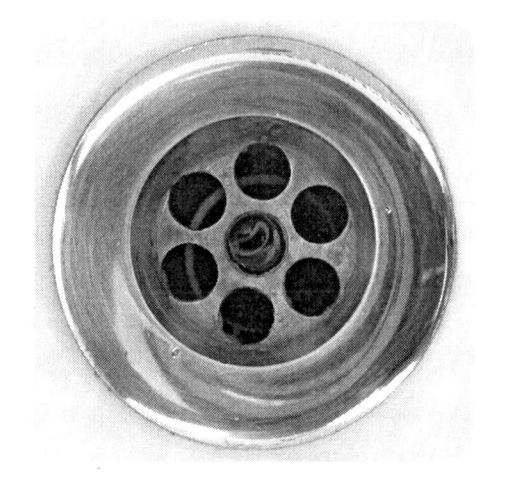

> **Obamacare will force the U.S. well of health to run dry**

patients in America. It would be unrealistic to think that doctors aren't concerned about money, especially when they spend so many years studying so they can live comfortable lives. And now that the government has limited their chances of making real money in the U.S., many of them will choose to practice abroad. Their alternative would be to stay in America and work themselves to death, earning money that is not commensurate with their workload, and being constantly burdened by inefficient medical resources and staff. The stress of having to deal with government interference all the time is also a persuasive factor. With government-controlled bodies always watching over their shoulders and limiting the quality of medical care, some doctors will choose to leave so that they can run their practices on their own. The healthcare bill offers no incentives for these medical professionals to stay, and instead forces them to comply – or leave. It is a sad truth that many of them will choose the latter option.

This bill goes even one step further, damaging America's future prospects in the medical industry. What young person, thinking of becoming a doctor, is going to spend nearly ten years studying and learning only to settle into a life like that? Obama has discouraged a whole new generation of American pre-meds from ever reaching the medical services industry. In a recent study published in the New England Journal of Medicine, 46.3% of all physicians feel that the bill will drive them out of practicing medicine. Nurses and other medical staff will also see a reduction in pay and an increase in workload. So, along with the already-burgeoning doctor shortage, even fewer nurses will be available to fill the gaps in service. Resources will be few and patients many. This is why there is so much fear about rationing medical care in America. If all the good doctors and nurses leave, and the rest are turned into government servants, it's only a matter of time before the effects hit the American family in a big way.

The Health Shortage

Because of unrealistic policies, overspending and the abusive treatment of our medical practitioners, America will experience a massive healthcare shortage. This shortage will lead to economic and social collapse in the U.S., with thousands of people dying due to neglect, long waiting periods and ineffective healthcare services. More and more Americans will be forced to seek medical services elsewhere, beyond U.S. borders. Unfortunately, the lower income group will suffer the most, as they are forced to either use the medical services provided or go without. The hard truth after all of this legislation is that America will not be able to handle the medical brain drain – which means that even though we now have blanket coverage, people still won't be able to get the medical services they need. Doctor's appointments will take weeks to book, operations will take months or years to schedule and, because of dire need, more pharmaceuticals will be handed out for serious illnesses that should be treated in hospitals. Obamacare will dry up the U.S. well of health. In a matter of years, our entire system will disintegrate around us.[93] It has been estimated that by 2019, over 700,000 jobs will have been lost as a result of this one piece of legislation. The economic effects of this bill will be far-reaching and will cripple industry in America, losing hundreds of millions of dollars for small businesses and the private sector. Over time, America will be severely weakened, perhaps enough for Obama to get what he wants – total control.

CHAPTER 3

ಸಾ•ಡಾ

FINDING A SOLUTION TO THIS LOOMING PROBLEM

Finding a Solution to this Looming Problem

୫୬•୦୪

With so many of President Obama's promises lying in pieces, we as a nation must pull together in order to come up with a solid plan to survive his socialist agenda. As the U.S. healthcare system travels on its slow path to destruction, we need to fully understand why trying to comply with his new system won't work. Because it was specifically designed to fail and to usher in a new nationalized America with a government-controlled medical services industry, your desperate attempts to pay all of his taxes and penalties still won't get you the medical services you need. Imagine yourself four years from now, with Obamacare in full effect. What happens if you are diagnosed with a life-threatening disease like cancer? Who will you turn to for help, when there are no more qualified doctors left in America?[94] When there are no new technological breakthroughs that could ease your pain? When chemotherapy takes months to book in advance? Not only will you be forced to buy overpriced pharmaceuticals that, but you'll also have to pay in cash whatever your useless insurance plan won't cover. Let's take a look at why getting a disease under Obamacare will end your life.

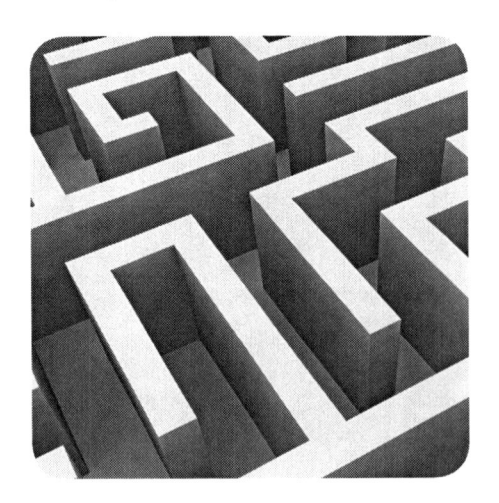

Chronic Disease Treatment – Why Low Cost Isn't an Option

Obamacare was supposed to make medicines less expensive and healthcare of a better quality than we have now. So far, these promises have amounted to nothing. One of the first horrible truths realized after the healthcare bill was passed was the enormous tax increase on everyday over-the-counter medicines. A whopping 40% tax increase on these drugs will affect those buyers paying cash, as well as those paying with a flexible spending or health savings account. Basically, it will affect everyone. With the limited coverage these new insurance plans offer, the elderly and people with chronic diseases will suffer most.[95] A very big part of Obama's plan to reduce the costs of healthcare is simply gutting part of the Medicare plan known as Medicare Advantage. This is despite the fact that over 10 million Americans are currently on this plan, and are benefiting from coverage for things like "care for chronic conditions," "hospitalization" and "prescription drugs." Take this coverage away from them and they lose their crucial, hard-earned medical benefits. It's back to square one, back to limited coverage and back to being bankrupted by the medical money-making machine. There is light at the end of the tunnel though, according to our President: the government will save $200 billion from the cuts. So while the federal government gets a nice bit of relief, 10 million people begin the trip down the long road of financial hardship and illness. The irony is that the new healthcare reform bill was supposed to help empty out emergency rooms, preventing unnecessary hospital admissions and thereby saving money. What the bill will actually do is create a system that severely punishes the disabled, the elderly and people with chronic health conditions. As standards fall, these people will have less access to the regular care that they need, and emergency rooms will start to fill up with the unwitting victims of this universal system. Let's take a look at the provisions in the new bill that prevent chronic disease patients from getting the affordable care they need.

Coverage for All Means Coverage for None

"Equal access to health insurance for all Americans" is just another way of saying that sick people and healthy people should all have the same benefits in their insurance plans. Take a minute to think about it. If healthy people have loads of additional benefits they don't need, but they still have to pay for them, who benefits? Insurance companies, of course.[96] If people with chronic conditions have limited coverage because the government wants to prevent "unnecessary" spending, who benefits? Insurance companies, pharmaceutical companies and large hospital groups that dictate prices for procedures. Where in this corrupt system do the people benefit at all? The young are forced to choose plans that are more expensive to cover the costs of the poor who can't afford insurance, and the old or sickly are forced to deal with thousands of dollars in additional costs out of their own pockets. Forget about the flexible spending accounts that helped them in the past – those have been capped. In other words, if your condition costs you $20,000 a year and your insurance only covers $5,000 of it, with your flexible spending account adding a grand total of $2,500 pre-tax dollars to the mix, you are left with a bill for $12,500. The healthcare reform bill is predicated on the notion that flexible spending accounts cause over-consumption of healthcare. It simply doesn't matter that you need the care, or that you'd die without it.

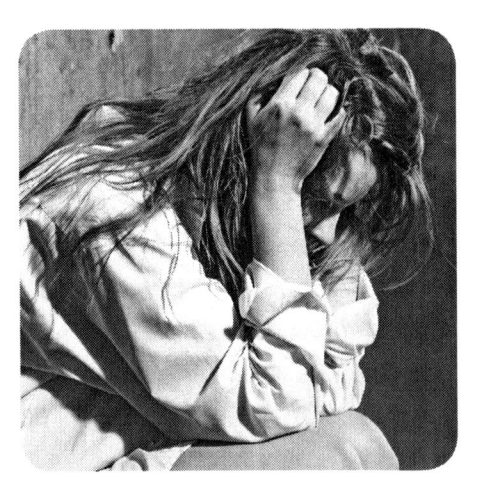

Take the average American diagnosed with severe depression or mental illness. Psychiatric treatment is not cheap, and medication for depression can easily rack up huge monthly bills for the patient. Take into consideration the fact that suicide is one of the ten leading causes of hospital admissions in America.[97] For serious treatment – attending psychiatry sessions or therapy on a weekly basis, coupled with hospital admissions and drugs – you're looking at thousands of dollars at the end of the year. Blanket insurance plans don't even come close to covering the costs that you would incur. Instead, to "help" you, the government capped your FSA, took away your comprehensive insurance plan and forced you into a system that demanded more taxes, more fees and gave less access to the medical care that you need. But don't worry – it's all in the name of better healthcare for everyone. It's a bitter pill to swallow. And people still believe that Obama's new healthcare plan will help them. It won't!

Rationing Your Healthcare

One of the loudest and most outrageous claims that Obama made was that the new healthcare system would not result in rationing – as though adding millions of extra people to the insurance pool wouldn't make it overflow. If you believe that, then the government really pulled the wool over your eyes. Rationing is fundamental to the new healthcare plan, especially with the government as desperate as it is to reduce costs.[98] President Obama himself stated that the plan is about limiting services to "healthcare that works" – a blanket statement that can be interpreted in a hundred

A socialized medical system requires rationing the amount of healthcare consumed by the general population

FINDING A SOLUTION TO THIS LOOMING PROBLEM

different ways. Of course, what he is indirectly saying is that certain services must be cut, limited or otherwise removed from the system. He wants you to believe that cuts + millions of new insurance plans + massive price hikes = better healthcare. In reality, it equals a flooded market, creating shortages and leading to severe rationing. Plus, with nearly half the population on the already-failed Medicare and Medicaid programs, we're facing a bleak future of long lines, never-ending waiting periods and outright denials of service to many patients with chronic conditions. A socialized medical system requires rationing the amount of healthcare consumed by the general population. Obama can't talk about limiting, controlling and redistributing services based on a government-run system of checks and balances and claim at the same time that we won't see rationing.[99]

Outright Denial of Treatment

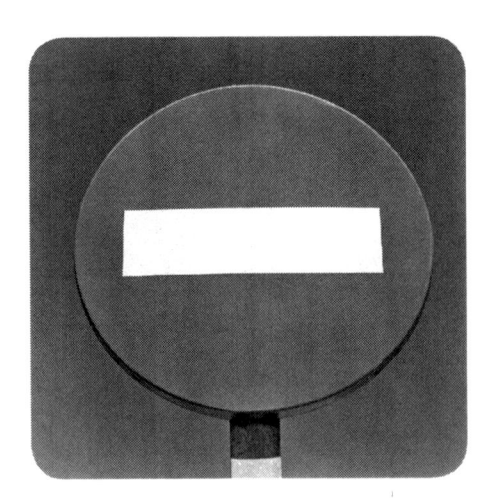

One very real problem in the near future will come from the harsh provisions that force doctors to accept low income patients on Medicare. The reimbursement rates in the Medicare system are so pathetic that the doctors who haven't fled the country are going to be extremely picky about who they choose to treat. Imagine for a moment that you are a patient on the new Medicare insurance plan.[100] You have been accepted despite the fact that you have a severe heart condition. How are you going to find a doctor who is willing to treat you and incur the costs of all of your expensive treatments? They know they won't be fully reimbursed for their time or for the procedures that you have to go through – not to mention all the ridiculous paperwork they have to complete in order to keep the government happy. The result will be that many doctors outright refuse to have you in their hospitals. As medical care begins to resemble a government bureaucracy because of this imposed control, healthcare will become more about the bottom line than about patient care. In Obama's world, this might be "unethical," but we can't be naïve and believe that it won't happen. Americans all over the country should get used to being sidelined so that hospitals can make ends meet.

Stunted Growth in Disease Treatment

America has always been a major contributor to the world's cutting-edge medical advances and methods of treating certain diseases more effectively. Under Obamacare, this will become a thing of the past. Hospital funding will be cut and research labs will be forced to downscale, with no hope for medical advances that aren't privately funded. This is because under the new law, hospitals take on the burden of research money. In the name of keeping costs low to balance out the many burdens hospitals will take on over the next few years, medical research will come to a grinding halt. Without all of the free market incentives that used to stimulate medical innovation, we can expect very little in the future. Research that could potentially save millions of lives will be curtailed as market experimentation ceases to exist. This is on top of falling healthcare standards, which will continue to plummet as long as the government puts costs ahead

> **With all the incentives that stimulate medical innovation gone, we have little to look forward to**

of public health. A drop in innovation means little future opportunity to lower fatality rates, develop safer treatments or find ways to diagnose people earlier than before.

Limited Access to Specialists and Medicine

Under Obamacare, access to medical treatment and drugs is restricted so that these services are not overused. What this means for chronic disease patients is that even if they are insured and eligible for treatment, the care they receive will be extremely limited. Under this new health regime, they will have to wait to see specialists – and even then, the specialists' hands will be tied by the government, limiting them on the kinds of services they provide their patients. Imagine having a cataract and suffering for months before seeing a specialist about it. Then you still have to schedule the procedure, which will take another few months. In the meantime, you'll be half-blind for a year because you can't find a doctor who has the time to treat you immediately. Or imagine having cancer and being forced to wait months for chemotherapy, when waiting a few months could be the difference between life and death. Our ability to find and treat or remove cancer in its early stages is why America has one of the best cancer survival rates in the world. Under this new healthcare system, these numbers will drop dramatically, putting our rate equal to or lower than that of nationalized systems like the UK and Canada. Cancer patients also have access to life-saving drugs here in the U.S., because drug companies knew they could recoup their initial expenses faster here than in price-controlled countries. Now that Big Pharma has the monopoly, we'll see less and less of these European drugs. And as a final blow, the doctor that the government assigns you to[101] might not be able to handle your specific chronic condition as well as others would, which could lead to life-long or even life-ending consequences.

Increase in Medical Malpractice

Medical malpractice has always been a sore point for doctors in America, as patients are quick to sue if something goes wrong during routine procedures or visits. In order to cover themselves and minimize the risk of lawsuits, doctors work tirelessly on patient health, ensuring that scans and tests are done even for the smallest problems. This is one of the reasons that serious illness is caught earlier in America than elsewhere. Unfortunately, this is all going to change. Because testing is going to fall outside of your medical coverage, doctors won't always have the option of sending you for testing due to financial reasons. This is just as well because under government control, hospitals won't be allowed to run scans or tests without a serious reason to do so. As these revealing preventative procedures disappear, many Americans will needlessly fall victim to ill health, disease and even death. To keep costs down, doctors will prescribe more medication rather than refer patients to specialists for tests. A patient who suffers from stomach pain, for example, will be put on several courses of medication before any additional steps are taken. If the problem persists, and the patient deteriorates to a point where he or she can hardly move, then the doctor will refer the patient to a specialist for testing. Stomach cancer left untreated and undiagnosed is a killer. A few months really do mean the difference between continuing a normal life and dying from the disease.

•

There is no doubt that this healthcare reform will irreparably damage the system and lead to thousands of unnecessary deaths. Chronic disease patients need to realize that they won't be getting the quality care that has helped them survive in the past. In order to stay healthy and alive, these Americans will have to look for medical services elsewhere, or become victims of the corrupt socialist system[102] that has invaded our shores. Those patients who decide to give the new system a shot will suffer the effects of limited medical access, enormous bills and an ever-decreasing quality of life. This extreme form of control that our federal government has exerted over our healthcare system will ruin doctor-patient relationships, bankrupt millions of families and lead to third-world medical care in the U.S. As more terrible effects of this new bill are realized, we will begin to understand the true meaning of a controlled healthcare system.

The United States of Controlled Healthcare

One of President Obama's boldest assertions about healthcare was the liberal notion that preventative medicine would lead to reduced costs and a healthier population.[103] What a load of rubbish. Preventative medicine has nothing to do with the general health of the population. All this reform bill has created is tighter government control. If a child grows up eating healthily, exercising regularly and receiving all of the government-sanctioned vaccinations, Obama believes that this child will end up costing the healthcare industry less. Though this may sound logical, let's take a closer look at the realities behind preventative medicine.

Controlled Health of the Public

The government has a goal of preventing "ill health" in the American population. This would essentially mean ending our right to eat, drink and smoke as much as we want. Say goodbye to your freedom of choice. Government-controlled health agencies will spring up, and each and every American will be forced to submit an annual fitness report to be analyzed by a government doctor. This doctor will then tell you what you need to do to get healthier – and you'll be forced to do it. These agencies will help you "prevent" ill health by telling you how to live.[104] If you're overweight, you'll be made to lose weight, either by attending a government-run "fat camp" or by losing the weight on your own under the careful supervision of your local doctor. If you have been cited as someone who will have major health problems in the future, expect to visit your doctor a lot more often.

If you think this weight monitoring is impossible, then perhaps you should take a look at the new weight laws for children.[105] Children already have to record their weight and fitness levels for inspection by government health agencies. Regular doctors' visits, mass vaccinations, dentists' visits, exercise programs and policing of the whole system will cost the government millions of dollars. So much for cheaper alternatives in the healthcare sector.

Of course, the most terrifying aspect of this preventative healthcare system is that no matter what we do, there will still be people who get cancer, diabetes and other chronic illnesses. It seems that the government just wants more control, not better health for the American population. We have seen it time and time again with this new healthcare reform: the government has a hidden agenda, one that doesn't promote health and wellbeing. During the debate leading up to this reform legislation, the issue boiled down to two choices: personal freedom[106] or government control. You can't have both. Either the government tells you what to do, or you decide for yourself. It's fitting that the government pushed through the vote for government control, because the American people certainly wouldn't have done it. No government-controlled system has ever worked efficiently, or in the interests of the population at large. With Obamacare, the government has destroyed our right to get quality healthcare.

Public Health Measures

When the government tells people that it is going to cut costs by reducing obesity and unhealthy lifestyles via the enactment of specific public health measures, alarm bells should go off around the country.[107]

FINDING A SOLUTION TO THIS LOOMING PROBLEM

> **No one has the right to tell you what to eat, what medicine to take and how to live your life**

What exactly does the administration mean by "public health measures"? It sounds as though they are going to try to change certain public behaviors. The only way they can do this is by regulating your physical condition, and forcing you to make changes they say are necessary. This is a scary thought. If we no longer possess the right to be as unhealthy as we want to be, then all hope really is lost. This scenario isn't that far removed from the new mandatory health insurance laws. First, we are forced to have government-controlled health insurance; then, we are forced to see certain doctors, forced to undergo certain tests, forced to get vaccinations and forced to take government medicine. Soon we'll have no choice but to comply. They will raise the banner that claims it's all for the good of the people, when really it's for the good of their social-control master plan. Don't forget that no one has the right to tell you what to eat, what medicine to take or how to live your life. That is what the government wants to control. They'll insist you take certain medications to keep healthy, and impose harsh fines if you don't. Then, when you're busy trying to keep up with everything you have to do, it'll transform into criminal law – so that the next time you don't comply, you go to jail.

This healthcare reform bill has extended the reach of Obama's socialist empire. Congressman John Dingell even announced when the bill passed: "The harsh fact of the matter is when you're going to pass legislation to cover 300 million people in different ways it takes a long time to do the necessary administrative steps that have to be taken to put the legislation together to control the people." You can only call control "regulation" for so long before people recognize it for what it is.

Mandatory Microchips

As if the power play of the massive healthcare bill wasn't horrible enough, Obama managed to sneak through a provision in the "Reconciliation Act of 2010" that provides for public micro-chipping. The bill refers to a class 2 implantable device. This device was recently approved by the FDA, which describes it as a radiofrequency transponder for patient identification and health information. Having a microchip implanted in your body might be convenient when doctors need to bring up your health records very quickly; but it also permanently allows the government to police you with a system that identifies your name and health status. Is the government preparing for further infringements of our rights in the future? Since only people on the government-controlled insurance system receive these chips, this explains why Obamacare forces people to switch from their personal plans to the "less expensive" government option. Critics don't want to talk about microchips, even though the provision does in fact appear in this second healthcare bill. Conspiracy theories aside – what right does the government have to mandate micro-chipping?

IRS and Control

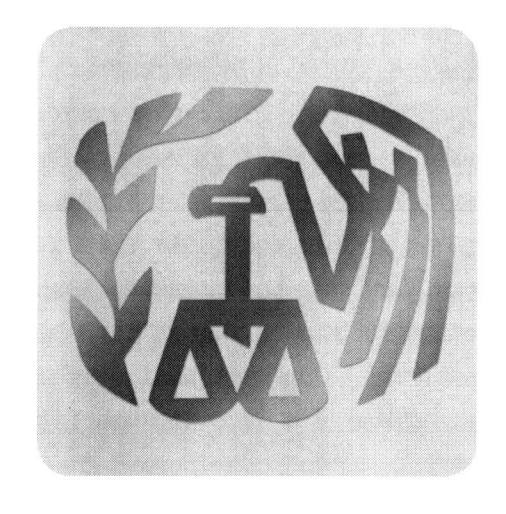

When the IRS has the power to put you in jail for failure to pay a government-imposed insurance charge, then something very wrong is happening in America. The IRS is known for poor quality service and inefficiency – except when you happen to skip a payment or two. The fact that the government is now burdening the IRS with a host of new taxes to enforce does not bode well for the general public. How many innocent people will be thrown in jail because they can't pay all of these ridiculous new healthcare taxes? More than anyone would like to admit. As America's new health law enforcer, the IRS will expand to include another 16,000 auditors, agents and staff to handle the increased workload and efficiently police the public. Now the IRS can reach everyone, regardless of race, class or income. They'll treat the American public with the same care and loving respect that they always have. We have a lot to look forward to with this new Obama-backed force.

Welcome to Big Brother

Obama and his administration have become the proverbial eye in the sky, and they want it all – control of your education, your industries, your money and your healthcare services. So far, they are doing pretty well for themselves. If you think that these new laws won't change your life, then you're in for a big surprise. Big Government is watching your every move. Think the IRS is going to overlook your failure to pay government-mandated taxes? You're wrong.[108] Obama's campaign slogan "Yes we can!" was obviously referring to the government, not the people. Can the government take even more of your hard-earned cash? Yes they can. Can they ruin your small business by forcing you to pay your employees' government-imposed insurance fees? Yes they can. Can they prevent you from getting a much-needed operation on your left foot? Yes, they totally can. In fact, as Big Government grows in power, soon they'll be able to do more about your health concerns than you can. That's the beauty of a socialist system: everyone is so busy being controlled that no one stands against it. Obama and his government really think they're entitled to redistribute the money that middle-class Americans earn. They want you to give what little you have to the poor so that everyone can enjoy a B-grade health system. "Yes I can!" screams

Obama, as the last vestiges of American freedom fall away. There will be serious consequences for everyone.

The Effects of a Failing Healthcare System

American politicians have a history of making bad policy decisions and then abandoning the general population to struggle with the consequences. Obamacare may just be the worst bill that Congress has ever passed, and will join the Patriot Act as one of the two bills that destroyed American freedom.[109] Let's take a look at some of the effects that the Obamacare system will have over the next few years.

The Short-term Effects of Obamacare

Many of the true effects of Obamacare will only be felt after the election in 2012. Clearly, government bureaucrats looked ahead at the damage that would occur and their potential plummeting poll numbers, and knew that it would be smart to postpone the worst for later, once they are reelected – and can do even more damage. They failed to foresee that the public would recognize this gambit for what it is: a blatant attempt to stay in power.[110] After everything that Obama has done with his term in office, he has no chance of being reelected – unless some catastrophe happens close to the election and he's able to "save the day." But the public is growing very weary of his half-truths and outright nonsense. If President Obama makes a promise, you can make a lot of money by betting that the exact opposite of that promise will materialize.

> **After everything that Obama has done with his term in office, he has no chance of being reelected**

No More Lifetime Coverage

The ban on lifetime limits on insurance plans is effective immediately.[111] This means that you can no longer get a cheaper deal by placing a cap on your coverage and then sticking with your insurer for life. Instead, you can enjoy standard insurance plans that will continue to push your premiums through the roof as time passes. Just another benefit brought to you courtesy of this draconian healthcare legislation.

Independent Appeals Process

This is your process for appealing medical decisions that government insurance companies make for you that go against your wishes. Unfortunately, because the government controls these bodies, your chances of ever getting them to change their decisions are slim to none. But, feel free to attempt to wade through the endless red tape that you will meet once you're there. Appealing your decision will also probably raise your premium. After all, government time is money!

Restructuring

You can expect to see a large-scale restructuring of the medical services industry as hospitals ready themselves for the implementation of the new system. Businesses will be forced to redraft their business plans, preparing to pay the new mandated employee insurance payments. This will result in immediate job losses in the medical and business sectors.

Overall, over the next year, we will slowly start to feel the ramifications of this flawed system.[112] As doctors become overburdened and underpaid, many will relocate or stop practicing altogether. You might have to change your doctor in the coming months, especially if you are uninsured and decide to start on the government insurance plan. Expect government bureaucracies to take hold, lines to build up and your general expenses to rise.

The Long-term Effects of Obamacare

If you compare our new healthcare system to the smaller model that Massachusetts instituted, then we are headed for the kind of insurance premiums that only celebrities and Bill Gates can afford to pay.[113] Obamacare is

> **Millions of Americans know how useless the government insurance will be**

built around the idea that anyone can get health coverage anytime, even if they just recently became ill or were in a serious accident. Because it is cheaper to pay the annual fine for not having insurance than to pay monthly health insurance premiums, it's obvious that millions of Americans will choose to pay the fine out of financial need – or because they know how useless the government insurance will be. The problem arises when people start signing up for insurance only when they really need the benefits – for an operation or for an expensive procedure. Once they get through the crisis, they drop their insurance and revert back to paying the less expensive annual penalty. Smart for the person involved, but terrible for people who need consistent insurance coverage, or for small businesses that are required to pay for their employees' plans. Who do you think is going to pick up the slack for the huge losses that the insurance companies start accumulating? The permanently insured. Premiums will keep rising[114] until Obama is forced to create another tax, then a government subsidy to re-inflate the insurance industry. But by this time, thousands of businesses will have closed because of rising premiums, thousands of families will have been forced into bankruptcy and the economy will have begun its rapid destabilization.

Unemployment for Young People

If you're young and are currently looking for a job, get one now – as soon as you can. When the healthcare bill takes full effect in 2014, employers will be forced to stop hiring temporary, unskilled or untrained employees. This means that young people who enter the job market around that time will suffer terribly as it becomes even more difficult to find a full-time job that pays well.[115] Starting in 2014, Obamacare mandates that employers must pay at least part of their temporary employees' insurance premiums. Many employers won't be excited to start paying that expense. Instead, they will fire all of their temporary staff, and hire a few skilled employees to assimilate the jobs once filled by temp or part-time workers. This will dramatically affect the retail industry and the hospitality industry, where young and unskilled employees could always find well-paying jobs in the past. In an already-icy job market, Obama has effectively sealed the fate of the unemployed for the next several years.

The Breakdown of Supply and Demand

Over the next ten years, the medical industry will be torn apart – resulting in the slow and painful breakdown of supply and demand in the healthcare sector. Millions of Americans will be in need of a primary care doctor, but there won't be enough left after many of them have been driven out by harsh restrictions and poor reimbursement plans. Seriously ill Americans will be forced to look for care elsewhere as the system suffers the effects of the specialist drain. Eventually, healthcare will not be available to anyone as the entire system falls apart. This is the shortage

> **Healthcare will not be available to anyone as the entire system falls apart**

that's coming. You can't expect a handful of doctors to satisfy the needs of over 300 million Americans, with at least 50 million who need constant medical attention. The long-term effects of a failing health system[116] include more taxes, harsher restrictions, and medical care that is so limited that you dare not get sick enough to go to a doctor.

Inflated Prices

As businesses all over America attempt to recover the losses that they will experience from taxes and insurance payments, prices will start to rise. This means that financial hardship is around the corner for many unprepared Americans. As businesses and families are forced to incur the costs of these new taxes, penalties and price hikes, many people will have to close shop, downscale or look for higher-paying jobs in a difficult market. God forbid you decide to get married in the next few years, because then you'd really feel the hurt.

If you wanted to create a painting depicting the effects of Obamacare, it would have to be an abstract piece with a lot of confusion, angry lines and red paint. There are so many problems that will result from this new bill that this text could be a work in progress for the next ten years. Nothing good can possibly come from a bill this power-hungry, which imposes extreme government control on an industry that needs to stay on the free market. The healthcare sector is going to undergo many changes.[117] Maybe that's what Obama meant when he shouted his slogan "Change We Can Believe In"! These days, the slogan should be "Change You Can't Believe!"

But there is hope, because even the stormiest cloud has a silver lining. You and your family can weather this dark time in U.S. history – if you know all of your options. We dedicate the rest of this book to helping you make the right choices in your medical care, so that you don't have to suffer under this draconian socialist healthcare regime.

FINDING A SOLUTION TO THIS LOOMING PROBLEM

Why Medical Tourism Is Your Cost-effective Healthcare Alternative

In the wake of the passage of Obamacare, Americans all over the country are looking for solutions to their growing healthcare worries.[118] With the financial stability of businesses and families at stake – not to mention the threat of serious illness that could strike at any time – more and more Americans are turning to affordable medical tourism. This will be your ticket to good health. For years, people have traveled overseas with a purpose – to find quality, cost-effective medical care from some of the best hospitals in the world. The U.S. healthcare system is so expensive that the cost of a plane ticket, travel insurance, hospital admission, treatment and rehabilitation actually saves you money.[119] With prices on the rise and a whole new host of taxes to pay, medical tourism may be your way out of this downward spiral. Imagine a clean, five-star hospital, with the best doctors in the region ready to tackle your medical troubles.

> **Imagine a clean, 5-star hospital, with the best doctors in the region ready to tackle your medical troubles**

That is what medical travel is all about – helping patients recover and find a better quality of life. Just because the U.S. healthcare system is failing doesn't mean we are doomed to endure neglect, malpractice and dirty, government-owned hospital beds. There is a better way!

Is It Really Cheaper to Get Medical Services Abroad?

Did you know that leaving the country for a medical procedure abroad can save you up to 80% of the costs you'd incur if you stayed here in America? It's no secret that over the past few years, medical costs in

Appendectomy Operation Cost

USA	$15 900
South Africa	$3 800

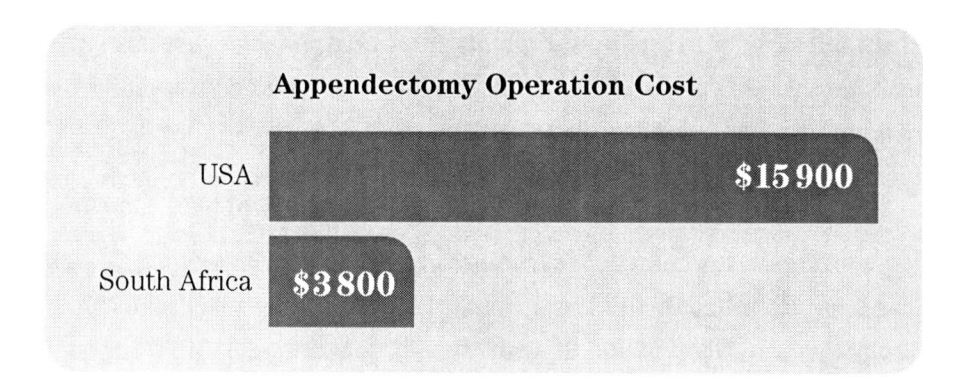

America have gone through the roof. Now, with Obamacare, you'll be paying even more – but losing the quality of service that the U.S. was once famous for. If you can afford to go to a hospital in America, then you can afford to fly overseas for that same procedure. Medical tourism has become a huge industry, and for good reason.[120] People are discovering that they can go on a "medical holiday," and save money at the same time.

Consider an average appendectomy. It's a fairly simple procedure that usually only requires a day or two in the hospital. But it's a necessary operation to have, especially if your appendix is inflamed. In America, let's say that the hospital admission comes to $12,500, with the operation itself costing around $3,400 (estimated national averages). Altogether, if everything goes according to plan, your simple procedure should set you back about $15,900. Of course, this is dependent on your location, which hospital you're in and who your doctor is. Sometimes appendectomies in America can cost as much as $60,000. If you travel to South Africa to have the procedure done, it will cost you around $2,000 for the entire operation and hospital stay, and about $1,800 for the plane tickets and insurance – and you're looking at savings of $12,100. Even if you incur additional expenses there, you still save thousands![121] Countries like Panama, Mexico, South Africa, Belize and Bali are just some of the beautiful medical tourism destinations. Whether you're looking to cut costs and save, or to find better quality treatment, medical tourism gives us hope that we can survive the U.S. healthcare system catastrophe. We need to educate ourselves about getting medical services abroad.

Discovering the Real Cost of Medical Tourism

It doesn't really matter where in America you live: anywhere you go, you'll find exorbitant healthcare costs, some that will cripple you financially if you are ever in the position to need them.[122] It's difficult to get hospitals in the U.S. to disclose how much an operation will cost, because there are too many factors to consider. Sometimes a patient will go in for a simple procedure, and complications will arise that extend the hospital stay for weeks. The costs can be astronomical. When you decide to travel abroad for medical attention, you must make provisions for a worst-case scenario. If you are stuck in a hospital at an affordable care center, you stand a chance of saving yourself from financial ruin. Any middle-class family can afford to fly overseas for medical attention. Even if you want elective cosmetic surgery, there are better alternatives abroad than the options we have here in the U.S.[123] It's all about perspective. There are many accredited hospitals in other countries that can offer you the individual care and attention that will vanish under our new healthcare system. This is especially true for chronic disease and elderly patients who need continuous care.

Imagine that your government insurance refuses to pay for your hip replacement surgery because you are deemed too old to have a prosthetic hip. Trying to pay for that same procedure outside of insurance would be near impossible. The costs are simply too great. Even if you have just enough money, the government still might prevent you from obtaining the much-needed replacement. So your choices are either to spend the next 20 years of your life in a wheelchair, or to start looking outside the U.S. borders. Flying to Mexico for a week to have the surgery done will not only save you money, but will prevent you from having to suffer from a great injustice of government bureaucracy. This is the major benefit of seeking medical services abroad: you will be able to overcome any government-imposed decision on your health and get the help you need. When you fly overseas, there is no Big Brother looking over your shoulder. No taxes to limit the quality of care that you can afford. No government doctors telling you that your procedure won't be done because it's too expensive for their hospital. You are free to choose what you need, when you need it. It's only a flight away.

> **You are free to choose what you need, when you need it. It's only a short flight away**

Saving Money the Smart Way

As your cost-effective healthcare alternative, medical tourism also offers you additional benefits that can help to lighten the load. Prescription or chronic medication in America is very expensive. It's so expensive that when people fly overseas for medical procedures, they are shocked at the affordable drugs they can now buy without insurance. You'll often find that in developing countries, there are cheaper generics that do exactly the same thing as the drug that's been costing you thousands of dollars a month.[124] It's a revelation that keeps international patients returning for low-cost, high-quality medical care outside of the U.S.

The general cost of living in other countries is also significantly lower than in the U.S. Products and services are more affordable, which helps to reduce the overhead cost of medical supplies, accommodations and medical staff. Private hospitals abroad offer international patients top-quality service, luxury and the best medical attention that your dollars can buy. And the savings are multiplied again by the fact that most currency conversion rates triple or even quadruple the value of our currency in other countries.[125]

If you're really looking to make a positive change, and to keep ahead of the crushing healthcare costs that will soon envelop large portions of the American population, then medical tourism is for you. Your health and the health of your family are more important than anything else in your life. Without proper medical care, you could experience the preventable early death of a family member. Don't let Obamacare ruin your chances of living a healthy, happy life. Medical tourism is out there, and it's getting bigger and bigger every year. Thousands of American families have already benefitted from the industry, coming home healthy – and still having enough money to live in comfort. You need to make the decision right now that you're not going to let a socialist president bring your family to ruin. Refuse to believe that getting medical services must bankrupt you. Refuse to believe that there is no way to get that operation you desperately need. You don't have to live under the tyranny of a corporate-controlled system that chews up the little guy. With all the injustice that the new U.S. healthcare legislation would bring to your business, your family, your life – you owe it to yourself to find a better solution. That solution is medical tourism, and we want you to spread the word so that every family is saved from Obama's medical tyranny.

Success Story:
Medical Tourism Changing Lives

Lynette Fletcher: Gastric Bypass Surgery
Lynette is a resident of Memphis, Tennessee, and also happens to work in the allied health field. As a surgical technician, she

knew she had to find someone to help her get the best surgery abroad, to save her the money and the headache of endless hospital bills. After struggling with her weight since childhood, Lynette decided to do something drastic and contacted the Medical Tourism Corporation about undergoing an inexpensive gastric bypass surgery.[126] The Corporation jumped into action and organized a surgery for her at a hospital in Puerto Vallarta, Mexico. Lynette was thrilled with the results of the surgery. The hospital was clean, the staff was dedicated and professional and she felt as though they really cared for her wellbeing during her stay. The surgery and experience was such a success that she plans on returning soon for breast augmentation surgery!

CHAPTER 4

INTRODUCTION TO GLOBAL MEDICAL TOURISM

Introduction to
Global Medical Tourism

ಶ್ರ • ೂ

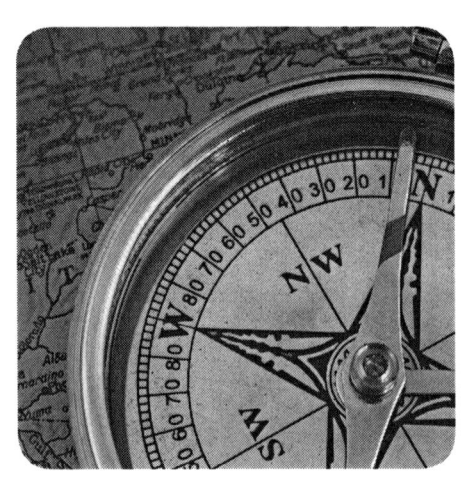

Medical tourism has been around for a long time, but it's only since the rise of the Internet and the fall of American healthcare services that people are starting to take notice of it. Health.com estimates that in the past year, over 6 million Americans chose to fly overseas for quality medical treatment rather than face the enormous bills they would accumulate here. There are currently more than 50 countries around the world that offer and market medical care for the discerning health traveler.[127] Whether you're going to Panama for open heart surgery, South Africa for a flawless nose job or Mexico for hip replacement surgery – there's always a better alternative abroad than here in America. Medical tourism has become even more important now that we are facing the implementation of Obamacare. As healthcare standards drop, more Americans will need to seek proper care elsewhere. American medical travelers are discovering the luxurious, cost-effective medical care that international hospitals can provide. Traveling to another country is no longer the scary, risky and unpredictable experience that it once was.[128] We're talking about hospitals equipped with the latest medical technology, doctors that are world-renowned and scores of highly-qualified nurses that attend to your every need. The medical tourism industry has grown in leaps and bounds over the past ten years. Now you can get low-cost medical care from some of the best medical institutions in the world. And the best part? You won't have to deal with the towering costs, neglectful service or the government bureaucracy that now runs our medical industry.

Global healthcare has enabled millions of people to get the services they need, when they need them. Whether you are looking for an affordable alternative to laser eye surgery or are in desperate need of a top-quality operation immediately – there is a global hospital that is fully prepared to satisfy your needs, even as you read this. Imagine going to Mexico to undergo a surgery that would have cost you $130,000 in the U.S., having the operation, and then staying for the rest of the month for a sunny vacation – all for under $10,000. That is what medical tourism now offers the U.S. citizen – a chance to get away from it all, return to good health, and enjoy a fantastic vacation.

Why Choose to Travel Abroad for Medical Services Now?

The healthcare reform bill puts greater stress on your pocketbook than ever before. Before Obamacare, many families were forced into bankruptcy over simple procedures that were exorbitantly priced. Now with the added taxes and increased government control, our fragile system – that was once admirable, though expensive – is lost forever. The personal attention and level of care that U.S. hospitals once stood for will be gone in a matter of years. Now, if you have an ailment, disease or procedure that requires medical care, your only option is to look beyond U.S. borders. It doesn't matter whether or not you are insured: there is a hospital abroad that can help you. Whenever medical tourism feeds a country's local economy, billions of dollars are passed on to that country's medical industry, encouraging medical advancements,

> **Medical centers in India, Thailand, South America and Europe would be delighted to have you**

hospital upgrades and well-paid staff who excel at what they do. This was one of the reasons the U.S. itself was a vibrant medical tourism destination in the past – because the free market encouraged an increase in the quality of care. Now that our free market system has been crushed, our only alternative is to benefit from other countries whose medical industries still strive for excellence because their doctors have enough incentive to do so.

If your new government insurance plan doesn't provide benefits for your condition, or outright denies you coverage for an operation you need, you don't have to give up on your healthcare. Medical centers in India, Thailand, South America and Europe would be delighted to have you. You stimulate their economy, provide jobs for their people and keep their medical services world-class, so when you go there as a patient, you are treated like an honored guest. Americans who have ventured overseas for their healthcare needs have been shocked at how personal and efficient these medical centers are. With direct access to your specialist, you are more informed about your procedure than you would be in a U.S. hospital; every detail is carefully covered so you get the best care for your money. Let's face it: no one likes to be ripped off, and that's exactly what you can expect from an American hospital. Instead, choose a location where your medical emergency will be solved without you going through the pain of waiting periods, rushed doctors and ever-decreasing standards of practice. You deserve to be pampered, looked after and healed – without being screwed by the system.

The Four Types of Medical Travel

There are a number of reasons why someone would choose to fly overseas for care. Sometimes Americans are surprised to find doctors in other countries who are better qualified to handle their specific healthcare needs than the doctors back home. You need to know: whatever your condition is, there is always a top-quality medical center abroad that can outdo U.S. services in every way. All in all, there are four main types of medical traveler, each with its own set of reasons to venture out into the world of medical travel. They are the elective surgery patient, the emergency surgery patient, the chronic disease patient, and the alternative medicine patient.

Elective Surgery

As the name implies, elective surgery is surgery that is not the result of an emergency medical situation. This doesn't mean that the elective surgery patient doesn't desperately need medical attention. An elderly man might need to have cataracts removed from his eyes in order to see again. This kind of procedure is classified as "elective" because the man could go without the surgery and still live for another 20 years. The fact that he would be blind during those years does not make it a life-threatening situation. One of the perks of being an elective surgery patient is that you have the time to research and organize your perfect medical trip abroad because it isn't time-sensitive. The category of elective surgery also covers cosmetic and dental surgery, though these procedures aren't usually performed to correct a medical problem.

Elective surgeries are the most common surgeries worldwide. They help to improve the mental or physical state of the patients who undergo the procedures. Something like a knee replacement could drastically improve a patient's quality of life as he or she is suddenly able to walk properly again. A large percentage of these surgeries are intended to relieve pain, or to help diagnose a potential future medical problem. Some are also carried out to change the physical appearance of the patient, as through plastic surgery.

Because elective surgery still requires patients to go under the knife and be put to sleep by an anesthesiologist, there are still serious risks involved with surgeries of this kind. Due to the invasive nature of many elective surgeries, it takes a fair amount of time to recover from them. Many kinds of surgeries fall into this category – and if you're thinking about pursuing these options, you should take the time to do the necessary research into exactly what will happen to you. Hospital stays vary depending on the kind of procedure you're receiving, where you are in the world and your doctor's recommendations for recovery time. Wherever you decide to go, make sure that you make the necessary arrangements to be gone for longer than the average recovery time in case any complications should arise.

Insurance Issues

Insurance companies love to get out of paying for elective procedures, and they often can if they determine that the procedure isn't absolutely necessary.[129] Of course what is inconsequential to your insurance company could be a life-changing moment for you. Consider facial reconstructive surgery, for example. What if you've spent your entire life scarred from a childhood accident, and you now have the opportunity to get it fixed? Your dreams will come crashing down when the insurance company denies you coverage. There's no way you can afford $60,000 on your own. So instead, you begin to explore your options overseas. You find a clinic in South Africa that offers the same surgery for only $4,000. Suddenly, the light is back in your eyes. That's what medical tourism can do for you, and indeed for all elective surgery patients. Despite what your insurance company says, you can still afford to get the procedure

– along with the much-needed rest and relaxation that comes with a trip to a beautiful foreign country, and make your recovery time a vacation to remember.

Cosmetic Surgery in the U.S.
The three most common types of elective surgery are all considered "cosmetic." In the United States, cosmetic surgery is a multibillion dollar industry. It costs a lot to look good, as they say. Procedures such as plastic surgery, dental surgery and laser eye surgery[130] are very costly here, and these are the procedures that insurance companies love to reject. According to research done by the American Society for Aesthetic Plastic Surgery, in 2008 alone, over 10.2 million Americans chose to have major work done on their bodies. Breast augmentation and liposuction top the charts as the most popular surgeries, with the traditional nose job being the most popular choice among men. Laser eye surgery is also a much-needed procedure for many Americans experiencing rapidly deteriorating vision. Often, the ophthalmologist who performs this simple surgery demands upfront payment because insurance companies don't pay for elective eye surgery. You need the cash – and it can get pricey.

The same goes for dentistry, a vital service for people who have dental problems, and yet still an elective that is scratched from insurance. Not being able to chew or speak properly because you have bad teeth – or no teeth at all – can be a humiliating and debilitating problem. Each tooth will cost as much as $3,000, with that amount escalating depend-

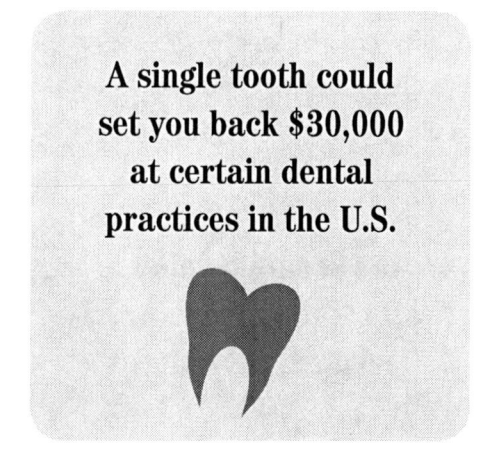

A single tooth could set you back $30,000 at certain dental practices in the U.S.

ing on where you go for dental care. According to DentalResources.com, a single tooth could set you back $30,000 at certain dental practices in the U.S. What chance is there of getting a set of new teeth when insurance won't cover the massive price tag? Each year, many patients fly overseas to seek quality dentistry, eye surgery and plastic surgery. They are able to save up to 70% of the initial cost quote they received in the U.S. Many even choose to go for two or more procedures on one trip, getting more bang for the buck.

Affordable Elective Surgery

In the past, many U.S. citizens would dip into their flexible spending accounts for elective surgeries – but now, with the $2,500 Obamacare cap, that option is out the window.[131] You now have two options: save as much money as you can and have the procedure done in the U.S., risking complications, additional expenses and financial hardship; or travel to Panama, Mexico or Belize for a third of the cost. Though the term "elective surgery" makes it sound as though you have a choice in the matter, this isn't true for many patients. Consider a couple who needs a particular fertility treatment in order to have a child, or a woman who wants a hysterectomy because an unwanted pregnancy could include deadly consequences. These deeply personal medical procedures are life-changing, and you should be able to afford them. Freedom of choice is all about deciding for yourself what the best course of action is for your family. Under Obamacare, you're faced instead with cost barriers, bureaucratic red tape and profit-hungry insurance companies – all preventing you from having the kind of life you deserve.

> **You should be able to afford the life changing medical procedures**

With medical travel, there is a safe and affordable way to get what you need. As an elective surgery patient, you can find the perfect location where all of these needs will be met. International hospitals offer medical travelers a variety of convenient payment options. This means that you can pay off your hospital bill over a period of a few months instead of having to pay it all at once. There are also several types of loans that you may be eligible for, especially if – even at a reduced cost – your surgery is still expensive. Find the best orthopedic medical care overseas and solve that nagging ankle pain; or go for a complete set of tests, including biopsies, scans and x-rays, that would usually cost you the earth and the sun. You can achieve the quality of life that you deserve without the flawed U.S. healthcare system draining all your money away. There's more to come on elective surgery, as we take a closer look at the various procedures you can get overseas, how much they will cost you and where you should go for your specific health concern.

Emergency Surgery

Emergency surgery is an unplanned medical procedure that needs to be done as soon as possible in order to prevent death or severe permanent damage. It begins with life-threatening situations like car accidents, violence, aneurisms, medical complications or heart attacks, or when people have broken bones or have collapsed for no particular reason. Emergency surgery patients are immediately transported to a hospital emergency room for treatment, where they are stabilized and assessed. This is the most challenging medical tourism scenario, because the patient isn't given much time to decide which overseas hospital he or she would like to be transported to once stabilized. Often, emergency patients need long-term care or repeated surgeries, which is why transport to a less expensive hospital across the border is necessary.

Emergency surgeries are the most life-threatening, and they require immediate medical attention for the patient involved. Whether you've just been involved in a traumatic attack or have suffered a stroke, when it comes to emergency surgery you need medical attention and you need it now. There is no way to plan for emergencies of this nature. In addition to the near-death experience, you'll be facing ridiculous medical bills as a result of being taken to the hospital closest to you, and you'll be paying for whatever surgery your doctors had to perform to keep you alive. Unfortunately, many American families won't be able to cope financially with emergency surgeries, especially because they often require long-term hospital stays and follow-up medical care. There are also other costs to consider, such as the ambulance ride, the paramedic treatment, tests, assessments and medications. All of these will add up to a bill that you can't afford to pay, even with your current medical plan. Therefore, it is often a viable "Plan B" to be air-lifted to a hospital abroad for long-term treatment.[132] Whatever surgeries, rehabilitation or critical care you are able to obtain overseas will greatly reduce your overall medical expenses.

Insurance Issues

If you are one of the millions of U.S. citizens who don't have medical insurance, then prepare for a rude awakening. You will be forced to take out personal loans to cover the costs of your medical care, and will spend the next ten years paying them off. Under Obamacare, if you do have medical insurance, prepare for something similar anyway. The standardized plans don't take into account the skyrocketing costs of healthcare, or the specialized treatment you might require to stay alive. Even though the new bill allows people with pre-existing conditions to get insurance, these plans won't cover nearly as much as they should and you won't get the long-term care you need. You'll be pushed out the door as soon as you're stable. Being sent home too soon is a serious concern, especially if you've just been through an experience that threatens your life. Your only option is to seek long-term medical care elsewhere.

What Happens in the ER?

When you arrive at the ER, the paramedics will hand you over to the hospital's trauma doctors. After a speedy initial diagnosis, they will start you on certain medication to stabilize your condition. You may then have to undergo some testing, depending on your emergency. If you have been shot, they may have to do x-rays, MRI scans and CT scans to make sure they know what they are dealing with internally.[133] You will then be rushed to an operating room where doctors and nurses will work to stop any bleeding and fix whatever damage has been done. Your surgery could take one hour or twelve – but you will be billed for every second you're under the knife. After they have saved your life, you will be put in the intensive care unit or in a private room to recover. But the nightmare doesn't end there. Once you are stable, you may still need further surgeries, more tests, extra medicine and around-the-clock care.

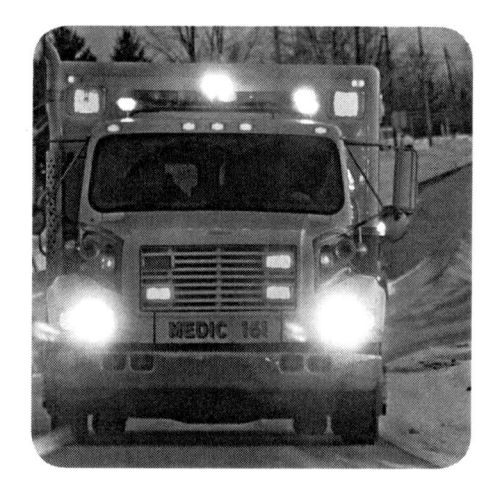

While America once had a reputation for having the best medical services in the world, this has all changed thanks to President Obama and his irrational health reform bill. Now Americans can expect to be treated by overworked doctors, ignored by neglectful nurses, given the wrong medication and subjected to terrible and unsanitary conditions at government-run hospitals. If you decide to leave, you can still get the quality, attentive care you deserve from doctors in free market systems overseas. The better quality care you receive, and the money you save on cheaper medicine and less expensive tests and procedures, will help you get your life back on track after your traumatic experience.

The Air Ambulance Option

Once you have woken up in the intensive care unit, you need to explore your options. Find a hospital just outside of the U.S. that can give you the care that you need without financially crippling you. Though there are additional costs involved with using an air ambulance, your decision to be moved to an alternative location will reap dividends in the end. An air ambulance has all the facilities necessary to transport you in a critical condition to another medical care center.[134] Trained emergency staff will monitor you all the way there, until you are handed over to your new doctors. If your condition is severe, you will need a friend or family member to make the arrangements for you. Though the transport can be risky, there is no reason not to do it if you are stabilized enough to be moved. As difficult as the decision will be to make, it's important that you think long and hard about it well before the emergency arises. Instead of leaving your future at the mercy of unscrupulous insurance companies and a hospital's enormous bills, be prepared to move so that you can recover financially as well as physically, in a safe, comfortable environment. The proof will come when you receive your two separate medical bills – one that will no doubt be huge, and the other much more reasonable, even if you ended up staying and having several more surgeries at your international hospital. Remember, most emergency situations

> **As soon as your U.S. doctor gives you the green light for travel, you need to go**

require several surgeries to correct, even if it's something as minor as a lacerated limb.

Look for private companies who offer Medevac services in the country you want to fly to. This might be the most affordable option. As soon as your U.S. doctor gives you the green light for travel, you need to go. Every day you spend in your hometown hospital is another few thousand dollars that you won't be able to pay. Countries like Mexico have special rehabilitation centers where skilled medical professionals monitor critical patients around the clock. You will even be assigned your own nurse, who knows your condition and can administer the right medication at the right time. Imagine recovering from a life-threatening medical emergency in an accredited overseas hospital that treats you like a special guest. That's what you want – the level of care, quality and attention that will help you through your difficult recovery period.

Treatment for Chronic Disease

Having a chronic disease means that you have had a specific disease for longer than three months, and it can't be cured outright.[135] Many chronic diseases are enormously expensive to live with and are debilitating for the patient. Treatment, surgeries and maintenance can create bills of up to a million dollars a year for these patients and their families. Chronic disease patients often choose to fly overseas for less expensive treatment, or for long-term care that won't bankrupt them. A family who has a daughter with cancer, for example, would take her to a dedicated care center in Mexico, where she would receive life-saving chemotherapy and surgeries at a greatly reduced cost, saving her family from financial ruin. Chronic diseases such as heart disease, cancer, cardiovascular disease, diabetes and arthritis can all be treated internationally.

Having a chronic disease is an emotional and vulnerable drain for the patient. When someone is diagnosed with a severe illness, his or her entire life changes – and becomes about beating the disease. Unfortunately, our new healthcare system is not designed to support people who are living through this kind of terrifying experience. A chronic disease affects more than the patient involved; it involves the entire family. Suddenly, your whole being is focused on staying as healthy as you can, so your body is able to fight off the illness for as long as possible. This requires a complete change in lifestyle that can become very expensive.[136] These complex conditions need to be managed and treated in a medical center that truly cares for the health and wellbeing of the patient. While in the past, the U.S. has had an incredible record of helping patients overcome and beat their chronic diseases, this won't be the case once Obamacare takes full effect.

Sometimes the patient is forced to live a lifetime with the disease, and it is never cured. Did you know that seven out of ten deaths in the U.S. are a result of chronic diseases? There are currently over 133 million Americans living with some form of chronic illness.[137] Many of these families suffer under the weight of the extreme costs these illnesses generate. The most common causes of recurring disease are physical inactivity, unhealthy lifestyle choices, smoking, drinking and pre-existing genetic markers. The most life-threatening chronic diseases are diabetes, cancer, AIDS, heart disease and arthritis. As people get older, they tend to acquire more conditions that need consistent care and monitoring, or treatment with medication.

Insurance Issues

One of the many pressures that the U.S. healthcare system has to contend with is the rising number of chronic disease patients, and their increasingly long life spans. Long-term care is now a vital feature of the medical industry, but it lacks adequate coverage and lower-cost medication. While you might think that insurance would cover chronic diseases, there are many conditions that are frequently left uncovered. High blood pressure, mental illness and addiction are all chronic diseases that are limited by the insurance industry. This is because medication is so costly, and these patients need to have it every day. Then there are those who are underinsured or not insured at all. They don't receive any kind of chronic disease treatment unless they pay for it themselves. This leads to many emergency rooms visits that could have been avoided if people had access to affordable, quality medical services. People with mental illness or a history of addiction often have to deal with increased insurance premiums, if they can get any coverage at all. Insurance companies are hesitant to cover these Americans because they have such a high hospital admission rate. Now, with the new system in place, more chronic disease patients will have access to healthcare, but it will be of an even lower quality than before. Even before Obamacare, there is evidence that many people with "comprehensive" coverage weren't getting the medical care they needed to stay healthy. This was especially true for the elderly and very young. Community Health Centers only offered quality care for half of their patients, while the rest had to live with substandard medical services.

Chronic Disease Patients

With one in every two adult Americans afflicted with some kind of chronic illness, there is a desperate need for better quality and more widespread medical treatment. Diabetes, for example, can lead to blindness, infection, amputation and death if not treated properly.[138] Unfortunately, Obamacare is going to crush the hopes of the afflicted, by saddling the already overburdened health services industry with more insured patients. At first glance, this may appear to be good news for patients living with disease; but in the long run, all it's going to lead to is a shortage of proper medical care for everyone. This blanket coverage

> **If you or a loved one suffers from a chronic disease—your best alternative is to explore medical tourism**

effectively ends the quality care that insured Americans have been receiving to make room for millions of new patients. If you or a loved one suffers from a chronic disease that costs you thousands of dollars every month, your best alternative is to explore medical tourism. Flying overseas for any of your chronic medical concerns allows you to experience the luxury of attentive care from some of the world's most outstanding treatment centers. You will also have the chance to receive specific treatments that may not be available in certain parts of the U.S., like stem cell therapy. Stem cells have been known to help patients with heart disease, diabetes, IBS, lupus and Parkinson's disease. These international chronic disease treatment centers have the latest technology, and at a fraction of the cost of an American hospital. Medical tourism provides the chronic disease patient with access to low-cost medication, tests and treatments whenever they are needed, which increases the patient's health and chance at a normal life. These centers offer controlled diets, exercise plans and relaxation techniques to assist the patient in overcoming the illness. You can recover knowing that when the pain is over, you still have some semblance of financial stability. For families, this makes all the difference. There is nothing worse than surviving cancer, then having to pay for it for the rest of your life – or worse, having to declare bankruptcy because of it. Financial limitations keep some patients from receiving the treatment they need – but it doesn't mean you can't get help. Researching about and traveling to an international destination could mean the difference between recovering from an illness... and dying from it.

Alternative Medical Treatment

Alternative medicine is defined as medicine or medical treatment that is not part of conventional medicine.[139] Treatments like homeopathy, alternative cancer treatment and acupuncture all fall within the realm of alternative medicine. The United States isn't big on alternative treatment, and insurance doesn't usually cover it because science says that it hasn't had a consistent success rate in healing people. But millions of Americans have been healed by alternative medicine, by traveling abroad to find the best and most effective treatments for their conditions. The alternative medicine patient can find an amazing variety of alternative medicines abroad that may help them where modern science has failed. This branch of medicine should never be ignored, and has been known to cure mental illness, cancer, chronic pain and fatigue.

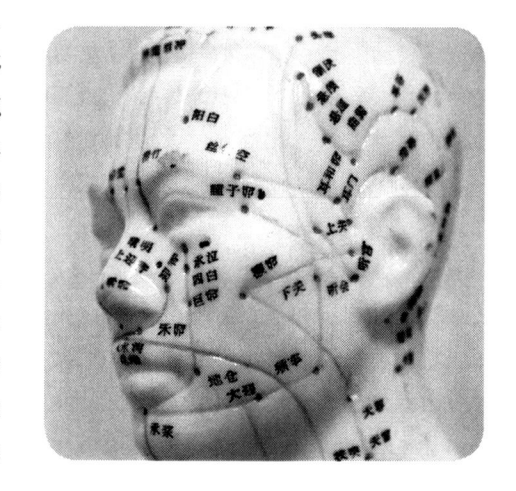

The United States has always been an advocate of modern, science-based medical technology.[140] As such, alternative medicine has been written off as a supplementary discipline that could help in pain or disease treatment but won't actually effect any real change in the body. If you understand that the body's natural defense systems are what keep a person healthy, then of course keeping these systems in top shape will help with any kind of illness. Doctors in the U.S. are hesitant to embrace natural healing methods, but these therapies have been known to reduce symptoms – and in some cases even cure diseases like cancer. Care for seriously ill patients should include an alternative medicine component, so that the patients' bodies increase the strength of their immune systems and have a greater chance of defeating disease. To cure these patients, going back to the basics of preventative and supportive care is sometimes exactly what is needed.

Whether you are experiencing medical issues from obesity, high cholesterol, emphysema or kidney disease, there is an alternative natural medicine that can help you. Doctors in Japan, for example, have been treating serious illness with acupuncture for thousands of years, with excellent results.[141] If you find that modern medicine is not working for you, or if you need more than what clinical medicine can provide, going on an affordable medical trip overseas for alternative treatment purposes is the way to go.

Insurance Issues

There are insurance companies in America that cover alternative medical treatment, but it is usually very limited. The coverage does not include long-term sessions, herbal medicines or beneficial exercise programs like yoga. If you find that you want to go the natural route, then you'll have to pay for it yourself. This would normally be an unrealistic goal if you had to have these treatments in America, but overseas it's a completely different story. There is a lot more respect for alternative medicine abroad, with many certified doctors providing these treatments in conjunction with modern medicine. Something as simple as the purifying properties of ionized water can boost your system enough to start helping to wage war against your disease or condition.

Alternative Medicine Patients

One of the best features of alternative or complementary medicine is that it often reduces the side effects of your traditional medication.[142] A cancer patient who goes for chemotherapy and radiation treatment might experience nausea, vomiting and fatigue. If this same patient is on a wellness program or a course of herbal medicines as well, these symptoms could be reduced and even eliminated because of the strengthened state of their body. Natural medicines are powerful, and they don't contain any of the harmful chemicals found in modern medicine.

> **Alternative medicine is especially beneficial to patients who experience chronic pain in their joints, back, neck and limbs**

Every treatment you undergo and every supplement you take builds up your body's resistance to the disease. Alternative medicine is especially beneficial for patients who experience chronic pain in their joints, back, neck and limbs. With massage therapy, chiropractic attention and acupuncture, this pain can be significantly reduced – without the terrible toll that prescribed pain medication would take on your body. International destinations like India, South Africa, Mexico and Thailand have many alternative treatment centers designed to help you return to good health naturally.

Alternative medicine also includes more daring studies on incurable diseases such as AIDS and cancer. There are clinics in Mexico, for example, that treat patients with alternative cancer treatments as well as chemotherapy. Natural medicine is less expensive than modern medicine, so developing countries like Panama and South Africa spend a lot of money on research into developing effective cures with herbal medicine. Many of these herbal medicines also detoxify the blood and help keep the patient's organs in good condition. Valerian root, for example, is used to treat central nervous system disorders, Pomorrosa leaves are great for diabetes, and Palco rids the body of unwanted parasites. It makes more economic sense for these countries to build their natural health industries, rather than pour millions of dollars into drug research.

There is also an emphasis on dietary wellness overseas that Americans seem to have lost. Tests are run in some health and wellness clinics to determine what kind of foods would suit a patient's body; then a diet is specially designed for that patient, which helps balance the body's healing powers with the additional medicines he or she is taking.

Moving Toward Greater Health

The natural medical tourism trade is booming, with thousands of Americans traveling all over the world in search of a healthy life, in spite of their conditions. There are various kinds of treatments, ranging from energy therapies to mind-body intervention therapies. No matter what condition you have, there is a natural solution that can help you live more comfortably with it, improving your quality of life. If you fly overseas for an operation or for medical treatment, you can enroll in one of these programs that will help you recover quicker. Non-Western medicine has its benefits, and you can discover them all while resting and recuperating in a spa-like environment abroad.[143] This is definitely something to look into if you are chronically plagued with pain, disease, disorders or addiction. There are testimonials all over the Internet from average Americans who have spent years fighting ill health, only to find the cure in a far-off land in the form of alternative medicine. It's not the crazy, anti-science health treatment it once was. You can now discover the affordable healing powers of alternative medicine in a beautiful setting abroad.

Why Your Doctor Thinks It's a Bad Idea

What happens if you speak to your doctor about medical tourism and he or she discourages you from going? This is not uncommon with medical practitioners in America, who don't like their business going elsewhere. Doctors who own small, private practices don't like to lose their patients – and all the cash benefits those patients mean to them – to medical tourism.[144] Until now, doctors have been willing to help their patients wherever they can, but some of them hold a true grudge against patients who choose to fly overseas for their surgeries and treatments. Others simply don't know enough about it to understand how beneficial it can be for their patients' health and wellbeing. You can see why large hospital groups would perceive medical tourism as a constant drain on their income. As millions of Americans flock to alternate destinations to get cheaper and more efficient medical care, many doctors are left feeling frustrated at their patients' lack of loyalty. But this cannot deter you from going, especially since most of these doctors are just interested in adding to their bottom line. We're not saying that all medical practitioners feel this way; on the contrary, many doctors openly support medical tourism and even do it themselves.

So what are the damaging things your doctor could say that would discourage you from going to a hospital abroad for your medical care needs?

Old-School Ideas of Medical Tourism

In the past, medical tourism had a dubious reputation, and a lot of horror stories were flying around about people going for simple procedures overseas and dying on the operating table. Of course, this is a risk people take wherever they go; but it should be noted that the incidence of patients dying for no reason on the operating table is significantly lower abroad than in the U.S. Visions of dirty, second-rate hospitals with bad equipment and even worse medical care might have stood up twenty years ago,

These days, many hospitals abroad are bigger and better than most hospitals in America

but not today.[145] These days, many hospitals abroad are bigger, better and employ more specialist doctors than most hospitals in America. These privately-owned hospitals offer only the best quality care, and maintain exemplary reputations in the global market – specifically to draw medical tourists to their doors.

What about Legal Issues?

Your doctor might bring up the fact that many countries lack strong enough laws to protect the patient if something goes wrong. If a doctor in Bali leaves a sponge in your stomach, for example, and you almost die – you can't sue them for it. While medical malpractice suits are not common overseas, they do happen. And there are laws to protect you, of course. Unfortunately, you probably won't be able to squeeze a large amount of money from an international hospital like you can here in the U.S. But there are global rules that doctors adhere to, and standards of practice that every medical care center has to follow. So, you don't have to worry about being mistreated, neglected or worse, and watching them get away scot-free. It just doesn't happen.

Higher Risk of Infection

One of the feeblest arguments made by some doctors hinges on the fact that when you are in a new country, you are not used to their water and food, and may not be immune to their native viruses. This makes you more likely to contract illnesses or an infection after an operation.[146] Any honest medical doctor will tell you that this is nonsense. If you take the required medication and give yourself time to recover before you travel, then there is no increased risk of infection at all. American doctors who use this argument just want to make you feel apprehensive about going. Your medical safety all depends on where you go and who treats you. Generalizing for the sake of a scare tactic is not going to help anyone. A medical tourist who checks into a quality, JCI-approved hospital abroad can look forward to all the perks their foreign doctor promised over the phone.

•

It's understandable that doctors in the U.S. feel threatened by medical tourism. The new healthcare system is bad enough, but the trickle-down effect will leave many small practices struggling to make ends meet. Even one of their patients deciding to go overseas for a procedure could be a nail in the coffin. If you plan your trip properly and thoroughly investigate your destination hospital, then there is no reason to be alarmed by anything your doctor might say. The doctor thinks it's a bad idea because for that practice, it is a bad idea. Less money means less income; and the more patients lost, the closer the practice is to closing.

Beat the Cost Barriers with Medical Benefits Abroad

We've already established that saving money is a huge incentive to go overseas for medical treatment – but what are the other reasons you should go?

Your Medical Vacation

The most attractive feature about medical tourism is that you are actually visiting another country. It's a vacation with a purpose. Once you have recovered from your treatment or operation, you get to explore the sights and sounds of a completely new place. Take some extra time to see the landmarks and special sites that your chosen country offers its tourists. This experience can be very positive, as you are able to get the medical care you need and the vacation you've been wanting all at once. Imagine sipping an iced drink in a five-star resort while recovering from your operation. Explore the local culture, try new foods and buy little trinkets that will remind you of your visit. A week in paradise is exactly what you need after your medical ordeal. It's physically and mentally rejuvenating, and you can enjoy it with your loved ones or your traveling companion.

Increasing Quality of Care

The doctors and nurses that you come across in your medical tourism destination are fully trained, some by medical facilities in the United States. This means that you still get the benefit of the best education and experience without having to deal with the rising prices that doctors demand in America. Money has been pumped into privately-owned hospitals by local investors, who recognize the tremendous opportunities that medical tourism brings to their shores.[147] With state-of-the-art facilities, new advancements in technology and immediate service, this is the preferred choice over Obama's new healthcare system. You won't have to wait months for a surgery, your doctor will help you from the first to the final stages of your treatment, and because everything is so affordable, you can do it all in style. Many of the hospital rooms are more like suites in a hotel!

Ease of Use

There are trained staff, 24-hour hotlines and even booking agents

It used to be a pain to get in touch with hospitals overseas. No one spoke English, contact details were scarce and trying to figure out exactly what you needed when you got there was a nightmare. These days, there are trained staff who speak your language, 24-hour hotlines to connect you with your hospital and doctor and even booking agents who will sort through the trip details for you. For the best international destinations, there are package deals offered by many medical tourism agents. These agents will take you through the process of planning and preparing for your stay, until you are completely prepared. Flight bookings, car rentals, accommodations, doctor's appointments, surgery bookings – everything is easy when you use one of these specialized agents.

Working Out the Exact Cost

A great benefit of getting medical services overseas is that even before you've left America, you know exactly how much everything is going to cost you. This allows you to work out how much you need to take, and how much extra to bring in case anything goes wrong. This is because international hospitals are very transparent about their costs. They will give you a complete price list so you can accurately assess the cost of your medical vacation. Accommodations, hospital stays, services and procedure prices are all included. This is in sharp contrast to hospitals in America, which only give you the surgical procedure costs. If you ask your doctor here, they have no idea what the bill will be so you almost always go in blind. This leads to additions, extras and amendments on your bill, until it's huge – and you have no idea how it got that way. But it's all in the name of good health, right?

> **Before you've left America you know exactly how much everything is going to cost you**

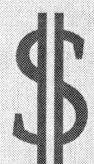

Licensed and JCI-approved

A JCI-accredited hospital is a hospital that exceeds the Joint Commission International's stringent set of regulations and standards of practice.[148] The JCI methods of evaluation involve only the best and most rigorous quality controls, ensuring that the hospital you visit is world-class. There are many JCI-approved hospitals around the world, and each of them has the level of care that you'd expect from a professional medical care center. When you decide to become a medical tourist, make sure your hospital is accredited by a governing body.

Competitive Care

> The competition inspires a level of care that America will soon lose

Because the market for medical tourism is so large, hospitals all over the world compete with each other to draw in new patients. This competition inspires productivity, and a level of care that America will soon lose due to our new socialized medical plan.[149] The global free-market system forces these incredible hospitals to lower their prices to be more competitive and to offer better services, luxury accommodations and round-the-clock nurses who ensure that you are always cared for. Their global reputation hinges on what you, the international patient, say about their hospital when you return home. As a result, they genuinely do everything they can to help you recover.

The Two-Way Street

International hospitals are more likely to go the extra mile because they understand the benefits of having you in their country. The more tourists that arrive in their country because of your good experience, the larger their hospital will grow, and the better their country's economy will get.

It's a two-way street that often results in both parties being thrilled at the outcome. A win-win situation!

Your First Steps to Improved Health and Wellness Abroad

You've thought about it endlessly, and you've made the right decision. You are going to become a medical tourist. If you thought that was the hard part, you were right. It's amazing how many people still accept the word of their primary care doctors as law. So many families have been hurt because of it.

But what in the world do you do now? It seems like a fairly insurmountable task – planning and then executing what will be your first medical jaunt abroad. Where the heck do you start? Well, start at the beginning.

Determining Your Immediate Need

Using the information in this chapter, determine what kind of medical tourist you are.

1. Are you an elective surgery patient looking to go overseas for rhinoplasty, a knee replacement, or a new set of teeth?
2. Are you an emergency surgery patient who is concerned about the standard of healthcare you are receiving, and the financial burden it's putting on your family?
3. Are you a chronic disease patient looking for a less expensive treatment for cancer, diabetes, heart disease or arthritis?
4. Are you are an alternative medicine patient looking for complementary medicine to ease your pain or chronic condition?

Once you have decided what kind of medical tourist you are, you can begin to make the right decisions about your trip. An elective surgery patient can go into great detail about where and when they want to venture overseas. The emergency surgery or chronic disease patient might want to call a medical travel agent to help them arrange the details as quickly as possible. Based on your needs, you will assess the right course of action for you and your family. Once you know exactly what procedure you need done, you can begin to make enquiries about it. There are three questions you must consider when calling around for advice:

1. Which international doctor is best suited for your particular condition?
2. What is the most convenient destination for you to travel to?
3. Where can you find the best quality medical care at the lowest price?

These three questions should be in your arsenal when searching for the ideal location, doctor, cost and medical care. Use the Internet to search for testimonials from people who have received care in the hospitals that you are interested in calling. Don't forget to ask your general practitioner whether they know of anyone who has had a successful experience abroad, or ask around your neighborhood for the same reason. A real person standing in front of you can give you a lot more details than a web page.

Destination Hospital

Once you have a general idea of where you want to go – directed by the three questions you've been asking people – then it's time to narrow down the choices. Visit these hospitals' websites to find contact details and locate a doctor in the department you need. Make sure that the hospitals you like most are JCI-accredited, or at least affiliated with an American hospital group of some sort. Hospital Punta Pacifica in Panama, for example, is affiliated with the Johns Hopkins Hospital Group, and will therefore be particularly in tune with your needs as an American medical tourist. Here's a tip: find images of the hospital before you call them. If the hospital looks well-cared for, modern and credible, then call. If it looks weather-beaten, old and care-worn, perhaps it's not the right choice. Once you reach the right specialist, you can begin to collect some specifics: how much will the procedure cost, how long will it take and what is that specialist's success rate with that procedure over the last two years. Ask the doctor how many international tourists he or she has helped before, and what that particular hospital can offer you as a medical tourist. If all goes well and you get a good feel for the hospital (even if you've had to speak to a few administrative staff and three nurses before reaching the doctor you need), then you are ready to begin planning your trip.

Doing It Alone

Find out from your chosen hospital exactly how much your procedure will cost. Then, add your flight costs, accommodation costs, insurance costs and at least $2,000 extra in spending money. Once you have all of your expenses in front of you, you can work on financing the trip. Get a loan from the bank, save, borrow or take out a second mortgage – whatever you do, keep in mind that you are saving yourself a whole lot more by becoming a medical tourist. We go into more detail about planning your trip later on in the book, but for now you have the money, the destination and the will to go – and that's enough.

Going Through a Medical Travel Agent

If you don't have the time to plan your trip on your own, you can hire a medical travel agent to do it for you. Medical travel agents will sort out your trip for you at an additional cost, and it's worth it if you are in a time crunch. They

Everything from A-Z is done for you

sort out tedious details like flight bookings, how much money you need to take, your accommodations, appointments to meet your doctor and how long the whole trip will take. Everything from A to Z is done for you. All you have to do is pack and go. These agencies often have offices in your destination country as well, so you won't be helpless when you get there. Make sure that your agency is full-service and not just a referral agency. Referral agencies help you plan for your trip, but they only offer certain services so you'll have to do some things yourself.

One Step Forward

Now that you know how to go about planning your trip, you need more information on the kinds of procedures and services offered by hospitals all over the world. The rest of this book is dedicated to informing you about various medical services and where you will find them on the global map. As an informed medical traveler, you should be able to find the best services in the world. Keep reading to learn more about medical tourism, hospitals and destination countries so that you can get the most out of this book, and the most out of your trip. Your medical travel journey starts now.

ಙ • ಜ

CHAPTER 5

AFFORDABLE ELECTIVE SURGERY ABROAD

Affordable Elective Surgery Abroad

If you're looking for an affordable location to get your elective procedure done, this section will recommend some of the world's best medical service destinations. Now that you've made the decision to go, there are a number of details that you need to sort out. The most important is getting more information about your specific surgery, and who in the world can do it for you at an affordable price. Elective surgery drives the medical tourism trade; with the right knowledge behind you, you'll be able to find the right country, hospital and doctor to suit your particular needs.

Questions You Should Ask Your Doctor

Calling, emailing and IMing will put you in contact with doctors who could potentially offer you the quality and affordability you're looking for in an elective surgical procedure. Here is a list of important questions to ask them, once you have them on the line.

Please tell me about your training and education

One of the best ways to make sure that your elective surgery will be done by an educated and experienced professional is to check out the doctor's credentials. Don't be afraid to ask your potential surgeon where he studied, and how qualified he is to carry out the elective procedure that you require. Doctors will often have an endless stream of qualifications behind their name – which is a good thing – but would be hopelessly average at performing your specific surgery. You don't want average. You want excellent. Talk to him about his training and education, and how prepared he is to perform your operation.

Would you send me your CV?

The next step might seem a little intrusive – but let's face it, we're talking about your life here, so the more information you can get on your doctor, the better. Ask the surgeons politely if they would be willing to send their CV to your email address. You might be surprised how common this request is in the industry; your potential doctor likely has one ready to send to curious international patients. If they are the best at what they do, then this shouldn't be a problem. If a doctor refuses to send you a résumé, then you should move on in search of one who will. Qualified professionals are proud of their medical achievements and won't mind letting you read about them. A giant red flag should pop up in front of you if the doctor becomes irritated or reluctant to help. This is not the kind of person you want to trust with your life. A great elective surgeon should also have a list of testimonials or references from patients he has operated on in the past. Ask the hospital if they would mind putting you in contact with a patient or two who had your specific surgery at that facility. This can prove to be most enlightening as you hear from an experienced patient about the entire process from beginning to end.

> **Qualified professionals are proud of their medical achievements**

Is your hospital accredited?

If you haven't already found out, ask the doctor you're speaking to if his hospital is accredited. Then ask which third-party agency has accredited the hospital so you can research the quality control standards that it abides by. Not all accreditations are equal, so make sure that you learn as much as you can about the agency before committing to a single doctor.

Do you agree on the surgical procedures I need done, or are there other alternatives?

You'll often find that different doctors recommend different procedures or surgeries for the same diagnosis. You may be lucky enough to avoid major surgery altogether because the doctor you've contacted has a very high success rate treating your medical problem with a less invasive procedure. For example, if you believe you need a certain type of cosmetic surgery, there may be a more simple procedure than the extensive surgery that your U.S. doctor recommended. It all depends on where you go, and how experienced your doctor is. If he is a world-renowned dental surgeon, and knows a method for giving you great teeth without removing all of your existing ones, then go for it! The surgery will be less expensive – and the recovery less painful – than you originally thought.

How safe is this elective procedure?

Many elective procedures are quite invasive, and can land you in the hospital for weeks. You need to ask your potential doctor how safe is the surgery, and what are the best and worst case scenarios? You also need to accurately describe your physical state so that they can make a true assessment of how your specific medical concerns will affect the safety of the surgery. Your age is also a factor, so be sure to mention it on the phone or in your email. An overweight, 64-year-old woman looking to have a face lift, for example, might have an increased level of risk during the procedure. Her age and fitness level could cause complications in even the simplest surgeries.

What is your personal success rate?

Ask your potential doctor for his success rate overall, and with the procedure you require. Often, a doctor who is quite good at general surgery doesn't have the necessary skill to perform complicated procedures. The same is true of specialists. To judge the performance of the doctor you have in mind, concentrate on the success rate for your specific elective procedure. Obviously, if the doctor's success rate is lower than average, you don't want to sign him on as your doctor. Keep your eyes open for specialists who have a great record in your specific area, and who have the credentials to match. You might also be interested in finding out how many errors, complications and problems that a surgeon has dealt with, and why. This information would be most helpful when you have narrowed your choices down to the final three. If your doctor can't give you his personal success rate, then ask for the hospital's rate instead. It should be noted: this step isn't necessary for patients who are flying abroad for minor cosmetic alterations, like skin treatments or tattoo removals.

How is the surgery performed?

Listening to your potential doctor describe your procedure can give you valuable insight into how he will communicate with you once you arrive. If he is detailed and honest about the surgery over the phone, then you can look forward to the same attention face-to-face. If he is dismissive and impatient about explaining it over the phone, then look for another doctor. The key here is to get an understanding of what will be happening to you from start to finish, throughout your stay in your destination country. Unfortunately, there can be a language barrier when traveling overseas for medical care, which is why it's so important to make sure that your doctor can communicate well. You don't want important details to be lost in translation. This is your chance to ask about the features of your operation – such as the anesthesia and medications that may be used during the procedure, and where the actual surgery will take place. Many specialists operate out of more than one hospital, especially those whose expertise is in high demand; you don't want to make preparations for one hospital, and then realize once you get there that it is more convenient for your doctor to perform the operation somewhere else.

How long does it take?

Knowing how long the actual surgery takes can help you do a cost analysis when comparing doctors and medical care centers. A procedure could take an hour in the hands of one surgeon, but two to four hours at a different hospital. If you find that the surgery takes particularly long in a hospital you are interested in, you can ask why, and mention that you've received other time estimates at other facilities. Also, it's very important to make sure that your doctor is the one doing the surgery. Surprising as it sounds, there have been instances of a surgeon neglecting to tell the patient that a team of residents who aren't as experienced as the surgeon will be involved in the surgery. This is especially true of teaching hospitals that attract new doctors. If an hour-long procedure takes two, ask why – it could reveal some hidden truth about the operation.

What is the average recovery time for the surgery?

Recovery time is important, and because you're heading overseas, you need to make time and cost preparations for your stay. Find out what the minimum and maximum stays have been for elective surgery patients who have undergone the same procedure. This can be enlightening, especially if you believed that you'd be recovering for a week but find out that 38% of patients who experience complications have to stay for an extra week before they can travel safely. Make the right preparations and you won't be surprised when it takes longer than you thought it would. Everybody recovers at his or her own pace, so allow for a week of extra recovery time, or at least a few extra days. This doesn't apply to patients who are traveling abroad for standard dental, fertility or cosmetic surgery. These procedures are very predictable, and it is rare indeed for complications to arise that would keep you bed-ridden after your surgery.

Keep these additional questions in mind[150] so you can successfully plan your visit abroad:
- Are there any side-effects associated with the surgery?
- What medications will be necessary after the surgery?
- How many American patients have you helped?
- Are you easily contactable?
- How much will the entire procedure cost?
- How much will a pre-surgical consultation cost?
- How much will post-surgical checkups cost?
- What pre-operative preparations should I keep in mind before the surgery?
- What medical records do you need from me?

These questions will give you a good idea of your specialist's skill level, communication skills, cost and quality of service. You should contact a minimum of three different doctors or hospitals in the location of your choice before making a decision. If you haven't yet decided which country you'll be visiting, then set a goal of contacting at least two hospitals per country so you gain a better idea of where you can find the best services at the lowest prices.

Cosmetic Surgery

Cosmetic surgery has become enormously popular in the world of medical travel because it's so expensive in the U.S. This branch of medical tourism is thriving as more and more Americans become aware of these "cosmetic vacations" that can improve the way they look and feel. Returning from a medical vacation like this can truly bring out the "new you" – younger, thinner, and better looking than ever before. Let's take a look at the five most popular cosmetic procedures offered in other countries.

#1 Breast Augmentation

Traveling abroad for breast augmentation[151] has become a massive trend for cosmetic surgery patients. According to Medicine.net, the procedure involves "enlargement of the breasts," which is achieved by gently inserting a silicone bag under the breast, or under both the breast and chest muscle. This bag is then filled with salt water to achieve the desired effect of fuller, more proportionate breasts. The patient also has the option of choosing a silicone gel implant, but saline is said to be safer and is therefore the more popular choice.

> *Tip!* Breast augmentation procedures do not come with a lifetime guarantee. If your goal is to get a new set of breasts, then expect to have a couple of extra surgical procedures throughout your life to maintain them. They do not last forever.

Benefits Include: A balancing of your figure with the size of your breasts, which makes for a better overall appearance. Reshaping removes any droop, sagging or scarring, and gives you more confidence in and out of your clothes.

Risks Include: A failed surgery, resulting in deformation or deflation, long-term pain and increased risk of infection. You might also experience a loss of sensation in your breasts, and not be able to breast feed after the operation. These risks can be eliminated with the right choice of plastic surgeon, and clean facilities during your recovery period.

Average Time of Procedure: Procedure times vary according to the medical care center and doctor you're using, but the average time is between one and three hours.

Recovery Time: Expect to be up and about after five days; but, due to the invasive nature of this procedure, a full recovery will take several months. This allows the marks to fade and the pain to subside. Exercise can resume after two months of rest.

Most Popular Medical Tourism Destinations for this Procedure: Costa Rica, Panama, Mexico and Thailand.

#2 Face and Neck Lift

A face and neck lift[152] is popular among older men and women, though women in their 30's have been known to have the procedure. The procedure repairs sagging, drooping or wrinkled skin of the face and neck. Your plastic surgeon makes small incisions above your hairline, behind your earlobes, and on your lower scalp – lifting your fatty facial tissue, tightening your muscles and removing loose skin. The result is a younger, thinner-looking face that has fewer wrinkles, and less skin damage and excess skin. There are a number of different facelifts, including standard, mini, deep-plane and mid-facelift.

> ***Tip!*** Ask your surgeon if you qualify for an outpatient procedure. They are less expensive as there is no hospital admission, and this is a fairly short, simple surgery that doesn't require full anesthesia.

Benefits Include: An immediate improvement in your facial contours, shaving off years and making you appear younger and healthier. It's a big confidence booster for older men and women who are looking to reclaim some of their former features. No more jowls, saggy eyes, wrinkled brows and turkey-neck problems.

Risks Include: Blood pockets under the skin, swelling, and nerve damage that can reduce facial movement for a few months after the surgery. These complications are easy to avoid, however, as long as you have a good surgeon and aren't on any serious medications that might increase the risk of side effects. Make sure you give your surgeon a list of all your medications prior to your procedure.

Average Time of Procedure: The average time is between two and three hours, depending on your plastic surgeon and the facilities at his disposal.

Recovery Time: Expect normal swelling and discomfort for two weeks after the operation. You will be fully recovered after a month or two. Make sure to follow your surgeon's medication regimen to reduce problems during your recovery time.

Most Popular Medical Tourism Destinations for this Procedure: India, Mexico and South Africa.

#3 Liposuction

Liposuction[153] is a favorite among Americans. Who wouldn't want to instantly lose weight without having to go to the gym or eat healthily? Not only does liposuction make you thinner, but it removes fat cells from your body so it is difficult for you to put the weight back on. According to Medicine.net, liposuction is the surgical suctioning of fat deposits from specific parts of the body. The most common areas to receive liposuction are the abdomen, the thighs, the upper arms and buttocks. Your surgeon will use an instrument called a *canula*, which he places under your skin to vacuum out the fat. This surgery is often used in conjunction with other procedures, like tucks and lifts. If the patient has excess skin after the vacuum procedure, that will also be removed.

> ***Tip!*** Inquire about advanced liposuction procedures that include techniques which shorten recovery times and have better results in the long run. Some of these techniques are the tumescent technique, ultrasound-assisted lipoplasty and the super-wet technique.

Benefits Include: Instant weight loss, improved confidence and a whole new lifestyle. There are also numerous health benefits that come from being thinner. This is the ultimate solution if, no matter how hard you've tried, you can't lose the weight on certain parts of your body. It's also excellent for grossly overweight patients, to help them get a fresh start and achieve permanent wellness.

Risks Include: Remaining pockets of uneven fat cells, excess skin, organ damage and infection. Like most procedures, these risks can be eliminated by choosing a qualified, reputable plastic surgeon.

Average Time of Procedure: Depending on the area or areas that need work, the procedure can take between one and four hours.

Recovery Time: Recovery time varies, but you can expect to be out and about in one week, and fully recovered after a month.

Most Popular Medical Tourism Destinations for this Procedure: Brazil, Thailand and Argentina.

#4 Rhinoplasty

Commonly known as the nose job, rhinoplasty[154] is one of the more complex cosmetic surgeries. If you have a misshapen or large nose, you can have it fixed and re-contoured by an international surgeon. A rhinoplasty can be defined as a facial procedure to enhance the appearance of the nose. Your surgeon will change the cartilage and tissue of your nose to make it look more attractive. It's also used to fix damaged or broken noses.

> ***Tip!*** After your nose job, it's better to sleep in an elevated position, to reduce the pain and discomfort you will experience for a few weeks after your procedure. Once you have healed fully, you can return to sleeping in your normal position.

Benefits Include: A more attractive nose, improved breathing, and greater confidence in your appearance.

Risks Include: Excessive bleeding from your nose and infection. These uncommon side effects can usually be remedied by going on a simple course of antibiotics after your surgery.

Average Time of Procedure: A nose job usually takes between one and two hours under the knife.

Recovery Time: It will take a week or two for the swelling and discomfort to go away, but you should be able to return to normal daily activities as soon as one week after the operation. Expect to be fully recovered after two months.

Most Popular Medical Tourism Destinations for this Procedure: Dubai, Croatia and Panama.

#5 Blepharoplasty

Often called eyelid surgery, this procedure is for older men and women who are looking to reduce the bags under their eyes and the puffy lids above their eyes. According to the Mayo Clinic, a blepharoplasty is a surgery used to repair droopy eyelids by removing excess skin, fat and muscle. Sometimes this surgery is necessary, as the sagging skin can impair your vision as your grow older. It's also a great complementary surgery to have with a facelift, for a younger overall look.

> *Tip!* If you suffer from high blood pressure or any other chronic conditions, speak to your doctor about the risks involved. This elective surgery is almost surely not worth having if it's going to put your life in danger.

Benefits Include: An immediate improvement in your appearance and confidence. Blepharoplasty is also extremely beneficial for people who struggle to see be-cause of fatty eyelids drooping and obscuring their vision.

Risks Include: Bruising, infection, bleeding, wound separation or excessive skin removal (which results in skin that is too tight around your eyes). You might have trouble sleeping because your eyelids won't stay closed. Choose the right plastic surgeon for this procedure to prevent these side effects.

Average Time of Procedure: Between one and three hours is the normal surgery time, depending on the amount of repair that has to be done.

Recovery Time: Bruising should heal within two weeks, and you can expect a full recovery in two months.

Most Popular Medical Tourism Destinations for this Procedure: Costa Rica, South Africa and South Korea.

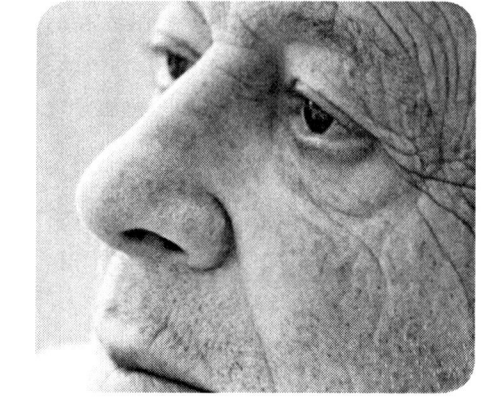

Dental Surgery

For many, dentistry is a four-letter word – but it can't be ignored. For some people, proper dentistry can mean the difference between an outgoing social life and the life of a hermit. Teeth matter, the position of teeth matters and nothing in the world is worse than tooth pain. This is why dental surgery abroad has become such a sought-after service. As far as U.S. dentists are concerned, it *pays* to look your best – or to be able to eat, close your mouth properly or live a pain-free life. If you are in need of affordable dental surgery, then medical tourism will open new doors for you. Many dental travelers choose to have several procedures done on one trip. Here are the top five dental surgeries in the world of medical travel.

#1 Dental Implants

Dental implants are extremely expensive in America, so most people go for dentures, bridges or crowns. But these can be painful to wear, and often make talking difficult and eating even worse. The most permanent and affordable solution if you are missing teeth is to go overseas for dental implants. An implant is an artificial tooth that replaces the one you are missing. Your dental surgeon will implant a titanium screw into your jawbone. Unfortunately, the crown or new tooth that will be inserted onto that screw can only be fitted several months later, so two trips are required.

> *Tip!* Why not get your titanium screws fitted in one country and then fly to another one when it's time to have your crowns put in? This way you get to experience two different countries and have two unique medical vacation experiences.

Benefits Include: Proper chewing functionality, prevention of bone loss and gum recession, and the confidence to smile again.

Risks Include: A 10% chance that the implants will fail and have to be removed. There is a risk of infection and tissue damage around the gums, and an upper implant can cause sinus problems. Most of these risks are easily corrected by the dental surgeon should they arise.

Average Time of Procedure: One dental implant takes an hour to fit. The more implants you have done, the longer the procedure will take.

Recovery Time: Pain usually vanishes after a week or two of the screw implantation; but there is a rest period of between three to seven months before the crowns are installed. This is because the screws have to settle and be accepted before any further action is taken.

Most Popular Medical Tourism Destinations for this Procedure: Mexico, Hungary and Peru.

#2 Jaw Bone Grafting

Bone grafting sounds terrifying, but it's necessary if you don't have enough bone in your jaw for the dental implant that you want. In that case, you will first have to undergo and recover from this surgical procedure, then proceed to the two-part implant procedure. Bone grafting basically involves putting new or synthetic bone into your jaw to create an anchor for your new implants. If real bone is used, very small bits of bone are taken from the pelvic region.

> ***Tip!*** An autograft, or bone taken from your body, is more likely to be compatible with your jaw bone and is therefore less likely to be rejected. It also reduces the risk of disease and encourages the growth of new bone.

Benefits Include: Being able to get implants once your bone is sufficiently healed, and therefore restoring your ability to chew, talk and have normal teeth again.

Risks Include: Rejection by your body, in the case of allograft, xenograft of alloplast grafts (donor, animal or inorganic grafts), in which case the graft must be removed. The risk of disease and infection also increases when these are used. The procedure itself is simple and there are not many risks involved other than potential reactions to the anesthetic.

Average Time of Procedure: The average time of the procedure depends entirely upon how much repair needs to be done.

Recovery Time: It will take you around three weeks to get back on your feet, depending on the kind of bone graft you had. Expect to wait three to six months for the graft to take. Once it does, you can move on to getting your implants.

Most Popular Medical Tourism Destinations for this Procedure: Hungary, Costa Rica, Mexico and Croatia.

#3 Endodontic Surgery

Endodontic surgery is really a banner term for procedures that involve the root canals of your teeth.[155] In the past, if one of your teeth was diseased or infected, it would have to be removed. These days, root canal treatment cleans out the infected area of the pulp chamber inside the tooth, and replaces it with filling material to save the tooth from extraction. During this procedure, the damaged nerve is also removed. Endodontic surgery is generally called for when you constantly experience pain but there is no evidence of a hole or infection on the exterior of the tooth. Surgery is also used when there are damaged root surfaces or problems with the surrounding bone.

> *Tip!* This tooth-saving surgery can spare you from needing to have your tooth extracted. When you ignore pain in your teeth, the infection could spread, and may result in the loss of a few of your teeth. Explore the options with your endodontist and decide whether the teeth are worth saving.

Benefits Include: Saving your tooth from extraction. This means that you won't have to pay for expensive dental surgery involving implants, dentures or bridges.

Risks Include: The chance that you might not be able to save your tooth, depending on how damaged it is inside. In this instance, your endodontic surgeon will simply remove the tooth. There are no other risks involved.

Average Time of Procedure: Altogether the procedure shouldn't take more than an hour or two, depending on how long it takes for the anesthetic to kick in.

Recovery Time: Varies according to the patient. Sometimes the discomfort goes away in a few days, sometimes weeks.

Most Popular Medical Tourism Destinations for this Procedure: India, Costa Rica and Hungary.

#4 Extraction

If your endodontic surgeon failed, or you have been found to have decayed, diseased teeth, you may have an extraction in your future.[156] A tooth extraction is needed when a tooth or set of teeth has been damaged – in an accident, by infection or because of neglect. Teeth may also be removed if they are in the way of other teeth or are impacted. An extraction is occasionally necessary to prepare for other orthodontic surgeries – to make room for implants or dentures, for example. The tooth is loosened using an instrument called an elevator while the patient is under local anesthesia. Once it is free from the bone, the surgeon can remove it.

> *Tip!* Extraction should be a last resort, or if you have your heart set on dental implants. Speak to your dental surgeon about being put to sleep instead of having to be awake through the pain of having a few teeth removed. It may be pricier, but you can afford it in another country!

Benefits Include: An end to your chronic tooth pain if root canals haven't helped. Extraction is also beneficial if you need extensive work done, including implants, dentures or bridges.

Risks Include: Complications with the anesthesia or an infection after the surgery. Further problems can be caused by a dry socket, or if the blood fails to form a clot after surgery.

Average Time of Procedure: Procedure times depend on the number of teeth that need to be pulled. Average time per tooth is under an hour.

Recovery Time: After two weeks, the swelling and pain should be gone. If pain persists, see your surgeon immediately. There may be a hidden infection.

Most Popular Medical Tourism Destinations for this Procedure: South Korea, Mexico and Costa Rica.

#5 Dental Bridge

A dental bridge is used to replace teeth that you have extracted or lost.[157] There are two types of dental bridges: fixed and removable. Fixed bridges may be conventional, resin-bonded or cantilever. Your dental surgeon will examine your teeth to see which bridge will suit you best. They will then prepare your teeth by shaving them with a bur. An impression will be made using dental putty, so that the surgeon can make a bridge for that comfortably fits you. In the meantime, you will be fitted with a temporary bridge that will probably be very uncomfortable. Once the final bridge is made, you return to have it fitted into place and cemented. You can choose to stay in your host country during the time in between, or go home and return at a later date. Bridges can be made from gold, porcelain or silver.

> *Tip!* Be very picky when trying on your permanent bridge for the first time. They generally need to be tweaked, until they are perfectly comfortable in the patient's mouth. It's best to stay for an extra week or two after the fitting so that these changes can be made if necessary.

Benefits Include: More natural-looking teeth, long lasting and reliable. Your bridge won't be noticeable (unless you've decided you want a gold tooth). Plus, the bridge relieves some of the pressure on your other teeth.

Risks Include: Cementing a completely painful bridge into your mouth, requiring a removal procedure. Also, if you don't clean it every day, infection may develop underneath the bridge.

Average Time of Procedure: Initial shaving and fitting shouldn't take more than an hour. Fittings after that may take longer depending on the severity of the problem that you are having with your permanent bridge.

Recovery Time: There is no recovery time for this particular procedure, though discomfort might endure for a few weeks until you become accustomed to your new bridge.

Most Popular Medical Tourism Destinations for this Procedure: Mexico, Costa Rica and Hungary.

Non-Surgical Dental Procedures

There are a number of non-surgical dental procedures available to you while on vacation in an exotic country. Routine dentistry and tooth improvement is still very expensive in the United States, so going for a check-up abroad could be a great way to save money and improve your smile. Imagine going abroad for two weeks... and coming back with perfect, pearly-white teeth! It's everything you've ever dreamed of, and now it's affordable too. You can even add a few of these enhancing dental procedures to your list when seeing your dental surgeon about something more serious. Let's take a look at the top five non-surgical dental procedures that draw Americans abroad.

#1 Whitening your Teeth

Bleaching or whitening your teeth is a simple, quick way to improve the appearance of your smile.[158] Having stained and discolored or yellow teeth can be very embarrassing, and it can't be cured with toothpaste or regular oral hygiene. As the years pass, many people's teeth naturally become discolored from use and wear. Your international dentist will whiten your teeth by applying a special whitening paste to them. Once the entire surface is covered, the dentist will put a gum mold in your mouth to shield your lips and gums, and use a bright light to activate the paste. This is known as light-activated tooth whitening. More traditional methods involve leaving a gel on the teeth for short intervals until white. It may take a few sessions, but soon your teeth will be baby white again.

Tip! Have your teeth whitened while you're in your destination country having another dental procedure done. It will give you the white teeth you've wanted, and save you hundreds of dollars at the same time.

Benefits Include: A blinding white smile that will light up your face, and bucket-loads of confidence.

Risks Include: A mild reaction to the paste, which may cause your gums to be a little tender after the procedure but it will soon pass.

Average Time of Procedure: Each session takes about an hour, and sometimes you only need one session to achieve the desired effect.

Recovery Time: There is no recovery time as this is a non-invasive procedure.

Most Popular Medical Tourism Destinations for this Procedure: Mexico, Argentina and Guatemala.

#2 Dental Veneers

According to WebMD, a dental veneer is a wafer-thin, custom-made tooth shell designed to improve your appearance.[159] People who have discolored, worn, chipped or badly aligned teeth can benefit from having veneers, as they fit around your teeth and improve the shape and color of them at the same time. A veneer is usually porcelain or composite, and can correct a person's smile without major surgery. Your dentist will shave the surface of your teeth with a bur to prepare them for the veneers. A mold will be taken, and when the veneers are ready, you go in for an appointment to have them cemented down.

> ***Tip!*** There is a time gap between having your teeth prepared for the veneers and getting them, so make sure that your dentist is willing to fit you with a temporary veneer during that time. Not all dentists will offer this, so you'd better ask!

Benefits Include: A drastic improvement in the shape, style and color of your teeth. Dental veneers literally transform your smile, and give you the opportunity to have perfect-looking teeth while still keeping the ones you have.

Risks Include: Incorrect bonding so that your veneers don't fit properly and shift; having too much of your tooth enamel removed; shattering your veneers, causing you to go back for a new set; and increased sensitivity to hot and cold foods. These are mostly the result of poor dentistry. Choose your international dentist wisely, and these won't happen.

Average Time of Procedure: Creating and fitting the veneers takes at least three appointments, each an hour or so long. The actual fitting might take between one and three hours, depending on the veneer fit and the corrections needed.

Recovery Time: No recovery time is needed from having veneers put in.

Most Popular Medical Tourism Destinations for this Procedure: South Korea, Costa Rica and Hungary.

#3 Dental Fillings

A filling is the most common dental procedure, and one that everyone has to get at some stage in their lives. When your tooth develops a cavity, it's your dentist's job to remove the bad part of the tooth and replace it with a filling. These fillings can be porcelain, silver amalgam, gold or composite resin. Fillings are also used to fix damaged teeth that have worn, cracked or broken. Your dentist will drill around the decayed area of your tooth, and then determine what damage has been done by probing around in the hole with an instrument. He will then clean it and fill it with your chosen material. A laser light will set the material and cause it to harden. Now your tooth is perfectly healthy again. Having fillings done overseas is perfect if you are in for a larger procedure. Each filling costs money, so if you need a few of them it will certainly pay to have them done abroad.

> *Tip!* The best looking dental material is porcelain, the strongest is silver amalgam and the most desired is gold. Choose the right filling for your needs and you won't be disappointed. In general, silver is great for back molars, while porcelain is more appropriate for your front teeth.

Benefits Include: Fixing your tooth so that it doesn't rot or decay. Different materials have different benefits; for example, composite resin is the least expensive, but it doesn't wear well. All filling materials can relieve toothache instantly.

Risks Include: Continued decay of the tooth if a cavity isn't cleaned out properly. A quick visit to your dentist will fix that.

Average Time of Procedure: A filling usually takes about an hour, depending on how long the local anesthetic takes to work.

Recovery Time: The numbing effect will disappear within a few hours after your dentist visit. Be careful not to bite into food when your lip is numb, as injury could result.

Most Popular Medical Tourism Destinations for this Procedure: Hungary, Costa Rica and South Korea.

#4 Dentures

A denture is described by MedicineNet.com as an artificial set of teeth that can be removed. They make up for lost teeth and surrounding tissue that has worn or has been extracted. There are two different kinds of denture – complete and partial. A complete denture set replaces all the teeth in your mouth, while partial dentures only replace a certain section of your mouth where teeth have been extracted. Low-cost dentures can be bought abroad that will fit you better and be of a higher quality than the ones you would have been forced to buy in the U.S. due to financial constraints. If you are traveling overseas for medical care anyway, a new set of comfortable dentures will complete your trip.

> *Tip!* You might want to think about replacing your dentures with dental implants so you can have your own set of permanent teeth again. At almost 70% less than the going price in the U.S., you can now afford a set of implants.

Benefits Include: A low-cost substitute for real teeth that improves your overall appearance, and helps you to chew and talk. They also offer structural support for your face. If you need a quality, low-cost set of dentures, you can find them through medical travel.

Risks Include: Mild discomfort, and they can be difficult to get used to.

Average Time of Procedure: It will take a minimum of three dentist appointments in order for your dentures to be made. Each appointment will last about an hour.

Recovery Time: No recovery time is needed, though it will take some time to get used to false teeth.

Most Popular Medical Tourism Destinations for this Procedure: Costa Rica, Mexico and Turkey.

#5 Gum Treatment

If you suffer from gum disease, there are treatments you can receive overseas that won't bankrupt you. Serious gum disease can result in the loss of your teeth if you let it get out of hand.[160] That's why gum treatment is so important. It can literally save you from having to wear dentures or get dental implants at a later age. Scaling and root planing help to remove bacteria from your gums. Your international dentist will scale your teeth to remove plaque buildup, and then plane the roots of your teeth. This essentially returns the gums to a healthy state, as they are given the chance to reattach to a healthy tooth. There are also various kinds of medications and laser treatments that can help you maintain healthy gums.

> *Tip!* Ask your dentist what you can do to keep your gums healthy. If necessary, repeat the treatment once a year in order to keep your gums in good condition.

Benefits Include: Reducing the signs of bacterial infection that causes serious gum disease; helping your gums attach naturally to healthy teeth; preventing gum recession; and improving breath.

Risks Include: Almost nothing. It's more risky to do without this treatment than to have it. There is no pain involved.

Average Time of Procedure: Scaling and planing can take up to three separate appointments of around an hour each. Laser treatment takes about twenty minutes.

Recovery Time: None.

Most Popular Medical Tourism Destinations for this Procedure: Mexico, Turkey and Costa Rica.

Medical Procedures

There are many elective medical procedures that can be done abroad, saving you a lot of money. Elective surgeries like hip replacements, hysterectomies, pacemaker implants and explorative tests can all be done by qualified international doctors who will give you the level of medical care that you deserve. Let's take a look at the top four medical procedures and what they have to offer you.

#1 Orthopedic Surgery: Hip Replacement

An orthopedic surgery like a hip replacement[161] could set you back a whopping $45,000 in the United States, and that's an average price. The most shocking of all is that under Obamacare, seniors who need this surgery may not always be able to get it. If the government insurance company denies your plea for approval, where are you going to go? Overseas, of course – and you'll be better for it. Even if the government gives you the go-ahead, you'll still incur huge costs. Traveling to another country for orthopedic surgery could save you as much as 86% of that cost. The smart choice is to find a widely respected orthopedic surgeon abroad. Hip replacement surgery involves replacement of the ends of the pelvis and femur in order to create new joint surfaces. Essentially, the upper end of the thigh bone is replaced with a metal ball, and the inside of the pelvic bone socket is resurfaced with metal and a plastic liner. This is a major surgery, and requires a skilled surgeon to complete successfully.

Benefits Include: Improved motor function; reduction or elimination of pain associated with arthritis; and a greater quality of life, as the patient is able to remain independent and enjoy normal activities.

Risks Include: Infection, blood clotting in the legs, stiffness and complete implant failure. This occurs when the joint loosens or wears out, which happens to all artificial joints eventually. If you take the right course of medication, you can avoid the clotting and infection.

Average Time of Procedure: The entire procedure from start to finish shouldn't take longer than three hours.

Recovery Time: Your movement will be very restricted in the first two months, but after six months you should be able to resume all of your normal daily activities.

Most Popular Medical Tourism Destinations for this Procedure: India, New Zealand and Taiwan.

#2 Cardiovascular Surgery: Pacemaker Implant

Non-emergency cardiovascular procedures are expensive, especially when they involve such specialist work. When your life is on the line, it's important to choose the right doctor; but it's also important to think about your financial future, and surgeries like this can be financially crippling. Open heart surgery can cost anywhere from $40,000 to $200,000, depending on your location. It's far less expensive overseas; and with such great risk involved, you don't want to survive the operation only to be put in jail because you can't pay the bills. Pacemaker surgery is very common overseas, with some of the best medical centers boasting higher success rates than American hospitals. For some, pacemaker surgery might not be urgent, but if they don't get it, they will die eventually as their heart rate continues to drop. When a person's heartbeat decreases to less than 60 beats per minute, a pacemaker must be installed – and fast. A pacemaker is a small medical instrument that is placed underneath your skin and near your heart to help it beat regularly. Though it is a fairly simple procedure these days, it's still a harrowing experience to live through. Small cameras are guided to your heart through a vein in your shoulder. This allows your surgeon to cut in the right place on your chest to insert the medical device. The pacemaker is then connected to your heart. Once it has been tested, you are sewn back up and the small device helps control your heartbeat.

Benefits Include: Regulated heartbeat that will prevent your heart from slowing. It adds years onto your life and keeps your heart strong.

Risks Include: Anything from a collapsed lung to bleeding and swelling under the pacemaker to nerve damage. This is a high-risk surgery as it involves the heart. On rare occasions the lead wires that connect to the heart may become dislodged or faulty.

Average Time of Procedure: The procedure usually takes about an hour, but no more than two.

Recovery Time: Swelling will go down within a week of the procedure. You should be fully recovered after a month.

Most Popular Medical Tourism Destinations for this Procedure:
India, Brazil and Mexico.

#3 Gynecological Surgery: Hysterectomy

Gynecological surgery is a huge industry overseas, with couples traveling together to have a vacation in the sun and to get a medical procedure done at the same time. If you need a hysterectomy, there are world-class facilities abroad that will help you through it in style. A hysterectomy[162] is a surgical procedure in which the surgeon removes a woman's uterus, and sometimes her cervix as well. This is usually done for the purpose of preventing further pregnancies, but is also fairly common in women who have uterine bleeding, fibroids or a cancerous cervix. This is a very invasive procedure that removes a very important part of the woman, and needs to be treated with care and compassion.

Benefits Include: Reduced risk of pre-cancers turning into actual cancer; reduction of certain health risks; elimination of any chance of further pregnancy; removal of all uterine pain.

Risks Include: Bleeding after surgery, injury to organs and tissue, urination problems, and damaged ureters. An abdominal incision might be necessary during surgery. This surgery can also bring on menopause if it includes an oophorectomy.

Average Time of Procedure: From one to three hours of surgery time.

Recovery Time: Can vary, but bet on at least four to six weeks of rest. Full recovery takes time, especially if cancer is involved.

Most Popular Medical Tourism Destinations for this Procedure:
India, Israel and Thailand.

#4 Diagnostic Surgery: Biopsy

Tests in the U.S. are expensive. In fact, they can be the reason that you can't afford to pay your medical bills. It all adds up in the end, and with diseases like cancer on the rise, you can't afford to leave your testing for another day. A biopsy is the perfect way to check whether you have a serious illness like cancer. Diagnostic surgery is used when a patient needs to have tissue looked at on a microscopic level. Once in front of a microscope and analyzed by the doctor, organ tissue can be identified as diseased. But first, a surgeon needs to surgically remove a few cells from the patient's organs. Other tests include MRI scans, CT scans and X-rays, but they are all overpriced. Countries outside of the U.S. offer you cheaper medical tests so you have the chance to beat cancer at an early stage, or to get a tumor removed before it does any real damage. A kidney biopsy, for example, would involve inserting a long needle into the back of the patient until it hits the kidney. A small scraping is taken, and the needle is removed for analysis. That tiny procedure can set you back as much as $10,000 in the States – and you haven't even been diagnosed yet.

Benefits Include: Early diagnosis of disease – or the great news that there is no problem. Either way, it's enormously important that you know as soon as possible so you can take steps to improve your health.

Risks Include: Infection from the needle or bleeding.

Average Time of Procedure: Some biopsies take longer than others, but most range from a few minutes to an hour.

Recovery Time: No real recovery time is needed, though the area where the biopsy took place might be tender for a while.

Most Popular Medical Tourism Destinations for this Procedure: Thailand, India and Panama.

Fertility Treatment

Not being able to have kids is something that affects thousands of Americans every year. Thanks to the kindness of insurance companies, fertility treatment isn't covered. Many potential parents have had to forgo having children because they can't afford the expensive therapies at fertility treatment centers in the U.S. But there is a way to increase your chances of starting a family – with medical fertility tourism. Here are the top five fertility treatments available abroad.

#1 In Vitro Fertilization

In Vitro Fertilization, or IVF, is the most successful way of increasing a couple's chances of having children.[163] IVF involves treatment in a medical care center, where sperm from the donor father is coupled with the egg from the donor mother in order to bring about fertilization outside of the body. The fertilized egg is then placed in the woman's uterus to grow naturally. This allows women who have damaged fallopian tubes to have kids. The process is often repeated several times in order for the fertilization to be successful. Each treatment can cost up to $15,000 in the U.S., which is financially impossible for struggling couples.

Benefits Include: A safe, reliable way to have a child when you wouldn't have been able to before. It's also not as invasive as many other fertility treatments.

Risks Include: Repeated failed attempts at pregnancy, and a chance that the woman could contract ovarian hyperstimulation syndrome, which can be painful.

Average Time of Procedure: IVF works in cycles according to the most fertile period for the woman involved. Each cycle takes four to six weeks.

Recovery Time: Very little recovery time is needed as this is a minimally invasive procedure. All that is required is patience and determination on the part of the potential parents.

Most Popular Medical Tourism Destinations for this Procedure: Barbados, South Korea and Argentina.

#2 Frozen Embryo Transfer

This is part of the IVF cycle, though a subsection all its own. Frozen

Embryo Transfer, or FET, is when an embryo is literally frozen and stored for the perfect moment of fertility. An FET cycle[164] is supported with medications or hormones to increase the natural fertility of the woman. The frozen embryo itself comes from a previous IVF cycle. Although the success rate drops, keeping healthy embryos this way can allow people to expand their families at a later point, especially if the quality of the woman's eggs is deteriorating. The surgical procedure of harvesting embryos from the woman can sometimes be too traumatizing to repeat. This is where FET comes in handy. The woman only has to experience this once for a few cycles.

Benefits Include: Less invasive embryo harvesting and repeated chances of becoming pregnant. Also, the process is somewhat less expensive than an entirely new IVF cycle.

Risks Include: Failed pregnancy. There is no risk to the child or the mother if the pregnancy is successful.

Average Time of Procedure: It varies, but it takes forty minutes for the embryo to thaw before being implanted in the woman's uterus.

Recovery Time: No recovery time needed.

Most Popular Medical Tourism Destinations for this Procedure: Barbados, Spain and Argentina.

#3 Intracytoplasmic Sperm Injection

An Intracytoplasmic Sperm Injection, or ICSI, is used when a couple is struggling with male infertility. An egg is held ready for a single sperm that is loaded into a tiny hollow needle. The sperm is carefully injected into the egg, past the shell and into the soft cytoplasm, where it fertilizes the egg. The fertilized egg is then placed inside the woman. This procedure is great for couples who are experiencing issues with low sperm count, sperm that can't get through the egg's outer shell or poor quality sperm. It enables them to have biological children.

Benefits Include: Increased chance of pregnancy for couples who have problems with male infertility.

Risks Include: Failed pregnancy; possible discomfort for the man, as sperm might have to be removed directly from the testicle if masturbation doesn't render the desired results.

Average Time of Procedure: Varies, though two weeks is needed prior to the procedure for monitoring the eggs.

Recovery Time: No recovery time needed.

Most Popular Medical Tourism Destinations for this Procedure: Barbados, Spain and Argentina.

#4 Gamete Intrafallopian Transfer

Gamete Intrafallopian Transfer, or GIFT,[165] involves taking a combination of male sperm and female eggs and injecting them into the woman's fallopian tubes where they can develop naturally. After fertilization takes place inside the body, then the egg will naturally move down to the uterus where it will begin to grow. This procedure is different from IVF in than it requires functional fallopian tubes to work. With IVF, the actual fertilization takes place outside the body, while GIFT takes place internally. This process is great for couples who want a more natural fertilization procedure but still can't conceive on their own.

Benefits Include: Increased chances of becoming pregnant. This is a non-surgical procedure and can be easily performed. This process excludes embryo culture so the couple doesn't have to create extra embryos for the treatment.

Risks Include: A much higher chance of multiple births and severe reactions to the hormone treatment.

Average Time of Procedure: Treatment varies from couple to couple.

Recovery Time: This non-surgical procedure doesn't require recovery time.

Most Popular Medical Tourism Destinations for this Procedure: Barbados, Argentina and Spain.

#5 Ovary Transplant

This is an experimental procedure that has helped some completely barren women give birth. An ovary transplant is when a woman has donor ovaries or ovarian tissue transplanted into her so that she can have children. Without healthy ovaries, a woman simply can't have children. With this new revolutionary surgery, every woman now has the chance to create a family of her own. Still very controversial, and not available in many hospitals, you can get this amazing new surgery overseas on your next medical vacation.

Benefits Include: The opportunity to have a child when it was previously thought impossible to do so.

Risks Include: All the normal surgical risks involved with a transplant procedure, and the chance that the woman's body might reject the ovaries.

Average Time of Procedure: Procedure times vary according to the location and doctor involved.

Recovery Time: It will take a couple weeks before you are back on your feet, and several months before the ovaries start working properly in your body.

Most Popular Medical Tourism Destination for this Procedure: Denmark.

Laser Eye Surgery

Laser eye surgery, also known as LASIK eye surgery, is the modern solution to bad eyesight.[166] The Mayo Clinic defines it as a procedure that corrects vision problems, reducing or eliminating the need for glasses or contact lenses. This is a refractive surgery that alters the shape of your cornea, instantly improving your vision. Imagine clearer, shaper images wherever you look, and never having to wear glasses again! It sounds like a dream – and it was for many Americans, who were forced to pay up to $3,000 per eye if they wanted the surgery. Until now, prices in the U.S. have simply been prohibitive. But now, you can get the surgery overseas for as little as $200, and enjoy the exact same results as you would have here. Laser eye surgery works for presbyopia, astigmatism, nearsightedness and farsightedness. LASIK surgery creates a circular flap inside your cornea with either a microkeratome or a secondary laser. The surgeon pulls the flap open and takes out some corneal tissue with an excimer laser. Ultraviolet light is then used to reshape the cornea as the laser shaves off little bits of your eye to achieve the desired focus. There is almost no pain involved in the procedure. After surgery, you will be required to take certain medication and rest for a few days.

Benefits Include: Instantly improved vision. Sharper images, better focus and clarity like you've never experienced before.

Risks Include: Astigmatism from unintentionally misshaping the eye during the procedure. Dry eyes can result, but they normalize after six months or so. Additional problems like blurred vision, double vision or glare issues may be found. There are many risks involved with LASIK eye surgery but they are rare. Make sure that your LASIK surgeon is genuinely qualified to handle the equipment, and nothing should go wrong.

Average Time of Procedure: The entire procedure is completed within 20 minutes.

Recovery Time: You have to wear protective goggles when you sleep for the first week after your surgery, but after that you can expect a full recovery within two months.

Most Popular Medical Tourism Destinations for this Procedure: Mexico, Brazil and Costa Rica.

●

Elective surgery doesn't have to be a nightmare. If you plan financially for the surgery, and find the right international medical center and surgeon to treat you, then you will have discovered a whole new frontier in medical care. You don't have to be afraid to improve your looks and self-esteem, or to get that knee replacement surgery you've always needed. Look forward to a better quality of life as a result of your new investment in global medical tourism. The returns far outweigh your costs, and you still get to enjoy a beautiful vacation while you're there. Why didn't anyone tell you sooner?

Testimonials from Elective Surgery Patients

Name: John B., Washington

Condition: None (Elective Plastic Surgery)
Surgery: Liposuction, Blepharoplasty and Tuck Procedure
Hospital: Hospital in India
Medical Travel Agency: Life Smile Healthcare
JOHN WENT SEARCHING FOR DETAILS on potential cosmetic surgery procedures he wanted to get done, and got some reliable information and very low cost quotes on the website of Life Smile Healthcare. He researched Internetall about India on the Internet and its healthcare facilities, and was fascinated by the technological advancements, culture and diversity. He was very pleased with Life Smile's care and attention in responding to his many questions, and eventually booked his healthcare tour through them. He underwent liposuction, a tuck procedure and a blepharoplasty, performed by a senior cosmetic surgeon (who had previously worked in Florida). Special care was taken since John had recently received a prosthetic hip. Everything – during the surgery, antibiotics, other medicines and the specialized after-care – went very well. Before the procedure, John traveled around India, visiting the Taj Mahal at Agra, and spending four

days at a Hindu monastery in the peaceful beauty of the Himalayas. While he was in the Himalayas, Life Smile booked him for a stay at a world-class spa, where he enjoyed a few Indian rejuvenation therapy sessions which were very effective and refreshing after the tour. He is planning his next visit to India for his other cosmetic surgery treatments.

Name: Ms. Ure O., Oklahoma

Condition: None (Elective Plastic Surgery)
Surgery: Rhinoplasty
Hospital: Hospital in New Delhi, India
Medical Travel Agency: Life Smile Healthcare
MS O. IS AN ESTABLISHED YOUNG MODEL, trying to maintain her career in an industry known to be critical when it comes to physical attributes. In other words, her job depends on her looks. Through Life Smile, she went to New Delhi for a traditional nose job. Life Smile connected her with a U.S.-trained, board certified plastic surgeon. He explained the process and told her exactly what he thought he could achieve – and then met those expectations. She made a vacation out of her recovery time, staying at a gorgeous, peaceful hotel, surrounded by greenery. Some of her favorite memories are the Bollywood movies, spicy Indian cuisine and the unending shopping excursions on the streets of New Delhi. Back in the States, she still finds herself listening to Indian music!

Name: Barbara Weightman, 65

Condition: None (Elective Plastic Surgery)
Surgery: Breast Lift and Tummy Tuck
Hospital: Netcare Rosebank Hospital
Medical Travel Agency: Surgeon and Safari
SOME PROCEDURES ARE BETTER DONE ABROAD. Several years ago, Barbara had an eye lift performed in the U.S. While the procedure was

successful, the pain was excruciating and the bruising took six weeks to dissipate. She had read about Surgeon and Safari in the Los Angeles Times and decided to investigate further. She went online, and was very impressed with the various procedures that were available for half the price she would pay in America. Then she read the resume of Dr. Rick van der Poel and was impressed even further – enough that she decided to go to South Africa for her next surgery. She was met at the airport and brought to a lovely home, where she had a private room prepared for her. Dr. van der Poel impressed her as a gentle and extremely competent physician. The surgery took place in a private hospital, where she was tended to by multiple nurses. After a breast lift and reduction, plus a tummy tuck, the pain and bruising were minimal. She recovered in luxury… and went shopping in Johannesburg's fabulous mall! She almost immediately planned her trip for the next year – this time, a face lift. Again, minimal pain and bruising.

Name: Charles Rychner, Milwaukee

Condition: Knee Pain
Surgery: Knee Replacement Surgery
Hospital: Hospital Clinica Biblica, Mexico
Medical Travel Agency: Medical Tourism Corporation

CHARLES WAS TOLD HE NEEDED knee replacement surgery, but he soon found out that his medical insurance wouldn't cover the cost of the surgery. He turned to medical tourism and spent some time researching hospitals abroad, settling on one he found particularly responsive – Hospital Clinica Biblica in San Jose, Mexico. After arriving at what could have been a resort by the sea, Charles was admitted into the hospital and had the procedure. If he had remained in the U.S. and fought to pay for a surgery here, it would have cost him $55,000 – no paradise included. Instead, the entire experience cost him a reasonable

$15,000, a fraction of the costs he would have had to deal with at home; and that included all hospital fees, flight costs and his stay in a luxury resort outside San Jose.

Price Chart – Surgical Procedures Only

Average cost of **BREAST AUGMENTATION**	U.S.	$6,500–$8,000
	Costa Rica	$3,000
	Mexico	$2,100–$3,000
	Panama	$2,150–$3,500
	Thailand	$2,600–$4,000
Average cost of **FACELIFT**	U.S.	$6,000–$15,000
	India	$3,000
	Mexico	$2,000–$2,500
	South Africa	$2,500–$3,000
Average cost of **LIPOSUCTION** (one area)	U.S.	$4,000–$8,000
	Argentina	$2,000
	Brazil	$1,200–$2,000
	Thailand	$1,200
Average cost of **RHINOPLASTY**	U.S.	$7,000
	Croatia	$2,500
	Dubai	$5,000
	Panama	$3,000

Average cost of **BLEPHAROPLASTY**	U.S.	$5,500
	Costa Rica	$1,350
	South Africa	$897
	South Korea	$1,650
Average cost of **DENTAL SURGERY** (each)	U.S.	$3,000–$4,000
	Hungary	$350–$2,000
	Mexico	$650–$3,000
	Peru	$350–$3,000
Average cost of **JAW BONE GRAFTING**	U.S.	$4,000–$7,000
	Costa Rica	$400–$750
	Croatia	$360–$500
	Hungary	$450–$700
	Mexico	$320–$750
Average cost of **ENDODONTIC SURGERY**	U.S.	$400–$1,500
	Costa Rica	$165–$250
	Hungary	$86–$120
	India	$75–$175
Average cost of **EXTRACTION**	U.S.	$300–$350
	Costa Rica	$120–$150
	Mexico	$120–$150
	South Korea	$120–$150

Average cost of **DENTAL BRIDGE**	U.S.	$1,500–$4,000
	Costa Rica	$250–$400
	Hungary	$250–$600
	Mexico	$250–$600
Average cost of **TEETH WHITENING**	U.S.	$2,300–$4,000
	Argentina	$650–$800
	Guatemala	$420–$600
	Mexico	$250–$400
Average cost of **DENTAL VENEERS**	U.S.	$1,850–$4,000
	Costa Rica	$320–$500
	Hungary	$350–$500
	South Korea	$60–$350
Average cost of **DENTAL FILLINGS**	U.S.	$170–$300
	Costa Rica	$85–$120
	Hungary	$80–$100
	South Korea	$70–$150
Average cost of **DENTURES**	U.S.	$2,700–$4,000
	Costa Rica	$500–$700
	Mexico	$700–$800
	Turkey	$680–$800

Average cost of **GUM TREATMENT**	U.S.	$400–$1,000
	Costa Rica	$80–$150
	Mexico	$80–$150
	Turkey	$50–$200
Average cost of **HIP REPLACEMENT SURGERY**	U.S.	$45,000
	India	$6500
	New Zealand	$14,000
	Taiwan	$7,000
Average cost of **PACEMAKER IMPLANT**	U.S.	$40,000
	Brazil	$8,900
	India	$7,000
	Mexico	$8,000
Average cost of **HYSTERECTOMY**	U.S.	$20,000
	India	$1,600
	Israel	$3,000
	Thailand	$4,600
Average cost of **BIOPSY**	U.S.	$500–$1,100
	India	$100–$150
	Panama	$150–$300
	Thailand	$150–$200

Average cost of **IN VITRO FERTILIZATION**	U.S.	$14,500
	Argentina	$4,000
	Barbados	$5,500
	South Korea	$5,000
Average cost of **FROZEN EMBRYO TRANSFER**	U.S.	$3,000
	Argentina	$1,000
	Barbados	$1,000
	Spain	$1,200
Average cost of **INTRACYTOPLASMIC SPERM INJECTION**	U.S.	$8,300
	Argentina	$4,000
	Barbados	$6,500
	Spain	$6,500
Average cost of **GAMETE INTRAFALLOPIAN TRANSFER**	U.S.	$10,000–$15,000
	Argentina	$8,000
	$8000	$7,500–$8,500
	Spain	$6,000
Average cost of **OVARY TRANSPLANT**	U.S.	Unavailable
	Denmark	$15,000–$50,000

Average cost of **LASER EYE SURGERY**	U.S.	$4,400
	Brazil	$350
	Costa Rica	$1,000
	Mexico	$400

ଚ୬ • ଚ୨

CHAPTER 6

AFFORDABLE EMERGENCY SURGERY ABROAD

Affordable Emergency Surgery Abroad

෨ • ෬

Emergency surgery is never planned. It can be needed at a moment's notice – anytime, anywhere. It happens whether you have insurance or not. Therein lies the problem: when you've been in a traumatic accident and rushed to the nearest hospital, the first thing on your mind is not "How much is this going to cost me?" But it will cost you – a lot. Emergency surgery often involves several surgeries in order to save the patient's life. For example, a car accident might leave you needing multiple fracture surgeries, open-heart surgery, organ repair and long-term physical therapy – not to mention weeks of intensive care in the hospital you were taken to. Emergency surgery is the most expensive type of medical service, specifically because it includes multiple branches of medical care. Thankfully, this is not always the case, as the emergency can also be related to one specific medical condition like a burst appendix. In this instance, the cost will still be great but there isn't much opportunity to be transported to a less expensive overseas hospital. This chapter deals with the time period after you have awoken from your initial life-saving medical treatment at your local hospital.

Questions You Should Ask Your Doctor in the Intensive Care Unit after Trauma Surgery

Once you have woken up in the ICU and the general anesthetic has worn off, you need to start asking some important questions about your condition, and about the cost that you have already built up by being transported to the nearest medical care center. If you are in too much pain or are completely unable to communicate, then a family member or

close friend needs to ask these questions for you. Here's why:
- Emergency surgeries often result in additional complications that can lead to more surgeries, tests and extended hospital stays.
- A one-day hospital stay in America can cost as much as $1,200, and that's just for the bed.
- A serious string of complications can push your bill over the million dollar mark.
- The quality of care in America is plummeting, and you need the best medical care you can get when your life is on the line.

What is my current condition?

Identifying exactly what your current condition is will help you determine whether or not you are able to travel. Sometimes a patient will be in such critical condition that he or she can't be moved for several days. If you're lucky, you'll be stable enough to move immediately.

Please give me a full description of the surgeries I've had.

Asking your doctor about the damage that was done to your body will help you determine the extent of your injuries. This is true whether the emergency was for one specific problem or for several. Be sure to make a list of the various surgeries that you've had so you can work out the costs involved. Don't be afraid to question your doctor about what happened to you when you arrived, and how long you were in the emergency room and on the operating table before arriving at your current location. This is also a good time to assess whether there were complications during surgery, and how serious they were.

What medications am I currently on?

You need to determine what medications your doctor has put you on so when you arrive at your new hospital, you can fill them in on your treatment history. Your international doctor might have less expensive generic versions of the same medication so you can continue healing – at a lower cost.

What additional procedures or surgeries do I still need?

Unfortunately, many emergency surgery cases require the patient to go in for more surgery after the body has had the opportunity to recover from the initial shock. For example, if you were shot in the shoulder, the doctors might take out the bullet and repair as much of the damage as they can, but there might still be nerve damage that would restrict your movement in that arm. You would need additional surgery so you can move your arm normally again. This surgery would require that you stay in the hospital for another few days, or maybe even weeks. A better option would be for you to travel across the border to Mexico, and get your extra surgeries there. It would literally save you thousands of dollars. Plus, you'd get the level of care you need from doctors who aren't overworked and underpaid.

What tests were performed, and what tests still need to be done?

Many emergency room admissions require quick tests – CT scans, MRI scans or X-rays – to determine exactly what is wrong with you. These tests can be costly, so you want to make sure that if you do need additional testing, it's done somewhere more affordable. You need to find a better location, especially if you have limited or no insurance. Under Obamacare, doctors in America will worry about getting reimbursement for any tests they give you, so they'll be less likely to recommend the testing in order to save themselves money. This will result in undiagnosed problems that can lead to serious health issues. In a free market economy like Mexico, the doctors would rather test you and give you a clean bill of health than risk missing something that could cost you your life. Keep this in mind when visiting your government-controlled hospital.

How long will I have to stay in the hospital?

This question helps you better understand your current condition and whether travel is a viable option. If you need to be in a hospital for another two weeks, then changing hospitals is a great idea. If you're only booked for another two days, then it's probably not worth the trip unless you have to have physical therapy or recuperative therapy after being released. There are several different kinds of after-care surgery that you might have to look into. Rehabilitation is needed for many forms of surgery, especially if an arm or leg has been removed or severely damaged. You need someone around the clock to help you get through this difficult time. That's the sort of dedication that American doctors will no longer be able to give.

What are the risks involved if I travel?

A good doctor should be able to tell you what the risks are if you travel in your condition. From here, you can talk to your doctor about traveling abroad for additional medical care, and which mode of transportation would best suit the situation. Air lifts and ambulances can both be hired from private companies, or you can often call ahead to your destination hospital and they will send transportation. The risk involved in travel is dependent on your condition. Medical transport services come fully equipped with trauma kits and medical staff so you should be secure all the way there.

How much will staying here cost?

It will be an uphill battle for you to find out exactly how much money your medical treatment is going to cost you, but you should try – just to put things in perspective. If you face a few more weeks of high medical bills, it will destroy you financially for years after your hospital stay. It may be a scary prospect to move once you've settled in somewhere and are frail due to your injuries, but you must force yourself to think of the future. After the ordeal is over and you are fully recovering on a tropical beach, you'll think back and be thankful that you made the move. Not only will your medical bills be half or less of what they could have been, but you received the kind of medical care that promotes healing and recovery. The new U.S. healthcare system will send you packing as soon as possible.

Hiring an Air Ambulance or Other Medical Transport

There are private global air ambulances for hire in the U.S. that will safely transport you to any country in the world. American Air Ambulance, for example, offers patients cost-effective emergency air travel to the hospital of their choosing. As fast transportation to your next hospital, you can't ask for anything better. Many of these medical transport services have flexible payment plans because they understand that your medical need is paramount when you have to be moved or rushed to a specialist hospital for care. These trips generally cost between $5,000 and $30,000. A private plane trip is a great idea if you realize that your medical fees will be astronomical. If you can't afford $30,000, then there are other alternatives. There are non-profit organizations that offer free air transport for patients who need to be moved but can't afford it. Lifeline Pilots and Angel Flight are two such free air ambulance organizations. If your child needs to be moved to a hospital abroad, there are also many organizations which provide free flight services and medical care en-route for children.

General Surgery

General surgery includes all types of surgery that involve the abdomen.[167] Many emergency surgeries are related to problems within the stomach, liver, appendix or intestines. These surgeries are fairly common, though they fix problems which would be life-threatening if not treated. Something as simple as a burst appendix leads to serious infection in the abdomen as bacteria leaks out of the ruptured organ. If you don't go to the hospital for treatment, you will die from this infection in a matter of days. General emergency surgeries might be easy to deal with when compared to their specialist counterparts, but many complications can arise from simple procedures. Internal bleeding is a common complication associated with general surgery and infection is always a risk as well. Countries all over the world offer general emergency surgeries, with advanced technology and highly experienced surgeons to help you through your recovery period. Many emergencies afford you a few days to organize a direct flight to an international hospital for surgery. For example, if you need to have your gall bladder removed "as soon as possible," you will generally have enough time to fly overseas and get it done.

With new technology in the world of general surgery, there are now less expensive ways to solve critical problems in your body. If you choose to have a procedure done at an accredited hospital abroad that has the latest technology, you will experience faster recovery times and shorter hospital stays. The goal is to always find the best medical care, at the best hospital abroad, for a fraction of the cost that you would pay in America. With Obamacare decimating our healthcare system and removing the free market incentives that made the U.S. a medically advanced nation, we can't expect to find the most advanced technology in our hospitals anymore. In order to keep costs low, more surgeries will be unnecessarily invasive as doctors are forced to rush through procedures. The incidence of surgical death will rise. We must look abroad. Let's take a look at some of the emergency surgeries you may someday need, and what your medical travel options are for each of them.

Emergency Gastrectomy

An emergency gastrectomy needs to be performed when a peptic ulcer becomes perforated, or when the patient has stomach cancer.[168] When a peptic ulcer is perforated, extreme pain and rigidity seize the patient around the abdomen. In cancer and ulcer cases, the stomach, small intestine, esophagus, pylorus and duodenum could be involved. The most common scenario is that a peptic ulcer perforates in the stomach. This is called a gastric ulcer and it needs to be removed immediately.

The emergency gastrectomy is also used to treat stomach bleeding, tumors and inflammation in that area. It involves the removal of part or all of the stomach. Total gastrectomy is when the entire stomach is removed, and the surgeon connects the intestines to the esophagus. A makeshift stomach is formed using tissue from the intestines. The much more common partial gastrectomy is when only part of the stomach is removed. Gastrectomy is a very serious emergency surgery that needs to be performed as soon as your doctor confirms that an ulcer is perforated. Once there is a perforation leading into your abdominal cavity, bacteria can get inside and cause severe illness or death.

This emergency surgery would have to be performed in the U.S. because it's so urgent; but, the fact that it requires a two-week hospital stay means that you could choose to fly abroad for most of your recovery time, reducing costs.

Urgency of Surgery: Within eight hours.
Average Time of Procedure: Full stomach removal requires between one and three hours of surgery.
Recovery Time: Expect to be in the hospital for at least two weeks. A full recovery will take approximately two months.
Best Medical Tourism Destinations for this Surgery: India, Mexico and South Korea.

> **Hospital Spotlight:**
> **Apollo Hospital in Chennai, India.**
> This JCI- and ISO-accredited hospital has private rooms, world-class service and room for families to stay with the patient on location.
> ***Estimated Travel Distance to India:*** 7,484 miles.
> ***Estimated Travel Time by Plane:*** 16 hours.

Emergency Gall Bladder Removal

Gall bladder removal surgery is also called cholecystectomy, and involves completely removing the gall bladder from your body.[169] Though the gall bladder stores bile from your liver, it's not a particularly necessary organ and there are no health implications from removing it. A large cut is made across your stomach, and your surgeon simply lifts the gall bladder out. Another method uses a laparoscope that is inserted inside your body so the surgeon can see the gall bladder on a screen. The gall bladder will then be removed through one of three smaller cuts on your stomach.

Emergency gall bladder surgery results from severe gallstone pain or the presence of cholecystitus. Gallstones are actually crystallized bile that has formed because of a chemical imbalance. These stones damage the gall bladder as they move around, and can cause horrible infection. They can even travel down the cystic duct and block up the liver. As with many abdomen-based problems, if bacteria leaks into the abdominal cavity, infection will result. Gallstones may cause perforations in the gall bladder. If this occurs, the gall bladder must be removed within eight hours. Alternatively, you might experience incredible pain from a gallstone, only to be told that you can schedule a surgery for the following week. In this instance, you'll have sufficient time to plan your trip and fly overseas for the operation. If it's acute cholecystitus, then you will have to have it removed within 48 hours.

Mexico is right on the U.S. border, which means that if you live in the southern part of the U.S., you can get there in no time at all. If you act quickly, you could even get to your destination within the eight-hour emergency period.

Urgency of Surgery: Within eight hours after perforation, or within a week after a severe gallstone attack.

Average Time of Procedure: Between one and two hours for open surgery, or one hour for the laparoscopic procedure.

Recovery Time: For traditional gall bladder removal surgery, hospital stays can be up to a week long. For laparoscopic gall bladder removal surgery, expect a day or two to heal. You should be fully recovered after two months, no matter which surgery you had.

Best Medical Tourism Destinations for this Surgery: Mexico, Panama and Brazil.

Hospital Spotlight:
Laparoscopic Solutions, Coahuila Mexico

This medical center deals specifically with laparoscopic technology, is JCI-approved and has private rooms where you can recover in peace. They even offer package deals for gall bladder removal surgeries at affordable prices.

Estimated Travel Distance to Mexico: 1,912 miles.

Estimated Travel Time by Plane: Between two and six hours, depending on your location in the U.S.

Emergency Appendectomy

An appendectomy is a common procedure; but, when you need emergency surgery, it's just as life-threatening as a heart attack.[170] When you contract appendicitis, your appendix becomes infected and inflamed. This inflammation can cause the appendix to burst, which will allow it to leak harmful bacteria into your body, causing severe illness and eventual death. The only way to cure appendicitis is to remove the entire appendix. Your surgeon does this by making a small incision on the right side of your abdomen, then tying off the appendix and cutting it out. If there is any damage to the blood vessels, or any bleeding in the cavity, the surgeon will repair it. In the event of an emergency appendectomy (i.e., after the appendix has burst), the surgeon will clean out the inside of your abdomen to prevent mass infection and illness.

If you've been diagnosed with appendicitis but your appendix has not yet burst, then you may have a few days to book your surgery. In this instance, medical tourism is a great option because you can quickly plan your trip with the help of a medical travel agent. Flying somewhere for a laparoscopic appendectomy will save you time and money. The procedure also allows you to heal faster because it's less invasive than open surgery – not to mention more cost-effective. It also lets you leave the hospital sooner, which is a further cost reduction considering the price of hospital stays. In a laparoscopic appendectomy, three small cuts are made along your lower stomach, and the laparoscope is inserted so that the surgeon can see your organs on a screen in front of him or her. The procedure is done through these small cuts, and the appendix is pulled out through one of them.

Urgency of Surgery: Up to a week for appendicitis; for a burst appendix, eight hours maximum.

Average Time of Procedure: Open surgery takes about two hours, while laparoscopic surgery takes an hour or so.

Recovery Time: You should be fully recovered after four to six weeks.
Best Medical Tourism Destinations for this Surgery: Thailand, Germany and India.

> **Hospital Spotlight:**
> **Bangkok Hospital Pattaya, Chonburi, Thailand**
> As the most technologically advanced hospital on the eastern seaboard of Thailand, this JCI-accredited hospital boasts top-quality medical facilities, luxurious private rooms and English-speaking doctors. If your appendix hasn't burst, book your ticket to Thailand for your medical vacation. In four days, you'll be back on your feet and seeing the sights of this culturally rich country.
> ***Travel Distance to Thailand:*** 8,791 miles.
> ***Estimated Travel Time by Plane:*** 18 hours, depending on your point of departure.

Emergency Inguinal Hernia Repair

There are many different types of hernia, but the most dangerous is an inguinal hernia that requires immediate surgery.[171] Over 770,000 Americans need this surgery every year, with men and children being affected disproportionately by this condition. A hernia occurs when soft tissue pushes through weak muscle, allowing an organ to poke through. They are found in the abdomen, and form as a result of strain to the body during exercise, coughing, defecation or urination. They are also common in people who are overweight and have naturally weak muscles. An inguinal hernia becomes an emergency situation when an intestine loop gets wrapped around the hernia and cuts off the blood supply to the small intestine. This is known as a strangulated hernia and can have serious effects on a man's testicles, damaging blood vessels and tissue. This is because the hernia can damage the tube that carries sperm to the urethra. As soon as serious symptoms manifest, you need to go to the hospital to get checked out.

The process of fixing an inguinal hernia involves making a large cut in your abdomen, pushing back the tissue that has spilled out and repairing the muscle wall. This is known as open hernia repair surgery. The more modern alternative involves the use of a laparoscope. Small cuts are made on the abdomen to allow the scope to slide in so that the surgeon can track his or her movements on the screen. The hernia is then repaired with other medical instruments through other cuts in the abdomen. These cuts are small and heal quickly.

If you have felt your hernia acting up recently, you might have time to fly across to Panama. If you have a bad hernia, you should always keep an eye on it and prepare for the day that you might need surgery. If your child has a hernia that makes him sick, act quickly. This digestive disorder affects a large number of children as young as a few months old, and kids can find the pain hard to endure. More emergency hernia repairs happen to male children than for any other demographic.

Urgency of Surgery: Emergency inguinal hernia repair should be performed as soon as possible, within one day of being diagnosed. Basic hernia repair to eliminate pain can be scheduled at the patient's convenience.

Average Time of Procedure: Between one and two hours for open surgery, and one hour for laparoscopic surgery.

Recovery Time: After two weeks, you should be able to resume normal daily activities. Expect a full recovery in two months.

Best Medical Tourism Destinations for this Surgery: Panama, Thailand and Costa Rica.

> **Hospital Spotlight:**
> **Hospital Punta Pacifica, Panama City, Panama**
> The only hospital in Panama affiliated with Johns Hopkins International, which means that many of their doctors were trained in the U.S. With private suites available and five-star treatment, you and your child are safe in the hands of these experienced professionals.
> ***Travel Distance to Panama:*** 2,071 miles.
> ***Estimated Travel Time by Plane:*** Four hours.

Emergency Mastectomy

When a woman has a very high risk of getting breast cancer, or already has breast cancer, then an emergency mastectomy could save her life.[172] This is an extraordinarily expensive procedure because it removes the breast, and many women choose to have breast reconstruction surgery immediately afterwards. Two costly surgeries mean that the total price tag can in fact exceed $100,000. For the woman who already has cancer, the price must be tightly controlled. Constant care and treatment may have already drained all of her insurance away, if she has insurance – and costs will be mounting. There are a few different kinds of mastectomy: total, radical and modified radical. Each removes specific parts of the breast, lymph nodes and muscles in order to save the patient from death. In the case of an emergency mastectomy, the patient usually has cancer, and has her breast, nipple and areola completely removed. The patient will certainly have the breast that contains the cancerous tumor removed; but, if the cancer is widespread, both breasts will be removed. This is an efficient procedure to use in conjunction with radiation therapy in order to beat the disease. This is one of those emergency operations that you simply need to have abroad. The need is pressing, but you can take a week to plan your overseas trip in order to save money. If you are suffering from breast cancer and don't have the time to organize a trip overseas to a better quality medical center, then at least get in contact with a hospital that will do everything for you.

Urgency of Surgery: This depends on the stage of the cancer, or your urgent need for preventative surgery. Essentially, you should get this surgery done as soon as you can, within three weeks of your recommendation.

Average Time of Procedure: Depending on your diagnosis and the extent of the surgery, it can take anywhere from one to three hours to complete, and a little more if you are having both breasts removed.

Recovery Time: About three to six weeks for a full recovery, but you'll be able to move around after a week of rest.

Best Medical Tourism Destinations for this Surgery: India, Mexico and Jordan.

Hospital Spotlight:
Apollo Gleneagles Hospital, Kolkota, India.
This ISO-approved hospital has an international patient services program and will organize your trip for you. With rooms for family members, private nurses and qualified English-speaking staff, this is the top-quality, affordable hospital you're looking for.
Travel Distance to India: 7,484 miles.
Estimated Travel Time by Plane: 16 hours.

Emergency Spleen Removal

The spleen is an organ that helps keep you healthy by fighting off infection and filtering your blood. Spleen removal is necessary when the spleen becomes diseased or damaged, or if there are tumors, cysts or abscesses inside it. Emergency spleen removal is generally called for when a patient has sustained severe abdominal trauma. If the spleen can't be repaired, then it has to be removed. It's difficult living without a spleen, because you become more prone to illness and infection that could cause you excessive health complications in the future and send your medical bills through the roof. Also called a splenectomy, this surgery can be done using either open surgery or laparoscopic surgery. The main goal of emergency spleen removal surgery is to stop internal bleeding and remove the damaged organ, which will be extracted from the upper left side of your body. A patient who has been in a car accident or suffered some other kind of bodily trauma will take longer to heal from a spleen removal because of the multiple internal repairs that are needed. This is one of those times when you can't prevent being taken to the nearest hospital, but you can decide to be moved elsewhere once you are in recovery. There are also very rare cases of a patient's spleen rupturing, which would also require immediate medical attention. Because the spleen has such a high density of blood vessels, it's easy for the patient to bleed to death if action isn't taken. The main artery must be tied off before the spleen can be removed.

Urgency of Surgery: Immediate, within an hour if possible.

Average Time of Procedure: This procedure takes about one hour, but the patient might be in surgery for a lot longer due to other internal damage.

Recovery Time: Hospital stays range from two days to two weeks, depending on the trauma you are recovering from. You will also have to stay for longer if complications arise.

Best Medical Tourism Destinations for this Surgery: Thailand, Malaysia and Singapore.

> **Hospital Spotlight: BNH Hospital, Thailand**
> A JCI- and ISO-accredited hospital with an outstanding international reputation for giving medical travelers the best possible service, this 100-year-old hospital offers private rooms, recovery facilities and even a restaurant on-site. Thailand also has facilities for trauma patients who need constant care or multiple surgeries, and a peaceful place to recuperate from their harrowing experience. Book a flight to this hospital once you have been cleared to travel, and enjoy affordable hospital accommodations and supportive staff.
> ***Travel Distance to Thailand:*** 8,791 miles.
> ***Estimated Travel Time by Plane:*** 18 hours, depending on your point of departure.

Lung Transplant

When a patient has lung disease, that person is in urgent need of a lung transplant. The clock is against the patient because donor lungs are in limited supply. Often, the patient will be hospitalized to manage the disease until a compatible donor lung is found. These patients go on a waiting list, and many of them die because lungs could not be found in time. The Scientific Registry of Transplant Recipients in the U.S. states that 2,500 Americans are on a waiting list at any given time, but only 1,500 ever have the procedure. Like most transplants, there is a specific timeframe in which to find the organs needed. As the American health system fails, transplants will be even more selective, with older patients being all but excluded from these lists. Finding a hospital internationally that can get you the donor lung or lungs should be your top priority. There are also procedures that involve a living donor giving you the lower lobe of one lung, extending your life until you can find a donor.

A lung transplant is needed when a patient is living with advanced lung disease. He or she may be put on a heart-lung machine during surgery to allow for continued breathing and blood flow. The surgeon will remove the lungs and replace them with compatible donor lungs by reattaching the new pair to the main airways and blood vessels.

Medical tourism is all about helping patients who need immediate medical treatment; when it comes to transplant surgery, no need is greater. If you go to the right hospital, flying abroad for your lung transplant could save you as much as $140,000.

Urgency of Surgery: As soon as donor lungs can be found.

Average Time of Procedure: The standard lung transplant usually takes around six hours for a single lung, and 12 hours for both. You will probably be in the hospital for two weeks; longer if your body rejects the lungs.

Recovery Time: The procedure takes about six months to recover from, depending on your progress and whether the immunosuppressive drugs work well.

Best Medical Tourism Destinations for this Surgery: Turkey, India and Singapore.

Hospital Spotlight:
Memorial Health Group, Istanbul, Turkey.

One of Turkey's leading hospitals specializing in affordable transplantation surgery, with JCI and ISO accreditations. With a hotel on premises for you and your family, this patient-centered hospital will help you through your lung transplant surgery, and the months before and after.

Travel Distance to Turkey: 5,450 miles.

Estimated Travel Time by Plane: 12 hours, depending on your point of departure.

Large Internal Hemorrhoid Surgery

A hemorrhoid is an enlarged vein around the rectum or in the lining of the anus.[173] There are 10 million Americans who suffer from hemorrhoids and seek medical treatment for them, but seeing a surgeon about this procedure can be very uncomfortable, especially when the condition has worsened to the point that the hemorrhoids are now protruding from the anus and bleeding profusely. People turn to surgery for the solution when all other methods of curing the hemorrhoids have failed. Emergency hemorrhoid surgery is performed when a patient is admitted into the hospital with severe rectal pain, bleeding and pus coming out of the anus. Often called a hemorrhoidectomy, this procedure involves the removal of the hemorrhoids by cutting them away. The incisions require stitches that will eventually dissolve as you heal. The patient is usually put under general anesthetic during the procedure. You also have the option of choosing laser therapy, which will burn and harden your internal hemorrhoids, or sclerotherapy, which uses a chemical to make the hemorrhoids shrink. External hemorrhoids may also be removed if you are already admitted for internal hemorrhoid surgery.

This is a particularly embarrassing surgery to seek medical attention for, and it should be handled by your surgeon with professionalism and efficiency. This makes it a great surgery to have overseas, in a private, relaxed environment where you can recover without having to answer uncomfortable questions about your condition. If you would like to get hemorrhoid surgery before it becomes a medical emergency, plan your trip to another country and book yourself for a week or two.

Urgency of Surgery: Depends on your level of pain and the condition of your hemorrhoids.
Average Time of Procedure: About an hour.
Recovery Time: Between two and six weeks for a full recovery.
Best Medical Tourism Destinations for this Surgery: Croatia, Mexico and Costa Rica.

> **Hospital Spotlight:**
> **Sinteza Health Centre, Zagreb, Croatia**
> A luxury private medical center where patients can enjoy hotel-like accommodations, consult with internationally renowned surgeons and take advantage of Croatia's modern diagnostic procedures.
> ***Travel Distance to Croatia:*** 7,231 miles.
> ***Estimated Travel Time by Plane:*** 14 hours.

Specialist Surgery

When doctors are in their final years of practical study at a teaching hospital, they may choose a specialty. Specialists focus on one specific branch of medicine. A heart surgeon would have specialized in cardiology, a brain surgeon in neurology, and so on. Specialist surgery encompasses all branches of medicine that don't fall under general surgery. In other words, these surgeries concentrate on specific parts of the body, like the bones, heart, veins, nerves and brain. A specialist can also favor a certain demographic: pediatric surgeons, for example, only operate on kids. Specialist surgery is much more expensive than general surgery, and many people don't have the money to get the medical care they need. Medical tourism offers patients the opportunity to get that care. The average cost of a coronary bypass in America is $54,115; in India, you can get the same procedure for as little as $9,206 and have better medical care. No wonder millions of U.S. citizens are choosing to fly overseas for their specialist surgeries. New Zealand, Thailand, Mexico, South Africa, Panama, Belize – they are all cheaper than the U.S., with equal or more advanced technology, patient care and medical services.

Check out these specialist surgeries available abroad and the huge savings you can accumulate if you decide to become a medical traveler.

Neurosurgery: Brain Tumor Surgery

Neurosurgery is considered one of the most difficult medical disciplines as it deals with delicate areas like the brain and the nervous system in the spine. The central nervous system of the human body is prone to a multitude of diseases, and many of them can be treated by a neurosurgeon. Neurosurgery treats movement issues, epilepsy, CNS infections, congenital abnormalities, spinal diseases and brain hemorrhages. A neurosurgeon studies for many years to be able to help patients defeat these life-threatening conditions.

One example of neurosurgery is brain tumor surgery.[174] When you are diagnosed with a brain tumor, you face multiple surgeries, crippling costs and endless bed rest as your tumor grows. A brain tumor is an abnormal growth in the brain, and tumors can be either cancerous or non-cancerous. Both are dangerous because they are growing next to the most vital organ in your body. While non-cancerous (or benign) tumors are fairly simple to remove, they are terribly painful and can cause permanent brain damage if they aren't removed immediately. These benign tumors sometimes become cancerous over time if they are left untreated. Cancerous (or malignant) tumors spread quickly and latch on to the spinal cord. These tumors are the most dangerous as they put enormous pressure on the brain, and can cause death if they aren't removed in time. Many people who have other forms of cancer end up getting brain tumors as the cancer spreads throughout their body. All brain surgery is classified as emergency surgery due to the threatening nature of the tumors themselves. The Gamma Knife Technique is a non-invasive brain surgery procedure in which your surgeon trains radiation beams at your tumor to kill it. Brain tumor surgery is possible overseas in clean, controlled hospitals with dedicated neurosurgical staff. When it comes to neurosurgery, there are better doctors internationally than there are available in America. These doctors don't overcharge you for treatment either, so you get both an increased survival rate and monetary savings.

Urgency of Surgery: Depending on the size of your tumor and whether it is benign or malignant, you'll need to have it out as soon as you can.

Average Time of Procedure: It depends – no two tumors are the same. Size, location and type all dictate how long the surgical procedure will take.

Recovery Time: If your tumor is benign, it will take you between four and eight weeks to fully recover from your surgery. Unfortunately, with a malignant tumor, recovery doesn't factor into the long-term treatment. You'll need aggressive surgery, radiation therapy and medicine for a very long time.

Best Medical Tourism Destinations for this Surgery: Germany, Costa Rica and South Korea.

Hospital Spotlight:
University Medical Center, Freiburg, Germany

As one of the most highly-regarded and largest medical centers in the world, this university-based medical center is a leader in neurological surgery and modern treatments. Their neurocenter will give you the best chance possible of surviving a brain tumor.

Travel Distance to Germany: 4,166 miles.
Estimated Travel Time by Plane: Six hours.

Orthopedic Surgery: Spinal Fusion

Orthopedics is the study of the human musculoskeletal system.[175] An orthopedic surgeon has therefore studied how to surgically treat diseases and disorders affecting the bones, ligaments and joints. Your orthopedic surgeon will be able to set broken bones, amputate limbs, replace joints, graft bones and perform spinal fusion. Many emergency room admissions are referred to the orthopedic surgeon for diagnosis and rehabilitation. For example, a woman who has fallen from a four-story balcony and has been transferred on a stretcher to the ER will have multiple fractures and lacerations, all of which can be fixed and reset by the orthopedic surgeon.

Spinal fusion is an excellent example of an orthopedic procedure. Spinal fusion is a procedure often performed to ease the pain of spinal stenosis.[176] Spinal stenosis occurs as a result of old age, arthritis or a serious spinal injury. Spinal fusion will often be performed in conjunction with other spinal procedures in order to correct damage and eliminate pain. Spinal fusion is the adjoining of vertebrae so that they no longer move in a way that causes the patient pain or discomfort. The surgery involves making a cut along the spine or neck, moving the muscle tissue aside and then fusing the two vertebrae together with a bone graft. The grafted vertebrae are held in place with screws until the wound has properly healed.

This kind of surgery can be both urgent and semi-urgent. Emergency spinal fusions happen when patient have damaged or crushed one or more of the vertebrae, and now have central nervous system damage. The surgery needs to be done as soon as possible, as spinal damage can be enormously painful and can render the patient paralyzed. If you need the operation, then you will be in pain until you get it, which makes finding an international hospital difficult. Work through a medical travel agent and hire an air ambulance if you must, but get your surgery done somewhere cheaper. Prices can be upwards of $100,000 for spinal fusion surgery in the U.S. Since you can get it done just across the border in Mexico for $12,000, you should live through the pain for the short amount of time it will take you to make travel arrangements.

Urgency of Surgery: Immediate in some cases; or as soon as you can get it.
Average Time of Procedure: Surgery takes between four and six hours.
Recovery Time: A week in a hospital to let your bone graft heal, and full recovery after one month.
Best Medical Tourism Destinations for this Surgery: Malaysia, India and Mexico.

> **Hospital Spotlight:**
> **Mahkota Medical Centre, Melaka, Malaysia**
> This private hospital has 50 specialists on staff ready to help you with your medical emergency. With private rooms, on-site accommodations for families and recovery facilities, you'll experience great medical care directly in the heart of Melaka's business district.
> ***Travel Distance to Malaysia:*** 9,527 miles.
> ***Estimated Travel Time by Plane:*** 19 hours.

Vascular Surgery: Abdominal Aortic Aneurysm Repair

A vascular surgeon deals with the vascular system, or the veins and arteries that carry blood around the body. Because vascular surgeons repair all blood transport systems, they also work in areas like neurosurgery and cardiac surgery. When arteries and veins become blocked, diseased, nicked or broken, this can have serious consequences for the patient. The vascular system provides oxygen and nutrients to your cells, and removes waste products from the body. If this system breaks down, the result could be a stroke or heart attack. Depending on the level of arterial damage when a stroke or heart attack occurs, the situation could be deadly for the patient. A damaged or clogged artery in the heart will cause the muscle to corrode and deteriorate because it's not getting what it needs to stay healthy. A vascular surgeon studies how to treat diseases that impair natural blood flow so the body can return to good health. Nothing in your body can function without the vascular system.

An abdominal aortic aneurysm can be defined as the enlargement of the large blood vessel that passes blood to your abdomen and legs. Many people who suffer from this type of aneurysm have no idea because it builds up over a few years without any symptoms. One day the aneurism ruptures and blood leaks out of it, causing extremely sharp pain in your groin area that may carry down to your legs. When your aneurism ruptures, you need to go to the hospital immediately for an open abdominal aortic aneurism repair. Fewer than 40% of patients survive a ruptured abdominal aneurism, so time is of the essence. If you know that you have a developing aneurism, schedule to have it fixed before it ruptures. Your vascular surgeon will make an incision in your abdomen and open your aorta where the aneurism is. They will then replace your aorta with a graft or another blood vessel, either taken from your body or made from synthetic material. This will stabilize the aneurism and prevent it from rupturing. If you survive the surgery to repair your aorta, you'll need to go somewhere to be monitored for a few weeks. Vascular surgery is available in many locations around the world. Vascular surgeons abroad are just as well trained as U.S. doctors.

Urgency of Surgery: If ruptured, immediately. If suspected, go and see your doctor for a consult.

Average Time of Procedure: Between three and four hours.

Recovery Time: A five-day hospital stay if there are no complications, and at least a month for recovery.

Best Medical Tourism Destinations for this Surgery: India, Mexico and Costa Rica.

> **Hospital Spotlight:**
> **Sahel General Hospital, Beirut, Lebanon**
> This ISO-certified hospital has 172 private rooms and fluent English-speaking staff trained to help you recover from vascular problems and disease. It's a must-see modern hospital in beautiful Lebanon.
> ***Travel Distance to Lebanon:*** 5,809 miles.
> ***Estimated Travel Time by Plane:*** 12 hours.

Cardiac Surgery: Aortic Valve Replacement

Cardiac surgery involves repairing the heart, one of the dominant organs in the body.[177] Without a healthy heart, your body can't pump blood to its organs and extremities. Your cardiologist will treat any heart conditions, traumas or diseases – these include heart disease, heart attack and atherosclerosis. Cardiologists also measure your heart's performance levels and test it to see if it's functioning properly. Heart surgeons study for ten or more years in order to work on hearts, and are some of the most disciplined professionals in the medical industry. Part of their job is to implant pacemakers and heart failure devices, and to repair clogged coronary or carotid arteries. They also perform heart transplants, bypass surgeries and heart valve replacements. Though cardiac surgeons may perform some of the same surgeries as vascular surgeons, they never stray far from the heart. Often patients only experience heart problems when it's something serious, say because of pain or an ER admission for a suspected heart attack. If you have been diagnosed with heart disease, you will be able to plan your treatment in another destination.

The heart has four valves that aid in pumping blood to the different regions of the muscle. The aortic valve is situated next to the aorta of the heart and pushes blood inside it, then prevents the blood from coming back out. When the aortic valve is diseased and needs to be replaced, the patient is at a high risk of heart failure. Emergency aortic valve replacement is necessary when a patient is admitted to the ER and is found to have valvular heart disease, or is experiencing labored breathing, heart palpitations and extreme fatigue. The cardiac surgeon will begin the surgery by making a long chest incision to expose the heart. The patient will be put on a heart-lung machine so vitals remain steady during the procedure. The heart is temporarily stopped so that the valve can be inserted safely and without any additional damage to the surrounding tissue. The aorta is then exposed and the malfunctioning valve is taken out. A prosthetic or animal replacement valve is secured in place of the diseased valve. This is a significant surgery and should not be taken lightly. Many complications can arise from open heart surgery, so take time to find the best possible international cardiothoracic surgeon when you need an aortic valve replacement.

Urgency of Surgery: Severe symptoms or disease need to be addressed with immediate surgery, on the day of admission.

Average Time of Procedure: Between two and five hours, depending on your surgeon.

Recovery Time: Recovery is expected within one to three months after the surgery.

Best Medical Tourism Destinations for this Surgery: India, New Zealand and Argentina.

> **Hospital Spotlight:**
> **Krishna Heart and Super Specialty Institute, Ghuma, India**
> This medical center has superb facilities and is ISO-certified. It specifically deals with heart disease and cardiac care, and is owned and run by specialists who studied in America. Its private rooms and recovery facilities are in serene surroundings. India has some of the world's finest cardiac facilities, with people flying there for the treatment quality – not the low cost benefits. India is heart surgery central.
> ***Travel Distance to India:*** Around 7,484 miles.
> ***Estimated Travel Time by Plane:*** 16 hours.

Pediatric Surgery: Pyloromyotomy

Pediatricians treat children who suffer from disease, injury or deformation. Pediatric surgery is therefore concerned with treating babies and children when they need surgical intervention.[178] There are many different types of pediatric surgeons, such as pediatric orthopedic surgeons and pediatric neurologists. These highly-talented individuals work with everything in miniature, and have to be emotionally strong and sympathetic. Because children's bodies are still developing, the pediatric surgeon adheres to certain protocols so the natural growth of the patient is not hampered in any way. Trauma surgery for children is the largest area of pediatric surgery, and accidents are the number one cause of death for kids under the age of fifteen. Parents will pay anything for the survival and health of their children. The best pediatric treatment can be found abroad at significantly lower rates than at U.S. hospitals.

Hypertrophic Pyloric Stenosis is a condition that obstructs the pyloric outlet of the stomach. This is common in babies who are between three and six weeks old. The symptoms include continuous vomiting and, as a result, extreme dehydration. The child is rushed to the emergency room, assessed and diagnosed with the condition, and then taken for fluid resuscitation and a procedure called a pyloromyotomy. The muscles in the pylorus of the child have become too large, and the pylorus is preventing food from entering the small intestine. The surgeon will create a small incision in the child's stomach and then proceed to cut the pylorus to loosen the muscle. The surgery can also be performed with a laparoscope.

Without this emergency surgery, your child could die from starvation or dehydration. Though the initial emergency surgery would have to be done locally, you can choose to get your follow-up treatment done overseas, especially if there are further complications or the enlarged pylorus comes back. Look for an accredited international children's hospital that performs laparoscopic procedures. They are easier on the child because they are less invasive, and the wounds heal faster than open surgery.

Urgency of Surgery: Immediate, or as soon as symptoms show.
Average Time of Procedure: About an hour.
Recovery Time: Your child should be fully healed within one month.
Best Medical Tourism Destinations for this Surgery: Singapore, India and Mexico.

Hospital Spotlight:
KK Women's and Children's Hospital, Singapore.

This JCI- and ISO-accredited hospital has excellent medical facilities for children. With 300 specialists on hand, and over 1,000 nurses for the 830-room hospital, this first-rate medical center provides 24-hour children's emergency service.

Travel Distance to Singapore: 9,649 miles.
Estimated Travel Time by Plane: 19-20 hours.

Testimonials from Emergency Surgery Patients

Name: Allen Miller, Washington

Condition: Severe Abdominal Pain from Gall Bladder
Surgery: Emergency Cholecystectomy (Gall Bladder Removal)
Hospital: Hospital Angeles, Mexico
Medical Travel Agency: WorldMed Assist

ALLEN MILLER HAD NO HEALTH INSURANCE after he quit his last job. When it came time to get private coverage, no insurance company would insure him because he was found to have Hepatitis C. After experiencing two solid months of agony in his abdomen, he went to his local doctor for some tests and found out that he needed to have his gall bladder removed – fast. The cost were more than Allen could handle: an estimated $20,000. He turned to the Internet and found WorldMed Assist, a medical tourism facilitator that could help him get the surgery he needed abroad. Once he made the decision and spoke to Dr. Ruiz about his surgery, he gave WorldMed the go-ahead and flew to Mexico for his surgery. WorldMed picked Allen and his wife up at the airport and took them to the hospital. After three days in the hospital, and three more days lazing in the sun, they went home. In total, the cost of the experience was only $6,000, far more affordable than $20,000! Altogether, a very enlightening and successful trip abroad.

Name: Sue Nagy, Illinois

Condition: Clogged Arteries in the Heart
Surgery: Emergency Angioplasty
Hospital: Hospital Angeles, Mexico
Medical Travel Agency: WorldMed Assist

SUE WAS RUSHED TO THE EMERGENCY ROOM after having what she thought was a heart attack – only to discover that 95% of her heart's arteries were seriously clogged. There was only one thing that would save her life – an enormously expensive angioplasty – and she didn't have insurance. After calling around, the cost of saving her life came to a nice round figure of $45,000. Like most new medical tourists, she turned to the Internet for advice, and she discovered WorldMed Assist.[179] Sue contacted them immediately, and together they set to work trying to find her the perfect hospital abroad. They settled on Mexico because it was the closest, and WorldMed Assist made all of the urgent arrangements for her. Ten days later, she woke up in a comfortable hospital bed in Mexico, with perfectly healthy arteries. Everything – the angioplasty, travel arrangements and expenses – cost her $13,000. Sue explained how thorough the cardiologist was before her procedure, walking her through what was going to happen step by step; and how very supportive he was once the procedure was complete. Her U.S. doctor even complimented her international doctor on his work! Nothing but quality healthcare, and lower costs as advertised.

Name: Conchetta Procopio, Arizona

Condition: Unknown
Surgery: Emergency Hysterectomy
Hospital: Hospital in Mexico
Medical Travel Agency: MedtoGo

DURING A ROUTINE CHECK-UP at her doctor's office, Conchetta was told that she needed a hysterectomy as soon as possible. A dedicated wife and mother of four children, Conchetta didn't have health insurance. She was told by a friend to investigate having the surgery done in Mexico through a company called MedtoGo.[180] With nothing to lose, she contacted the company – and was so impressed with their services that she eventually hired them for the job. Convinced that the surgery in Mexico would be top-quality, and that she'd save a ton of

AFFORDABLE ELECTIVE SURGERY ABROAD

money, Conchetta left for her medical destination. After a brief meet and greet at the airport, she was taken to the hospital and attended to by a highly qualified surgeon. Even the post-operative care was taken care of by MedtoGo. All in all, the surgery went exceptionally well, and Conchetta made a full recovery at home.

Price Chart – Surgical Procedures Only

Average cost of **EMERGENCY GASTRECTOMY**	U.S.	$50,000–$67,000
	India	$8,000–$10,000
	Mexico	$10,000–$13,000
	South Korea	$10,000–$15,000
Average cost of **EMERGENCY GALLBLADDER REMOVAL SURGERY**	U.S.	$8,000–$10,000
	Brazil	$3,000–$4,000
	Mexico	$5,000–$6,000
	Panama	$3,000–$4,000
Average cost of **EMERGENCY APPENDECTOMY**	U.S.	$17,000–$20,000
	Germany	$5,000–$6,000
	India	$2,000–$3,000
	Thailand	$2,000–$4,000
Average cost of **EMERGENCY INGUINAL HERNIA REPAIR**	U.S.	$23,000–$30,000
	Costa Rica	$4,000–$6,000
	Panama	$4,000–$6,000
	Thailand	$5,000–$7,000

Average cost of **EMERGENCY MASTECTOMY**	U.S.	$12,000–$35,000
	India	$1,000–$3,000
	Mexico	$1,000–$2,000
	Jordan	$2,000–$4,000
Average cost of **EMERGENCY SPLEEN REMOVAL**	U.S.	$3,000–$6,000
	Malaysia	$1,000–$2,000
	Singapore	$1,000–$2,000
	Thailand	$800–$1,500
Average cost of **LUNG TRANSPLANT**	U.S.	$400,000
	India	$40,000
	Singapore	$50,000
	Turkey	$30,000
Average cost of **LARGE INTERNAL HEMORRHOID SURGERY**	U.S.	$5,000–$10,000
	Costa Rica	$2,000–$3,000
	Croatia	$800–$1,000
	Mexico	$1,400–$2,000
Average cost of **BRAIN TUMOR SURGERY**	U.S.	$45,000
	Costa Rica	$35,000
	Germany	$30,000
	South Korea	$30,000

Average cost of **SPINAL FUSION**	U.S.	$55,000–$65,000
	India	$9,000–$11,000
	Malaysia	$6,000–$7,000
	Mexico	$12,000–$15,000
Average cost of **OPEN ABDOMINAL AORTIC ANEURYSM REPAIR**	U.S.	$20,000
	Costa Rica	$7,000–$10,000
	India	$5,000–$6,000
	Mexico	$3,000–$4,000
Average cost of **EMERGENCY AORTIC VALVE REPLACEMENT**	U.S.	$70,000
	Argentina	$16,000–$18,000
	India	$10,000–$12,000
	New Zealand	$30,000–$35,000
Average cost of **EMERGENCY AORTIC VALVE REPLACEMENT**	U.S.	$7,500
	India	$800–$2,000
	Mexico	$1,500–$3,000
	Singapore	$1,500–$2,000

ಸಾ • ಛಿ

CHAPTER 7

AFFORDABLE CHRONIC DISEASE TREATMENT ABROAD

Affordable Chronic Disease Treatment Abroad

ℰ•ℛ

Chronic diseases have escalated over the last fifty years, thanks to our modern diet and inactive lifestyles; and this trend is only going to put more strain on an already bursting healthcare system. Dr. James Marks, Director of the CDC's National Health Center for Chronic Disease Prevention and Health Promotion, commented that "If we are concerned about the rising costs of healthcare, we will have to learn how to better deal with chronic diseases." Unfortunately, it looks as though that will never happen now that we have a socialist healthcare system in place. Instead, millions of Americans will be diagnosed with diseases like cancer, heart disease and mental illness, and be cast out to sea, left to deal with their health problems alone. This news is somewhat dire as the most recent CDC report states that almost half of the American population has one or more chronic disease. Of these people, there are millions who don't fully understand the extent of their disease, or how they can help themselves through various medical and natural means. In fact, a large percentage of Americans are completely unaware that they have life-threatening illnesses. With the rise of Obamacare, and the testing restrictions placed on U.S. hospitals, what are the chances that these Americans will discover the truth about their ill health – before it's too late? Chronic diseases kill more Americans every year than any other medical condition. This chapter is designed to give you all the options when it comes to

> **Almost half of the American population has one or more chronic disease**

the main chronic diseases that affect the American population. Learn about treatments and their costs abroad, and where you can get long-term medical help when you need it most. If you're one of the many Americans who suffer from chronic illness, you need to pay special attention to this chapter. It could save your life.

Questions You Should Ask Your Doctor

It doesn't matter what kind of chronic illness you have – only that you have decided to take a leap of faith and find a doctor or hospital overseas that can help you get well again or effectively manage your disease. When shopping abroad for a doctor, there are certain questions that you need to ask concerning each facility's level of care and the treatment options they offer. Not only will you be saving yourself a lot of money, but you'll be introducing yourself to treatments that aren't available in America. The American Cancer Society reported that families with health insurance have still gone bankrupt because of the astronomical costs of treatment in America. Cancer patients and their families have lost their homes, jobs and cars. Many have become completely destitute at some point during their treatment.

You can avoid this fate if you plan to get treatment abroad. Let's look at some of the most important questions you should ask your potential international doctor when seeking medical care for your chronic disease. Refer also to Chapter 5, which lists "Questions to Ask Your Doctor," for the broad introductory questions you should ask when searching for a qualified medical practitioner.

Do you regularly provide treatment for my condition?

The first thing you should ask your potential doctor and medical care center is how prepared they are to handle your chronic disease. You will find that there are certain hospitals that specialize in specific treatments and provide cutting-edge care in those areas. Cancer treatment centers abroad, for example, are well equipped to handle the full range of cancer, with its 120 variants. On the other hand, a hospital in Mexico might have a cancer wing, but tends to be more advanced in the area of kidney disease and has a very high success rate at treating foreign patients for that specific ailment. Do your research.

Do you have facilities for long-term care?

Many chronic diseases progress into a need for constant medical attention in order for the patient to survive. Ask your doctor if there are facilities in the medical care center that are meant for long-term stays; and ask about special features, such as the opportunity to hire private nurses to care for you while you are there. Also, many hospitals abroad have on-location accommodations for families so you can all stay together during this trying time.

Is your surgical unit prepared for emergency surgeries arising from a chronic disease?

Often, an extended stay at an international hospital for chronic disease treatment will end up including emergency surgery. A type 2 diabetes patient, for example, might have a heart attack while abroad, or might suffer from kidney damage that can only be corrected through surgery. You want to make sure that the hospital you're in is not only suited for long-term care, but can also handle complications that may arise from your condition. This is also your opportunity to discuss the severity of your disease, and what surgeries are likely in the future should your health continue to deteriorate.

Does your hospital provide any alternative treatments in conjunction with mainstream modern medicine?

There have been many cases of patients who had all but given up hope – until they traveled abroad for medical care, including additional alternative treatment, and overcame their diseases as a result. Alternative treatment is becoming more important for chronic disease patients, and a strengthened immune system might be exactly what you need to conquer your illness. Inquire about non-pharmaceutical-based treatment that you can get abroad. If the hospital doesn't provide it directly, then they should be able to refer you to an alternative health practitioner with a track record of helping people with your condition.

Do you offer counseling for patients and families dealing with my condition?

Having a chronic disease is life-defining, and can be extremely painful for patients and their loved ones. Most hospitals support the needs of their patients by employing qualified counselors who can guide them through the emotional aspects of chronic disease. There are many benefits to counseling, including learning the coping mechanisms needed when facing surgery, treatment, pain and hopelessness. This is why counseling facilities are so important.

Are there any clinical trials I can participate in?

Participating in a clinical trial can be very beneficial, especially when many other methods of treatment have failed to cure you or control your symptoms. Often, the most advanced, cutting-edge medicine is being tested in clinical trials – and the cost of taking part in trials, and gaining access to these new treatments, is significantly reduced overseas. According to an article published in Medical News Today, most clinical trials occur outside of the U.S. While a top-rated medical care center in India would charge you $2,000 to take part in a trial, it would cost as much as $20,000 to take part in that same trial in America. Make sure you investigate what chronic medication trials your potential hospital is participating in. It could be your reason to fly to that specific center.

What can I expect when I arrive for my treatment?

Doctors abroad are very willing to explain to you the process of getting settled in at your new treatment center. For a patient who is already suffering from severe illness, it helps relieve the stress of traveling. Knowing what to expect allows you to prepare physically and mentally for your arrival, and helps you make the necessary arrangements for your family. Depending on the extent of your illness, the first things you have to look forward to when you arrive are admission, accommodations and initial testing.

What medical records and test results should I bring with me?

You will have to make sure that all of the required medical records and test results come with you to your new hospital. This means that you will have to submit a written request to your U.S. doctor or hospital. They will produce copies of all the data you need in order to continue your medical treatment overseas. This might cost you some money, but it's necessary. Based on these scans, X-rays and other diagnostic test results, your international doctor will be able to assess your medical condition and make plans for any further tests that are needed.

How much will my treatment cost?

All potential patients have the right to request a full breakdown of the costs involved when choosing a medical center abroad. Asking for a cost breakdown will help you plan for the long term and make the necessary financial arrangements or loans for your trip. It's also helpful when you are comparing hospitals, doctors and success rates, trying to get the best quality medical care for the lowest possible price. If you're traveling to a mental health treatment center, for example, you can likely calculate the exact costs that you will incur on a monthly basis. For more uncertain diseases like cancer and heart disease, ask about average procedure costs, how much testing will set you back and what the price of surgery will be if it becomes necessary. Let's examine the main chronic diseases that Americans have to deal with, and reveal some enlightening facts about costs, facilities and treatment.

Cancer

Roughly 1,500 people die every day in the United States from cancer, and over a million new cases of the disease are reported every year. The American Cancer Society, the National Cancer Institute and the Centers for Disease Control and Prevention carefully track these numbers, and though the overall survival rate is increasing, so is prevalence of the disease. This is largely due to exposure to carcinogens, inherited genetic characteristics and lifestyle choices like smoking and drinking. Cancer is a disease that causes an abnormal growth of cells which sometimes spreads all over the body from the point of origin. Certain types of cancer[181] are gender-specific, like ovarian and prostate cancers, but most forms of the disease can affect anyone – across race, age and gender. Many of the world's best cancer treatment facilities are overseas, and offer affordable, quality care for patients suffering from specific types of cancer.

Main Variants of Cancer

Breast Cancer: An abnormal growth that starts in the tissue of the breast. One in eight women in the U.S. will be diagnosed with breast cancer.

Hematologic Cancers: Cancer that occurs in the bone marrow or blood. Of 35,070 reported hematologic cancer deaths in America, 22,280 died of leukemia.

Lung Cancer: Cancer that occurs in the air passages or tissue of the lung. Of 196,454 Americans who contracted lung cancer, 158,599 died.

Prostate Cancer: Malignant cell growth in the prostate gland. One in six men in the U.S. will be diagnosed with prostate cancer.

Skin Cancer: One of several types of cancer that form in skin tissue. One in five Americans will develop skin cancer during their lifetime.

Endometrial (Uterine) Cancer: Abnormal growth of cells in the uterus. In 2009, 42,160 women were diagnosed with uterine cancer. Of that number, 7,780 died.

Colon Cancer: A malignant cell growth on the inner lining of the colon. Of the 106,100 Americans who were diagnosed with this cancer in 2009, 40,870 died.

Pancreatic Cancer: Cancer of the pancreatic tissue. Of 42,470 Americans who developed pancreatic cancer in 2009, 35,240 died.

Treatment Options

Surgery

Surgery is often the only way that doctors can remove a cancerous growth and see how far it has spread in your body.[182] If you have been diagnosed with cancer, then you will have surgery at some point during your treatment. There are three main types of cancer surgery: diagnostic, staging and curative. These represent the testing, explorative and healing stages of your treatment. There are several other reasons for which you could need surgery during your treatment, so it's important to find a great surgeon who can help you beat this disease.

Radiation Therapy

Radiation treatment will help disrupt or damage your cancer cells, and is therefore a vital part of most curative cancer protocols. If your cancer is dividing and spreading, radiation may be effective enough to prevent or at least curb the disease from attacking other parts of your body. Radiation therapy does not kill cancer cells – it mostly keeps healthy cells near the affected area from becoming cancerous. It is also useful at shrinking cells during early stage cancer, or at preventing cancer from returning after it has been surgically removed.

Chemotherapy
Chemotherapy is the most common form of cancer treatment, and involves systematically taking in certain drugs to treat the disease. Chemotherapy can be light or intensive, and may mean getting injections from your doctor or taking pills every day. Often mistaken for radiation therapy, this non-invasive form of cancer treatment has had the best results worldwide. It is often used in conjunction with surgery and radiation therapy.

Targeted Therapy
Targeted therapy is relatively new and can be used to treat a multitude of diseases. There are many variants of this kind of treatment, but they all involve using drugs to attack diseased cells. Instead of damaging all cells, they specifically target the sick ones – hence the name. They effectively prevent these cancerous cells from growing and spreading. Various types of targeted therapy include the drugs Iressa, Sutent, Gleevec and Mylotarg.

There are also many other forms of cancer treatment, partly because there is no definitive cure for the disease. These include: immunotherapy, proton therapy, antiangiogenesis therapy and photodynamic therapy.

Long-term Medical Care

Most medical procedures only require short-term care in a hospital abroad, but this is not true of a disease like cancer. Treatment can often last several months, which could be a serious problem for the patient and his or her family. Go overseas. Find an inexpensive apartment near your treatment center and work from there. It will save you money, even if members of your family have to fly back home a few times. Savings of 40-80% can accumulate over these months.

Duration of Stay: Between four and ten months, depending on the level of treatment required.

> **Hospital Showcase:**
> **Bumrungrad International Hospital, Thailand**
> This is a state-of-the-art cancer care facility that treats every stage of the disease, from diagnosis to recovery. The medical staff was trained in the U.S., and the center is one of the most complete and prestigious cancer care facilities in Asia.

Type 2 Diabetes

Diabetes affects millions of Americans, with type 2 being the most common, accounting for 90 to 95% of all reported cases. Also known as adult-onset diabetes, this chronic disease forces your body to resist insulin, which feeds your cells with much-needed sugar. Sugar is the main source of fuel for your body. The combination of high levels of glucose in your blood plus your body's inability to use any of it can lead to serious medical problems, and sometimes even death. The buildup of sugar in your body is called hyperglycemia. Untreated type 2 diabetes has been known to cause kidney failure, heart disease, blindness and the loss of limbs. There are many Americans who have this chronic disease and don't know about it, because they haven't yet developed any real symptoms. Type 2 can be managed from home with good exercise and eating regimes. It's generally when this condition isn't treated that complications arise. Medical tourists travel to other countries for diabetes-related surgeries, treatments and even stem cell therapy. Data shows that in 2006, over 72,507 Americans died from diabetes-related issues. If you have type 2 diabetes and are running into all kinds of medical problems, then perhaps it's time to fly overseas for some real, affordable treatment.

Other Main Variants of Diabetes

Type 1 Diabetes: An autoimmune disease most typical in children, this form of diabetes causes the body to destroy beta cells. Patients are dependent on insulin injections because the pancreas, where insulin is made and where the beta cells live, stops working.

Pregestational Diabetes: Diabetes that exists in a woman before she gives birth causes some risk to the baby's health if the condition is not properly treated.

Gestational Diabetes: Diabetes that occurs during pregnancy. In other words, the woman's blood sugar levels rise while she is pregnant. This occurs because the placenta is preventing the woman's body from making enough insulin.

Pre-Diabetes: The condition prior to developing type 2 diabetes, when your blood sugar levels are higher than normal.

Treatment Options

Choosing the Right Diet

Approaching a dietician is crucial when you have been diagnosed with type 2 diabetes. He or she will help you pick the right foods to eat and help you monitor your daily intake. Food is one of the biggest contributors to rising blood sugar levels, so be sure to eat properly all the time or you could gain weight and worsen your condition.

Monitoring Blood Sugar Levels

Your doctor will give you a comprehensive treatment plan that will include exercise, your medication regimen and what you can and can't do. Stress can often cause insulin reduction in the blood, so you'll need to take it easy whenever you can. Alcohol will be removed from your diet, and any medications that contradict your treatment will be removed from your medical routine. International hospitals often have dieticians on staff who specially create these new lifestyle plans for patients. Following such a plan should prevent any future complications from the disease.

Medication and Insulin

When you begin your new lifestyle, you will also be given any medicine that you need to take on a daily basis. For patients with type 2 diabetes, Metformin is a common medication used to lower the glucose production in your body. Insulin therapy might also be required and involves a series of injections that keep your insulin levels up. If these two treatments aren't enough, and your health continues to deteriorate, then an insulin pump may be attached to your body. The catheter leading from the external pump will be inserted under your skin and will feed your body insulin when it needs it.

Surgery

There are certain kinds of preventative surgery that can help keep diabetes under control. Bariatric or weight loss surgery will effectively reduce the size of your stomach, and will force you to lose weight as a result. This surgery has had amazing results with patients suffering from high blood sugar levels. Patients' glucose levels stabilize after the surgery and unpleasant symptoms stop. This type of surgery is usually very expensive, so flying overseas for this diabetes treatment will correct your health problems and save you a lot of money at the same time.

Long-term Medical Care

Your goal during long-term treatment is to continue taking your medication and living a healthy lifestyle. If you do, you won't have to endure the many complications of this disease. If you choose to fly overseas for treatment, you'll get medicine for less and have the opportunity to get the surgery you've wanted. Hospitals abroad offer the finest medical care and recovery centers, with private dieticians to cater to your every need. Plus, they offer a range of alternative treatments and relaxing spa therapies to help you recover and rejuvenate on your medical vacation.

Duration of Stay: If you are traveling for type 2 diabetes treatment, your times are flexible. Because you are there for a combined treatment/vacation, you can determine the length of your stay. If you go for bariatric surgery, however, you're looking at a minimum stay of three weeks before you are ready to travel.

> **Hospital Showcase:**
> **American Hospital, Dubai**
> This hospital has a world-class diabetes center dedicated to helping patients manage their disease. These "diabetologists" offer diabetics truly specialized medical care. All doctors are board-certified, and have spent years educating and supporting patients with all forms of diabetes.

Heart Disease

Heart disease is really a banner term for diseases that affect the heart. These diseases are the number one cause of death in America, eclipsing cancer, diabetes and accidental death. Most heart disease also involves the blood vessels in and around the heart. Emergency situations like heart attacks and strokes occur when these blood vessels become diseased, clogged or narrowed. Different types of coronary disease have different symptoms. If you begin to experience chest pain, or you ache regularly, then it's time to schedule an appointment with your local medical center. If you are diagnosed with heart disease, fly abroad to have it treated. Heart disease includes conditions such as an enlarged heart, high blood pressure, aortic aneurysm and congenital heart disease. Many of these sneak up on undiagnosed patients and end their lives prematurely. Every 34 seconds, an American dies from a heart-related condition. A disease of this severity requires treatment – now. There are a wide variety of treatment options abroad.

Main Variants of Heart Disease

Heart Attack: The coronary artery becomes clogged, the blood supply is cut off to the heart and parts of the muscle die. A heart attack is also called a myocardial infarction. More than 1 million Americans have a heart attack every year.

Coronary Artery Disease: A general build-up of plaque and cholesterol is deposited in the coronary artery. If this disease degenerates, it causes a heart attack. More than 13 million Americans currently have this disease.

Cardiomyopathy: The myocardium in the heart becomes diseased, which results in an enlarged heart. As a result, the heart stops pumping blood efficiently, and heart failure occurs. Over 50,000 people in the U.S. are affected by this disease every year.

Atrial Fibrillation: This condition involves an irregular heartbeat that increases the risk of a stroke and of developing heart disease. By 2025, 3.3 million people will end up in the hospital because of this condition. One in every 136 people has it right now.

Heart Valve Disease: A disease that causes the valves in the heart to work irregularly. Improper heart function can lead to failure. Over 5 million

Americans are diagnosed with this disease each year.

Pericarditis: A disease that causes the pericardium around your heart to become inflamed. It's rare – but when diagnosed, it needs to be treated immediately.

Treatment Options

Surgery

Many forms of heart disease require some sort of cardiac surgery. This might include pacemaker installation, angioplasty, valve replacement, heart transplant or defibrillator implant. Each has its own risks, but they are ultimately required if you're going to beat the disease. Finding the right cardiac center abroad is very important in this instance because the surgery is so specialized and your life hangs in the balance.

Other Medical Procedures

Short of these highly invasive surgeries, your surgeon might recommend one of several less invasive procedures. For example, your surgeon might suggest a catheterization, in which he unblocks your clogged arteries and insert a stent. A stent is a small tube that is meant to keep the arteries clear. By entering through the arteries in your limbs, the surgeon is able to complete this procedure without opening your abdomen or chest. Other less invasive procedures include a valvuloplasty and an endoluminal graft.

Medication and Diet

There are many medications that you may have to take when diagnosed with a heart disease. They will help manage and improve your condition as time passes. This medication might include aspirin because it thins the blood so it flows more readily and easily through the arteries. Cholesterol medication will prevent your arteries from becoming clogged with plaque; beta blockers will keep your blood pressure low; and ACE inhibitors prevent the production of the substance that narrows the arteries in your body. As for your diet, your new doctor will prescribe a strict eating plan of healthy foods and plenty of exercise. Medication for patients with heart disease can be found all over the world, in some of the best cardiac hospitals outside the U.S. With cheaper medication, you'll have more incentive to enjoy life despite the fact that you have this serious illness.

Long-term Medical Care

The nature of heart disease makes it very urgent; the sooner you get to your five-star international hospital, the sooner you can recover and go home with a clean bill of health, or at least with a stabilized and manageable condition. It takes a long time to recover from surgeries of this type, so it's best to count on staying a few months in your chosen destination. You will also need constant medical care as you are nursed back to health.

Duration of Stay: Most open-heart surgeries take around six to eight weeks for recovery but you won't be able to travel until after four months so count on an extended medical vacation.

Hospital Showcase:
Medi-Clinic Heart Hospital, South Africa

This private hospital specializes in the treatment of heart conditions and disease. As a world-class center situated in the country where the first heart transplant was accomplished in 1967, the Medi-Clinic Heart Hospital is one of the best. With high care, an ICU, and medical and surgical units, you'll find all the quality treatment you could ever want for your heart.

Kidney Disease

In 2008, there were over 77,000 Americans waiting to receive a kidney transplant because their kidneys had failed. Kidney disease is a term used for any serious disease that affects the kidneys. All of them are life-threatening, chronic illnesses that are difficult to live with – and often result in kidney failure. The kidneys are vital to bodily function, as they remove waste products and help to balance vital nutrients in your blood. When you develop kidney disease in any form, your kidneys either slow down or stop cleansing your blood, and waste begins to accumulate in your body. Kidney disease is often the result of other chronic conditions like heart disease or diabetes. This makes patients even more unstable as the families juggle health problems and mounting medical bills. If you develop kidney disease, you need to get to a specialist treatment center as soon as possible, where you can remain on dialysis and experience the level of care that you need to survive.

Main Variants of Kidney Disease

Renal Tubular Acidosis (RTA): Acid buildup in the blood excreted from a kidney, caused by an improper metabolic acid balance. This is a precursor for bigger kidney problems on the way.

Polycystic Kidney Disease: A disease that causes cysts to grow on the kidneys. This could lead to kidney failure as the cysts grow. One in every 453 Americans will develop cysts on their kidneys.

Alport Syndrome: A hereditary condition that causes renal failure, similar to an auto-immune disease. About 5,000 Americans are living with this disease.

Kidney Reflux: Also known as renal nephropathy; urine flows into the kidney, causing it damage. Left untreated, this causes urinary problems and potential further kidney issues.

Chronic Renal Insufficiency: A chronic lack of renal activity that results in eventual kidney failure.

Treatment Options

Surgery

Kidney diseases can be life-threatening, so if you are fortunate enough to be appropriate for surgery to correct or remove the problem, that's exactly what you should do. There are a number of surgeries that can save your kidneys from complete failure or further damage. For example, surgery can unblock a part of your urinary tract that has become clogged with a kidney stone.[183] That stone needs to be removed immediately or it could severely damage your urinary tract. Cyst removal is the same concept – taking the dangerous, bleeding growth away in order to save the kidney. There are also a few less invasive procedures that you can consider for many kidney disease problems. Speak to your doctor about your surgical options, and you might be able to save yourself the pain and recovery time associated with open surgery.

Dialysis and Transplantation

When you have experienced kidney failure, you will be put on a dialysis machine until you find a pair of donor kidneys, if you opt for the transplant.[184] A dialysis machine is a machine that controls and cleans your blood, taking the place of your renal system. There are two main kinds of dialysis: peritoneal dialysis and hemodialysis. When you are hooked up to a dialysis machine, you have to be very careful about infection and the foods you eat. A kidney transplant is a big surgery. New kidneys will be put in your abdomen and connected to an artery and a vein. They should then be able to create urine like your failed kidneys once did. Kidney transplants have a high success rate but you'll have to wait for a donor, which could take some time.

Kidney Medication

If your condition isn't far advanced, it can be managed with medication and a healthy lifestyle. Kidney disease is often the result of a pre-existing condition or another degenerative disease. Medication may be able to control your kidney disease or the underlying cause. Medications might include beta blockers for high blood pressure, diabetic medication or cancer treatment.

Long-term Medical Care

Kidney disease is very serious, and requires long-term support and medical care. If you have progressed to the point where you need to be put on dialysis to wait for a transplant, your best option is to look overseas. There's no point getting a new pair of kidneys in the U.S., and then having to sell everything you own to pay your exorbitant medical bills.

Duration of Stay: When traveling overseas for kidney disease treatment, expect to be there for a few months, especially if you are in the advanced stages of the disease. A transplant will keep you in the hospital and recovery center for at least eight weeks. With other surgeries, recovery time depends on whether you're having open or laparoscopic surgery. An average surgery will have you in and out of the country in under a month.

Hospital Showcase:
Fortis Kidney Institute, India

Part of the prestigious Harvard Medical International Hospital in the U.S., this hospital specializes in the treatment of kidney diseases. With research, the best modern technology and the latest medical breakthroughs, this team of doctors will support you through every step of your treatment – all the way back to wellness.

Chronic Respiratory Illness

Chronic respiratory illness is also known as chronic obstructive pulmonary disease (COPD). Any disease that obstructs the airways and causes labored breathing is called a chronic respiratory illness. This term encompasses diseases like asthma, emphysema and chronic bronchitis. According to the World Health Organization, more than 500 million people worldwide suffer from one of these health complications.[185] Chronic lower respiratory illness alone claimed 107,679 lives in 2006. You may develop one or more of these conditions, and they can't be cured – only managed. The worst part of chronic respiratory illness is that the symptoms become progressively worse and can prevent you from exercising, working or accomplishing simple tasks. Your health declines as you gain weight, and further medical problems arise. If you are diagnosed with this chronic illness, you need to get treatment as soon as possible or your lungs will be damaged beyond repair, and you might have to wait in line for a lung transplant. There are international hospitals that cater to foreign patients who are suffering from advanced COPD and other respiratory diseases. There, you will get the medical attention you need, without having to file for bankruptcy after repeated visits to your local hospital.

Main Variants of Chronic Respiratory Illness

Asthma: Recurring inflammation of the bronchi that causes the airways to narrow. In America, 63% of parents who both have asthma will pass it on to their kids.

Pulmonary Arterial Hypertension: High blood pressure in the pulmonary artery that leads to a damaged lung. Three hundred cases of this condition are reported in the U.S. each year.

Emphysema: A lung disease that accumulates air in the alveoli and causes them to rupture or become enlarged. Eventually, this prevents the patient from being able to breathe independently. Over 2 million Americans suffer from this disease.

Chronic Bronchitis: A cough that doesn't go away after 3 months, and that brings up sputum. This is caused by inflammation of the airways, and can lead to emphysema – and eventually lung failure. Each year, over 12.2 million Americans contract chronic bronchitis.

Treatment Options

Medication

You will need medication to treat your lung disease, depending on the symptoms you're experiencing.[186] If you are in the advanced stages of one of these diseases, you will be given a bronchodilator to use when you're at the hospital. You can also get one for your home, but they are expensive. Filled with anticholinergic agents that will relax the muscles in your lungs, this breathing machine helps you enjoy a better quality of life. You will be put on a strong course of antibiotics to kill all infection, and given medication to loosen your sputum and ease your pain. The most common anti-inflammatory drugs are called corticosteroids, and are used after surgery. Stick to your medication and it could improve your chances of avoiding surgery altogether.

Surgery

After going through a large battery of tests, you may be told that surgery is your best option for treating your severe lung disease.[187] Surgeries to treat emphysema include lung volume reduction surgery (LVRS), which removes parts of the damaged tissue in your lungs. For less invasive surgery, your surgeon may install bronchial stents to improve the function of your lungs. For the worst kinds of lung disease, you might have to endure a lung transplant or a lung resection. The resection removes one lung or parts of your lung in order to heal diseases like cancer and emphysema or other advanced lung disease.

Long-term Medical Care

If you have been diagnosed with a respiratory illness, then you need to seek professional medical help from a specialist. Many types of lung disease require constant medication, treatment and repeated surgeries. Treatment for lung disease can be either supportive or intensive. In either case, flying abroad to a treatment center is the best option because it won't cost you a fortune – and you'll get the world's best lung specialists working on bringing you back to health.

Duration of Stay: This depends on the extent of your disease and the treatment you need. After a lung transplant, expect to stay in the country of your choice for around six months while you heal properly and get the support you require.

> **Hospital Showcase:**
> **The Beijing Anzhen Hospital,**
> **including the Beijing Institute of Heart,**
> **Lung and Blood Vessel Diseases, China**
> This advanced medical treatment facility has a department dedicated to respiratory health. Fully equipped with a lung function, blood gas and bronchoscope laboratory, this is the ideal location for patients dealing with any stage of lung disease.

Obesity

Did you know that 66% of Americans are obese? Obesity is the leading cause of a multitude of chronic conditions. The National Institutes of Health define obesity as being more than 30 pounds overweight. Obesity in America affects people of all ages, with 25% of children already suffering from this condition. Most people who are obese don't have to undergo a body mass index test to realize that their weight is causing medical problems. If you are so overweight that are you medically classified as obese, you don't exercise enough or eat the right healthy foods. Obesity is caused by a combination of genetic factors and bad lifestyle choices, and is the precursor for a lifetime of serious conditions. Obese people can develop diabetes, cancer, heart disease and gall bladder disease. Morbid obesity is a medical term that describes someone who is so overweight that the body isn't able to function normally anymore. If you or a loved one is obese or morbidly so, you need to seek medical attention before you develop these life-threatening illnesses. If you already have one or more of these chronic conditions, then traveling overseas for medical care will help you to manage both your weight and the conditions caused by your weight.

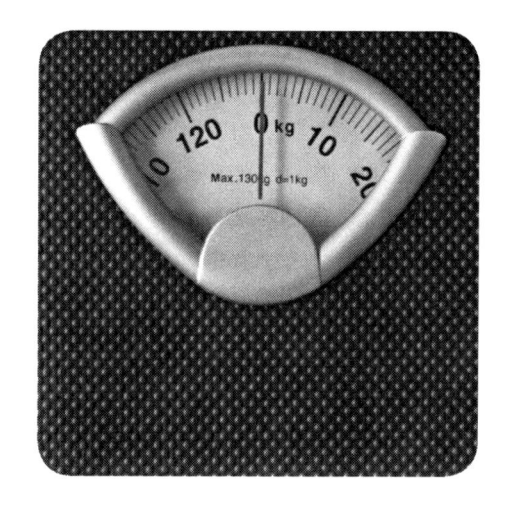

Main Diseases Linked to Obesity

Stroke: When an artery to the brain becomes blocked, the supply of oxygen is cut off, which results in the death of brain cells.

High Blood Pressure: A buildup of pressure in the arteries that can affect the vital organs of your body, resulting in death.

Gallstones: Bile that has crystallized to form a "stone" that can cause damage to the gall bladder.

Sleep Apnea: Your breathing is repeatedly interrupted during sleep, causing poor sleep and fatigue.

Heart Failure: When the heart becomes unable to keep up with the demands of the body, and oxygen supply to vital organs is cut off.
Cancer: A malignant growth of cells that spreads inside the body in a specific organ or location.
Pickwickian Syndrome: A combination of hypoventilation, red skin, drowsiness and twitching.

Treatment Options

A Lifestyle Change

If you are obese but you don't have any serious medical complications just yet, then your doctor should guide you through a lifestyle change. This will be a long-term plan, during which you progressively lose your excess weight. A rigorous exercise regime will be part of the treatment, as well as a daily menu of calorie-restricted foods. These lifestyle changes are important. Many surgeons will only give you surgical options if you are in serious medical need, or if you can prove you tried to lose weight and failed. If you need a structured plan, then visit a dietician – or give yourself a head start at an obesity center abroad that specializes in helping people lose weight.

Medications

In order to prevent illness, you might be given a course of medication that helps your body burn fat, prevents you from absorbing fat from food or makes you feel full after you've eaten a small amount.[188] Therapeutic counseling may also be in order if your obesity is connected to a psychological dependency on food. You can experience all of this at a spa-like weight control center abroad.

Gastric Bypass Surgery

If you can't lose the weight no matter how hard you try, and you are suffering from diabetes or heart disease, you could opt for a gastric bypass. This surgery effectively changes the way you digest food by limiting the amount of food you can consume. In addition, there are other forms of bariatric surgery that remove part of your stomach, so that you are forced to eat a little throughout the day. Either of these surgeries will achieve the desired result of helping you lose weight – and improving your health.

Long-term Medical Care

Because obesity has so many fatal medical side effects if left untreated, many people decide to travel abroad to obesity treatment centers. These centers teach these patients discipline and healthy lifestyles, and give them a good head-start on their weight loss journey. Enjoy long-term help from teams of dieticians, gastroenterologists, cardiologists and psychologists, who are all there for you.

Duration of Stay: If you want to attend an obesity center, you'll have to call ahead and ask them their individual program dates. A one-month stay focusing on lifestyle changes and exercise may be exactly what you need to get back to better health. Expect to be inactive for six weeks after any surgery – but during that time, you can learn all you need to know about staying thin. And you'll be enjoying a beautiful vacation.

Hospital Showcase:
365MC Obesity Clinic, Korea

If you are obese then you'll find friends at this center, where they deal with the issues of obesity on a daily basis. With first-class medical care, a range of weight reduction surgeries and supportive technologies to enhance your experience, this is the best place in Korea for obesity treatment.

Stem Cell Treatment

The controversial and hotly debated use of stem cell therapy is worth mentioning in this chapter, due to its revolutionary healing abilities.[189] A stem cell is a master cell that can grow into any other important cell in the body. Stem cell treatment enables a patient's body to repair "irreparably damaged" tissue, or simply re-grow it. Once introduced into a body, the stem cell begins to divide and replenish or replace damaged tissue. There are fundamentally two different types of stem cells: fetal stem cells and adult stem cells. Modern medicine is finding new uses for stem cells all the time. These cells are already used to treat disease; in the future, the possibilities might include being able to re-grow an organ, or at least fully regenerate diseased tissue. Stem cell treatments offer new hope to patients who have tried everything else and still suffer from the symptoms of their illnesses. These treatments have helped cancer patients, people needing bone marrow transplants and cerebral palsy patients. There are great stem cell treatment centers abroad, where you or a family member can receive cutting-edge treatments.

Main Diseases That Can Be Treated with Stem Cells:

Crohn's Disease: A disease in which the intestines become inflamed, negatively affecting the digestive system.

Hodgkin's Lymphoma: Lymphatic system cancer that damages your immune system.

Parkinson's Disease: A neurologic disease that gets progressively worse, causing tremors, muscle weakness, stiff facial features and slow muscular movements.

Osteoporosis: A disease causing the progressive reduction of bone mass because of a reduction in the body's calcium and bone protein levels.

Multiple Sclerosis: A central nervous system disease that causes problems with muscle coordination, bladder control, speech and vision.

Cancer Stem Cell Transplantation

Stem cell treatments for cancer patients make it possible for them to receive higher doses than normal of radiation and chemotherapy. The stem cells effectively replace the damaged bone marrow cells needed to carry oxygen and prevent infection. An autologous stem cell transplant involves the donation of your own cells that can then be put back after treatment. Allogenic stem cell treatment does the same but with another person's donor cells. The rarest form is the syngeneic stem cell transplant, in which the cells are harvested from a twin. All of these treatments work to keep your body healthy after cancer treatment.

Stem Cell Treatment You Can't Get in the U.S.

Overseas, you can get an injection of stem cells into a targeted area of your body that needs to regenerate. This treatment has been known to cure Parkinson's disease and a variety of other serious illnesses. President Obama has lifted the ban on stem cell research, but America won't see any advances in this area for years, if ever. Germany, on the other hand, has been working with stem cells since they were first found to have restorative properties. It's simply not true that all stem cells come from live embryos. They can be harvested from your own body, from blood, or from umbilical cord blood. The cells have even been found to slow the progression of irreparable conditions like Alzheimer's disease.

Long-term Medical Care

Stem cell therapy can occur once or multiple times, depending on the severity of the disease you are trying to treat. Expect to stay in your host country for at least two weeks when you receive the transplant. Recovery time is minimal: you'll be up and around in a day or two.
Duration of Stay: Between one and two weeks, depending on your condition.

> **Hospital Showcase:**
> **Emcell Clinic, Ukraine**
> This stem cell transplant and treatment clinic has served over 6,000 patients in urgent need of medical care. Having conducted some of the most advanced research and development in the world on stem cells, this clinic is the global leader for all of your stem cell needs.

Mental Illness

More than 57.7 million Americans suffer from some form of mental illness. As an often underappreciated medical condition, mental illness has plagued U.S. society for a very long time.[190] For example, a high percentage of emergency room admissions involve people with mental illness who have tried to commit suicide or who have hurt others. Mental illness is a banner term for all disorders and conditions affecting your mind. This includes instability in behavior, thinking and mood. There are certain types of chronic mental illness that completely debilitate the patient and prevent him or her from leading a normal life. Just like physical diseases, disorders affecting the mind can have a huge impact both on patients who have been diagnosed with the illness and on their families. The most common mental illness is depression, which in turn can cause additional mental illnesses such as eating disorders, masochism and phobias.

Getting treatment for mental illness in the U.S. is very expensive, and patients often have to visit their psychiatrists twice a week or more. Even if insurance covers some of the financial burden, the remaining bills can still be astronomical. Finding a mental illness treatment center abroad is a great way to ensure that you can work your way back to mental health.

Main Variants of Mental Illness

Impulse Control Disorders: An inability to resist acting on impulses that often leads to destructive behaviors. Gambling obsession is an impulse control problem that 2.5 million Americans live with every day.

Anxiety Disorders: This general term encompasses things like phobias: the patient overreacts to certain stimuli, causing mental and physical symptoms. Around 5.3 million Americans have social phobias, 3.2 million have agoraphobia and 6.3 million have a variety of other phobias.

Psychotic Disorders: Unusual, skewed or distorted thoughts that cause the patient to experience visual and auditory hallucinations, and to perceive imagined things. Nearly 2.2 million Americans suffer from schizophrenia, one of the psychotic disorders.

Mood Disorders: Unstable moods that swing to extremes, either very happy or completely depressed. As an example, roughly 5.7 million Americans are affected by bipolar disorder.

Personality Disorders: Strange fixed personality traits that cause patients problems in their daily lives, and which force them to have thought patterns outside of the normal realm of perception. Nearly 2% of adults are said to have borderline personality disorder.

Eating Disorders: Emotional involvement with food to such an extent that it causes the patient's life to be ruled by impulse, fear and a distorted attitude about normal eating patterns. About 20% of all Americans with eating disorders die of complications related to the disorder.

Treatment Options

Medication and Behavioral Therapy

Most mental illnesses can be managed with a combination of drugs and intensive cognitive behavioral therapy. The medication that you take depends on your specific illness and how bad it is.[191] The same pill may be given to two patients with the same disorder, but one may take a higher dosage because he or she experiences worse symptoms than the other patient. Medication does not cure the chronic illness, but it suppresses the symptoms. These medications can include anti-depressants, mood stabilizers, antipsychotic medication and sedatives to relieve anxiety. Finding the right psychotherapist can be difficult, especially when the patient or family member does not want to be involved in treatment of the illness. Mental illness centers abroad will help you understand your disease and will teach you how to cope with it, with or without medication.

Electroconvulsive Therapy
This harsh but sometimes necessary procedure causes temporary seizures as electrical currents are passed through the patient's brain. The goal of such drastic therapy is to alter the brain's natural chemistry, and to therefore reduce or eliminate the symptoms of mental illness. This is a preferred method of therapy only when a patient does not respond well to medication and is difficult to treat via psychotherapy.

Hospitalization
Patients with mental illness often degenerate and pose an immediate threat to themselves and to other people. They become suicidal or disassociated, or can no longer think clearly about the consequences of their actions. When it reaches this point, hospitalization will keep them safe and will provide a secure environment for their recovery, both mentally and physically. There are great mental health institutions abroad that are more like five-star hotels than treatment centers.

Long-term Medical Care

When flying abroad for mental health treatment, the timeframe can vary depending on the reason for going and the extent of the illness. If you are looking for a top-quality mental health facility, you'll find them all over the place. Patients can be rehabilitated and then released when they have worked through the program.

Duration of Stay: Varies widely. Some people go for cheap medication and two months of psychotherapy, while others are admitted into mental health institutions for many months.

> **Hospital Showcase:**
> **Life Path Health Group, South Africa**
> This HASA-accredited group of mental health clinics offers highly specialized treatment programs. Patients are assessed and then referred to the clinic that will best suit them. These clinics promise peace of mind and dignity to all of their patients as they help them recover.

Addiction

Addiction in all its forms affects millions of people in America, disrupting families and causing an emotional drain on everyone involved in the addict's life.[192] Did you know that one in every eight Americans has a drug or alcohol problem? Substance abuse has been said to cost America $250 billion each year. Addiction is a chronic disease that needs to be handled by either a medical care center or a rehabilitation center. Both are very costly, and many Americans simply can't afford it. So life goes on, and the addiction continues – leading to additional health problems like kidney failure, heart attacks and mental illness. Addiction is an epidemic that manifests itself in various forms. Drug and alcohol abuse are the two most common, with gambling and sexual addictions not far behind. People who are caught up in addiction need to seek medical help or rehabilitation in some form. There are many rehab centers abroad that cater to international patients who are fighting addictions.

Main Variants of Addiction

Drug and Alcohol Abuse: A physical and mental dependency on drugs or alcohol. It's estimated that over 4 million women in the U.S. currently need treatment for drug abuse.

Gambling Addiction: An inability to stop gambling or a strong compulsion to gamble.

Sexual Addiction: An intimacy disorder that causes obsessive thoughts about sexual activity and can lead to compulsive sexual acts. Nearly 5% of the U.S. population suffers from sexual addiction.

Treatment Options

Counseling or Group Therapy

One of the healthiest ways to recover from addiction is to become accountable for your actions. This is why people join groups like Alcoholics Anonymous or Gamblers Anonymous. Sometimes, making the decision to quit and to join a support group is all that is needed for an addict to fully recover from the illness.

Rehabilitation

Alcohol and drug abuse, the two most common forms of addiction, are usually treated in rehabilitation centers. These centers offer detox facilities to help the patient recover from physical dependence, and then provide support in the form of one-on-one and group counseling until the patient is ready to go home. Many of these centers also provide options for multiple dependencies.

Prescribed Medication

Giving an addict more drugs? Not exactly. Science has found a way to help addicts shake the addiction to drugs or alcohol by replacing these substances with harmless medical alternatives. Drugs like Suboxone are prescribed to help addicts get off Oxycontin or heroin. Because it's available over-the-counter, you can get it anywhere – for a price, of course. Many of these medications used for treating addiction, both prescribed and over-the-counter, can be bought in other countries for next to nothing. Taking a vacation to Brazil with your addict son, for example, would be a great time to buy these cheap alternatives and wean him off illicit drugs.

Long-term Medical Care

Rehabilitation for addiction usually takes about a month of intensive care. If you're going to go abroad for treatment, then make sure the facility is reputable and has a glowing track record.

Duration of Stay: One week to one month, depending on the treatment.

> **Hospital Showcase:**
> **Nova Vida Recovery Center, Portugal**
> This privately-owned luxury rehab center treats addictions of all kinds, and is small enough for the therapy to be personal and intensive. With four world-class doctors treating the patients, you are guaranteed better results than you would receive from a large rehabilitation center. Nestled in a stunning, secluded setting, this center will arrange your medical recovery trip for you.

Chronic Disease Care

If you have a chronic disease and you need affordable treatment abroad, there are exceptional treatment centers all around the globe at your disposal. For most chronic diseases, there are strict rules that you have to abide by in order to keep yourself as healthy as possible. Pay attention.

Prevent Illness

Make sure that if you are genetically predisposed to a specific chronic illness, you take the necessary steps to avoid contracting it. The hard truth is that most chronic diseases can be prevented if you live a healthy lifestyle.[193] Make the decision to become a healthier person – or call a medical care center abroad to discuss the many options available to you. There's no excuse for forgetting to prevent disease. Millions of Americans every year die from these diseases – and all one of them wished that they could go back in time and change the way they lived. There are health centers abroad that can teach you about being healthy, and teams of dieticians just waiting to turn you into a health nut.

Get Regular Diagnostic Testing

Any disease diagnosed early is a curable disease – that is the mantra you should live by. If regular preventative testing is too expensive in the U.S., plan a week away every year to an affordable location, and get a series of tests done there. Most diseases caught at an early stage can be treated with light medication or surgically removed. Don't be one of those people who ignore their chest pain and then get rushed to the hospital with advanced heart disease they didn't know they had.

Follow Your Doctor's Plan

Your international doctor knows a thing or two about chronic diseases, which is why he or she works at a hospital or treatment center that specializes in treating your disease. Listen to what your doctors, nurses, therapists and dieticians have to say, and follow their treatment plan to the letter. This effort could reduce surgery time and future complications. Most importantly, don't think for one second that you can't get better treatment overseas for your disease. The doctors abroad are highly qualified, highly compassionate people who care about your health –

even after you've paid them. Reject the new U.S. healthcare system and save your own life – by flying overseas for quality medical treatment.

Testimonials from Chronic Disease Patients

Name: Rand Loftness, WA

Condition: Wolff Parkinson White Syndrome
Treatment: Radiofrequency Ablation
Hospital: Apollo Hospital, Delhi
Medical Travel Agency: WorldMed Assist

RAND HAD LIVED HIS LIFE with a rare heart disease that caused the electrical impulses between his heart chambers to misfire. As he grew older, he could barely do anything without feeling weak, dizzy and exhausted. Desperate for a solution to this life-threatening problem, Rand went to the University of Washington looking for answers. To his dismay, he discovered that the recommended treatment would cost him over $70,000 – a gigantic price tag for such a small procedure. While Rand was a successful self-employed businessman, he still knew that this was far too much to pay for treatment. So, he turned to the Internet and found WorldMed Assist. After some discussion and searching, WorldMed found a hospital in India that would perform the radiofrequency ablation he needed for only $3,300. He arrived at the Apollo Hospital in Delhi with his friend Bill. He was released after three days in the hospital, and toured all around the country while waiting to attend his final two check-ups. His stay was excellent, and he has now returned to an active lifestyle.

Name: Dr. O, Oklahoma

Condition: Morbid Obesity; High Risk of Contracting Diabetes Mellitus
Treatment: Laparoscopic Adjustable Gastric Banding
Hospital: Accredited Hospital in India

Medical Travel Agency: Life Smile India

DR. O. IS A PRACTICING OPHTHALMOLOGIST. For years, he tried every diet plan and weight loss product, spending a significant amount of money in the process. He was making no progress with losing weight and keeping it off, and was in fact steadily gaining more weight for about 15 years. By his 54th birthday, he was morbidly obese on a 5'10" frame. He knew he needed to explore other possibilities for weight loss, especially as he had a very strong family history of diabetes mellitus. After thorough research for solutions, he chose laparoscopic adjustable gastric banding surgery and looked for locations overseas. India is known for highly skilled doctors and world-class medical facilities, providing reliable healthcare at an affordable cost –a mere fraction of the price tag in the U.S. He admits that, being a doctor himself, choosing an overseas destination for his own surgery was initially a difficult decision. But in December 2006, with excellent healthcare tour facilitation by Life Smile, he underwent a complication-free laparoscopic gastric banding procedure, performed at an accredited hospital by one of the most experienced laparoscopy surgeons in India. Dr. O. regards his obesity surgery as the best investment he ever made. He lost weight, and is healthier, happier, slimmer and younger. He's also saving money on diets that ultimately don't work, and on future treatments on the co-morbidities that would surely have developed with his obesity – diabetes mellitus, hypertension and heart disease. He was very happy with the staff at Life Smile India, who he described as efficient and caring. They booked his hotel, met him at the airport, arranged all of his hospital appointments, communicated with his doctors throughout and arranged sightseeing and shopping trips. They made a potentially scary trip extremely rewarding.

Price Chart

Average cost of **CANCER SURGERY**	U.S.	$15,000–$18,000
	India	$1,500–$3,000
	Mexico	$5,000–$6,000
	Thailand	$4,000–$5,000
Average cost of **CHEMOTHERAPY PROCEDURE**	U.S.	$15,000–$30,000
	India	$3,000–$6,000
	Mexico	$5,500–$9,000
	Thailand	$5,000–$10,000
Average cost of **RADIATION TREATMENT**	U.S.	$10,000–$15,000
	India	$3,000–$4,000
	Mexico	$7,500–$8,500
	Thailand	$7,000–$9,000
Average cost of **DIABETIC GASTRECTOMY**	U.S.	$30,000–$40,000
	Costa Rica	$12,000–$13,000
	Dubai	$10,000–$13,000
	Panama	$9,000–$11,000

Average cost of **PACEMAKER IMPLANT**	U.S.	$40,000–$50,000
	South Africa	$6,000–$10,000
	South Korea	$5,000–$6,000
	Thailand	$5,000–$7,000
Average cost of **HEART VALVE REPLACEMENT**	U.S.	$60,000–$80,000
	South Africa	$20,000–$25,000
	South Korea	$24,000–$26,000
	Thailand	$20,000–$25,000
Average cost of **ANGIOPLASTY WITH STENT**	U.S.	$45,000–$50,000
	South Africa	$7,000–$10,000
	South Korea	$8,000–$10,000
	Thailand	$7,000–$9,000
Average cost of **KIDNEY STONE SURGERY**	U.S.	$12,000–$15,000
	Costa Rica	$5,000–$7,000
	India	$3,000–$4,000
	Mexico	$4,000–$6,000

Average cost of **KIDNEY TRANSPLANT**	U.S.	$100,000–$120,000
	Costa Rica	$20,000–$30,000
	India	$19,000–$25,000
	Mexico	$20,000–$25,000
Average cost of **LUNG DISEASE TREATMENT**	U.S.	$30,000–$150,000
	China	$4,000–$5,000
	India	$2,000–$5,000
	Mexico	$5,000–$7,000
Average cost of **SURGICAL OBESITY TREATMENT**	U.S.	$55,000 -$65,000
	Mexico	$12,000–$15,000
	Panama	$16,000–$17,000
	South Korea	$16,000–$20,000
Average cost of **NON-SURGICAL OBESITY TREATMENT**	U.S.	$5,000–$10,000pm
	Mexico	$1,500–$3,000pm
	Panama	$2,500–$5,000pm
	South Korea	$1,000–$2,000pm

Average cost of **STEM CELL TREATMENT**	U.S.	Not Available
	China	$25,000–$45,000
	Germany	$5,000–$30,000
	Ukraine	$8,000–$25,000
Average cost of **MENTAL ILLNESS TREATMENT**	U.S.	$15,000–$25,000
	India	$2,000–$3,000
	Mexico	$1,200–$2,500
	South Africa	$2500–$3,000
Average cost of **ADDICTION TREATMENT**	U.S.	$30,000
	Mexico	$7,000
	Portugal	$8,000
	Russia	$5,000

୫ଠ • ୠଷ

CHAPTER 8

ಶು•ಲ

AFFORDABLE ALTERNATIVE MEDICINE ABROAD

Affordable Alternative Medicine Abroad

ℰ • ℛ

Alternative medicine has always been portrayed as an old form of medicine that can't possibly work as well as modern medicine does. But the fact remains that these natural forms of medicine have helped millions of people regain their health after terrible accidents, chronic disease and surgical treatments. Also known as complementary medicine as many patients worldwide like to use it in conjunction with modern medicine, natural healing could be the key to your full recovery. Alternative medicine includes herbal supplements, exercise and specialized techniques to help your body heal. These methods strengthen your immune system and the overall wellness of your internal systems, and have helped people beat cancer, recover speedily after transplant surgery and bring mental illness under control. Natural medicine is strong and should be treated with respect. Its side effects can be just as harsh as the effects of traditional chemical-based pharmaceuticals. You need to find a gentle balance between undergoing modern forms of treatment and encouraging a healthy body with alternative medicine and lifestyle changes. Keeping your body in top condition can often be the deciding factor between defeating or succumbing to your illness or injury. In this chapter, we explore the many different kinds of alternative treatments and how they can complement your modern medical procedures.

> **Natural medicine is strong and should be treated with respect**

Questions You Should Ask Your Doctor

Every modern physician has his or her own ideas about alternative medicine. Some think it's nothing more than a way to get healthier; others think it has the potential to succeed where pharmaceutical medicine and surgery have failed. Whatever ideas your local physician has, this age-old branch of medicine should not be ignored. Many have found pain relief from acupuncture, after all but giving up on pain medication; others have fully recovered from serious illness with the help of alternative treatments like Ayurvedic medicine and biofeedback therapy. Alternative medicine is as diverse as the kind of medicine practiced by licensed physicians; you simply need to find the right kind to complement your medical treatment. When shopping around for the right complementary therapy, there are certain questions that you should ask your international doctor. Doctors abroad are more inclined to see the beneficial effects of alternative medicine than American doctors, either because it is a part of their culture or because it has made an impact on the sick in their country. Here are few important questions you should ask when looking into a specific treatment.

> **Doctors abroad are more inclined to see the beneficial effects of alternative medicine than American doctors**

Which alternative treatments do you specialize in?

This may seem like an obvious question, because when you contact a specific doctor about alternative treatments you should already know that doctor's specialty. But asking this question can be helpful nevertheless. An alternative medicine practitioner will often choose one main treatment, and then complement that treatment with other forms of natural medicine. By asking doctors which treatments they specialize in, you are essentially asking them exactly what they can do to help your condition – with whatever medicines, treatments and therapies they have to offer. For example, an acupuncturist in China may also see fit to introduce you to Chinese herbal medicine, and perhaps an exercise form such as Tai Chi. The right combination of complementary treatments will improve your health far quicker than just one form.

Tell me about the process. How does it work?

Learning the process step-by-step over the phone or by email can help put your mind at ease before you travel. There are some alternative medical treatments that are uncomfortable or downright unpleasant. You need to decide which will be the best option for you. This question will also give you insight into the amount of time it takes to complete your complementary therapy. Some treatments might take a session or two; others might have to be repeated over the course of a few months. Either way, in order for it to work, you have to be prepared to stick it out until the end.

What benefits can I expect from this treatment?

Like modern medicine, some forms of alternative treatment can be intensive – so you have to know how you're going to benefit from it in the short and long terms. Your international doctor will be able to describe how the treatment will help with your illness. and will also be able to direct you to clinical studies, case studies or scientific research that serves to validate the therapy. It's important to know as much as you can about the treatment before embarking on your natural health journey. Some therapies work better than others – and some are useless, creating false hope. This happens most often with new "revolutionary" herbal drugs that claim to do things like cure cancer and AIDS when, in fact, they don't – and never will. Become a savvy natural medicine traveler by looking into each treatment yourself.

Will I be given herbal medicine, and if so, what are the side effects?

In a perfect world, "natural" would mean untouched by chemicals or toxins. But this is not always the case when dealing with herbal medicines. Many unscrupulous sellers of herbal products don't tell you that there are strong pharmaceuticals hidden within the natural-sounding supplements. Make sure that you know exactly what you're putting in your body, or you could be in for some serious side effects. Imagine that a patient has been put on extreme pain medication for a spinal injury, and then decides to start a course of "natural" medicine to help with healing. What happens if there are unlisted chemicals in the herbal supplements that interact badly with the pain medication? Most worries can be eliminated by making sure that your natural health practitioner is licensed and sells approved herbal medicines and supplements. If the products really are natural, then you won't suffer from any surprise side effects.

What kind of facilities do you have?

The mark of a practiced, successful alternative health practitioner is the private facility, with all of the latest technological bells and whistles to help with treatment endeavors. Many overseas treatment facilities also have accommodations on the premises, helping you relax and rejuvenate during your stay. It's a vacation with a purpose, in a five-star luxury facility that will ease you back to good health. As the staff at the facility brings your mind and body back into balance, you will be prepared to face the physical and mental demands of your illness. If you opt for a live-in establishment, they will prepare your meals for you and offer you a range of other pampering treatments, like hot rock therapy and massages. Make sure you compare at least three alternative treatment facilities, getting a better idea of cost, quality and schedule, before deciding on one.

How are you uniquely qualified to do these treatments?

A good alternative health practitioner will have many qualifications in everything from their specialist treatment to similar treatments to herbal medicine. Because of the popularity of complementary medicine these days, you have to be careful about the doctor you pick to perform these treatments. Write down each doctor's list of qualifications and research the details on the Internet. The Internet will tell you exactly how long someone had to study for such a qualification, and how relevant it is in the market. A three-week course is not much of a certification; but these days, doctors can choose to study branches of medicine like acupuncture and naturopathic medicine when getting their doctorate. Take this opportunity to ask for references from past clients. A great doctor will be only too pleased to accommodate you, and speaking with past clients will give you a better idea of the doctor's treatments as well as that former patient's general experience – information that can't be gleaned from e-mail or phone conversations with the actual doctor.

Have you treated anyone with my specific condition before?

If your doctor claims to be able to help you and yet admits to never having treated anyone with your condition before, that should set off warning bells. Just like every qualified medical practitioner, you want your natural health therapist to be experienced so he or she knows how to handle your illness. Speak to your international doctor about past success rates, and talk frankly about the results the treatment has achieved for other patients.

After these pertinent questions, you should have a clearer perspective on the doctor, the treatment and the facility you will be traveling to. Arm yourself with as much information as possible so you can ask more questions as they arise during your treatment. Walking blindly into alternative medical treatment is not an option. You need to know all the facts before setting out so you can come back healthy and ready to move on with your life. This is true for all patients flying abroad, whether for medical or complementary treatment. Both types of treatment are important – and can be used as a one-two punch to beat your illness or injury. Let's take a closer look at the various forms of alternative medical treatment, and how they can help you.

Alternative Cancer Treatments

There are many forms of alternative cancer treatment, and each has something unique to offer.[194] If you or a loved one has cancer, you realize how important it is for a patient to do everything possible to survive. People all over the world have discovered that one or more of the treatments listed below can be an invaluable accompaniment to modern cancer protocols. After surgery, chemotherapy and radiation therapy – where can you turn to find help when all else has failed? Take a look at these modern naturalistic cancer treatments.

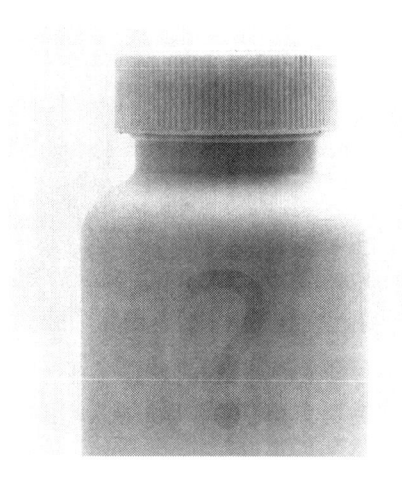

Immunotherapy

Immunotherapy strengthens the weakened immune system of the patient; and, as a result, the body's natural resistance to cancer grows stronger. There are two main types of immunotherapy – Immuno-Augmentative Therapy (IAT), and Issels Whole Body Immunotherapy.

Immuno-Augmentative Therapy

This therapy includes mixing protein with blood and then injecting this antitumor concoction into the cancer patient's bloodstream on a daily basis. This is not a cure for cancer, though specialists claim that it can cause the disease to go into remission by strengthening the immune system. Though there is no clinical evidence that this method works, it remains one of the most popular – and controversial – alternative cancer treatments.

Issels Whole-Body Immunotherapy

This alternative cancer treatment uses cancer vaccine protocols, stimulating the body's natural immune system to kill cancer cells in the patient's body. People often turn to Issels for results when all other treatments have failed. Thousands of patients in advanced stages of cancer have been restored to good health with this treatment.

Nutritional Therapies

Nutritional therapy treats cancer based on nutrients introduced into the body through the right diet. This kind of therapy has been known to help cancer patients recover from surgery or chemotherapy faster than usual, which contributes to their overall wellness.

Macrobiotic Nutrition

This form of cancer treatment uses specific combinations of food to increase life expectancy and maintain wellness, even during time periods of aggressive forms of modern treatment. There are many examples of people who have been cured of cancer who attribute it to their macrobiotic diet of vegetables, whole grains and fibrous foods.

Wheatgrass Therapy

Wheatgrass is full of chlorophyll, which stimulates blood production and in turn creates more room for oxygen to circulate in the blood. Wheatgrass therapy treats cancer by causing more oxygen to reach healthy cells. Wheatgrass also contains anticancer agents like selenium, which helps to combat the disease.

Adjunctive Therapies

An adjunctive therapy is literally a treatment used in conjunction with the primary therapy. In other words, it is an alternative medicine used to complement a modern medical treatment. These therapies include treatments such as hyperthermia and DMSO therapy.

Hyperthermia

The concept of hyperthermia cancer treatment is to modify the body's cells through heat exposure.[195] This change in cellular structure makes the cells more susceptible to radiation and chemotherapy. There has been documented success with treating targeted areas of the body to reduce tumors and otherwise aid in the primary treatments.

DMSO therapy

DMSO, or dimethylsulfoxide, works by binding to your chemotherapy drugs then forcing the cancer cells to absorb the drugs, thereby making the chemo drugs more potent. It is an effective way of making the chemotherapy drugs target cancer cells instead of the normal cells in your body.

Biological Therapies

Biological therapy works to boost your immune system. It helps reduce the effects of the damaging chemotherapy medication and can prepare your body to fight the disease. It has also been known to prevent the spread of cancer, and to slow the growth of already existing cancer cells.

Revici Therapy

Revici works as an alternative form of chemotherapy: instead of using chemicals, Revici uses lipids, sulfur, caffeine and lithium to kill cancer cells. The concept hinges on the theory that cancer forms as a result of a fat (or lipid) imbalance. Each Revici therapy is tailor-made for the patient once he or she has been analyzed.

Antineoplastons

Antineoplaston therapy uses chemicals called antineoplastons to defend the body from cancer. These chemicals build up your body's bio-defense systems and help prevent further growth of the disease. This treatment is taken intravenously or in pill form, and has been said to restore the body's natural ability to fend off disease.

> **Hospital Showcase:**
> **The Budwig Center, Spain**
> This state-of-the-art alternative cancer treatment facility boasts 30 years of experience, and can offer you thousands of testimonials to back up their reputation. They provide their patients with a variety of treatments, including hyperthermia, cleansing therapies, herbal medications and their "Budwig protocol," which claims a 90% success rate.

Homeopathy

Homeopathy is the practice of giving a patient a small amount of illness in order to invoke the body's natural healing system.[196] Homeopaths believe that the human body is stronger than modern medicine gives it credit for, and that with the right prompting, it can fix itself all on its own.

When your body manifests an illness in the form of symptoms, homeopaths believe that these symptoms are the body's way of kicking into action to fight off the problem. Homeopathy is also used to maintain health so healing doesn't become necessary.

Among the branches of alternative medicine, homeopathy has received the worst press, and yet it has a proven track record of helping people. In Cincinnati, a cholera outbreak in 1849 resulted in a death rate of 50% for those people treated by modern medicine; and yet those who went to homoeopaths for help recorded a survival rate of over 97%. There are medical doctors all over the world who refer their patients to homeopathy practitioners, or prescribe remedies themselves. In countries like India, Germany, Australia and Argentina, this branch of medicine is held in high regard, with around 42% of all doctors saying they would use homeopathic medicine.

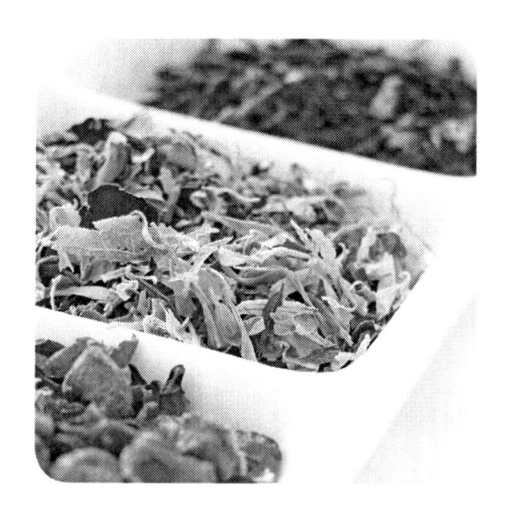

Classical Medicine

Homeopathic remedies in this group match a patient's symptoms to an image. The patient will need to go in for a consultation and speak extensively about his or her symptoms. The homeopath will then prescribe a remedy based on the condition diagnosed. Most homeopathic medicines are classic in nature, which means that they are from a single ingredient. They include remedies like Arnica Montana and hawthorn.

Constitutional Medicine

Homeopaths take into account how patients react to certain medication, what age they are – even their gender. Constitutional medicine is literally an observation of the surrounding factors that have caused the illness, and then matching that patient up to the appropriate cure. Because this is such a personal kind of medicine, the homeopath needs to know as much about the patient's mental and physical state as possible. Remedies usually include a combination of two or more substances to treat the overall health condition of the patient.

Polychrests

Polychrests are a type of constitutional medicine so easy to prescribe that they have been integrated into over-the-counter medicine. Archetypes are used to match symptoms with conditions, and then the diagnosis is made. Great examples of polychrest medicines are Ipecac, belladonna and aconite.

Allergodes, Nosodes and Sarcodes

An allergode is used to treat an allergy that flares up in the patient, while nosodes and sarcodes respectively deal with diseases and immunities. They have been called vaccines because they deliver a little of what the patient is allergic to or ill from, creating a natural immunity. Snake venoms, influenza and German measles are examples of illnesses treated with these medications.

Complex Medicine

A complex homeopathic medicine is created when a cure is mixed from different substances at different potencies to treat a certain condition. Their creation is dependent on the skill of the homeopath, and it takes a vast knowledge of natural medicine in order to achieve a good result. Most of these high-potency mixtures are only available overseas.

Homeopathy Abroad

Compared to modern medicine, homeopathy is inexpensive and effective. It is successfully administered all over the world in a variety of ways. Because it is based in nature, there are few or no side effects when taking this medication. It can be very beneficial for patients who are looking to regain some of their overall health or to fight an illness. Unlike traditional medicine, it builds the immune system up by using the body's natural healing processes. Homeopathic practitioners always try to find the best route from your current condition to health. Even if you have a severe illness like Parkinson's disease, there is something in the homeopath's arsenal of remedies that will help you. The most common remedies are for pain relief, stress reduction and energy enhancement.

> **Hospital Showcase:**
> **The Australian Homeopathic Society, Australia**
> Australia is home to some of the world's best homeopathy centers, where patients receive treatment for a host of various conditions, diseases and illnesses. Their mission at the Australian Homeopathic Society is to spread the word about the benefits of homeopathy, and to help people who suffer with health issues find natural cures for their conditions. The Fountain Center in New South Wales is part of this association, and offers comprehensive natural healthcare solutions to their patients.

Chelation Therapy

Chelation therapy is best known for treating heart disease, but it is most commonly used as a method of treating mercury poisoning. The process usually involves binding metals in the body via an intravenous injection so they don't do any damage. EDTA versenate is the chemical used to treat mercury poisoning, while EDTA endrate has been said to be effective against diseases like heart disease, cancer, multiple sclerosis, schizophrenia and autism. The therapy works by cleaning out your clogged arteries, preventing heart attacks or stroke. The main component of plaque in your arteries is calcium, which is what the EDTA endrate binds to and removes. The chemical cleans out the system of the sufferer, thereby easing symptoms and improving his or her quality of life. This systematic treatment involves a series of visits to the doctor's office in order to get the injections. It may take up to 40 weeks for the treatment to be complete. Chelators also come in pill form but these aren't as effective as the injections. This means that if you're flying abroad to get chelation therapy, you may have to choose: go for up to ten months, or opt for the pill form.

The Controversy

Many people feel that chelation therapy was the reason they survived their advanced heart disease.[197] The question remains: why has this method of curing disease not been explored further? Why hasn't the FDA tested it in clinical trials? They say that it will be too expensive; but let's face it, if a miracle cure came along that had the potential to cure heart disease, a lot of medical professionals would be out of work. If this is your last option, and all other treatment has failed – then do it, on the off chance that it saves your life.

Hospital Showcase:
Advanced Medical Group, Mexico
With a comprehensive range of chelation therapies, this facility will provide you with the treatment you deserve at an affordable price.

Naturopathic Medicine

Naturopathic medicine is a system of healthcare that relies on prevention and natural therapies to relieve pain, disorder or disease. Many naturopaths don't believe in pharmaceutical medicine, or in the healing properties of herbal medicine. However, there are some licensed naturopaths that do prescribe medicines, whether they are from natural sources or chemicals. The foundations of this medical system are a healthy diet and physical treatments like acupuncture, heat therapy, and water and light therapy. Like homeopathy, this system treats the entire person – physical, mental and social. This is because they believe that disease or illness is not exclusively a physical concern, but also has to do with the patient's state of mind and lifestyle choices. A naturopath believes in the healing power of the human body, and that by removing features of a person's life that cause illness – like smoking, bad diet, excess weight and stress – they can cure any ailment. This branch of alternative medicine is very focused on completely removing any reason for your body to be sick – which often leads to major life changes. If you have a chronic disease and follow a naturopathic way of life, your symptoms could be greatly reduced or you could be cured altogether. There are seven subsections that make up naturopathic medicine.

Physical Medicine

This refers to treatments that affect the body. These procedures can include massage therapy, heat and light therapy and electric therapy. A physical need might prompt the naturopath to change your exercise regime, and to suggest that you undergo chiropractic muscle and bone manipulation.

Psychological Medicine

Naturopaths believe that the mind is a powerful tool, and that it can cause illness if left unchecked. As your "psychological medicine," you will be required to change your thoughts and patterns of behavior by engaging in counseling, hypnosis or anxiety management classes.

Light Surgery

Many naturopaths are qualified physicians, and can therefore operate on you if need be. They never do complex, specialist surgeries because they try to keep treatment as minimally invasive as possible. However, if a patient has a cyst on her ovary, the doctor may go in and remove it before it enlarges or becomes cancerous.

Nutrition

An important part of receiving naturopathic treatment is learning to change your eating habits. Your naturopathic doctor believes that the fuel you put in your body is equal to the effort you get out. What this means is, if you're not putting the right healthy food in your body, you can't expect it to function properly. The result of a poor diet is disease. Treating medical problems with the right diet is a great way to reduce side effects and return the patient to good health.

Homeopathic Medicine

Homeopathic medicine supports the naturopathic philosophy that natural cures are better than modern medical treatments. Homeopathy allows the naturopathic doctor to treat illness with natural substances, triggering the body's innate healing abilities. If a patient suffers from headaches, for example, she may be given an herbal supplement rather than a painkiller.

Botanical Medicine

Plants have been the source of all good medicines for thousands of years. A medicinal plant offers the user a chance to experience multiple benefits – not just one, as in modern chemical-based medicines. Plants are better for you than chemicals, and are not rejected by your body. Naturopaths use botanical medicine to heal, calm and even cure.

Naturopathic Obstetrics

Your naturopathic doctor will help you deliver your child the way nature intended. Combined with modern methods of monitoring the growing baby, naturopathic obstetrics focuses on strengthening the mother so that the birth goes well. If you're looking to travel abroad to have your baby naturally, a naturopathic doctor is your best choice.

> **If you're looking to travel abroad to have your baby naturally, a naturopathic doctor is your best choice**

Naturopaths also have a certain fondness for eastern medicine because the two traditions share many beliefs in how to keep a person healthy. You might find that your naturopathic doctor practices eastern medicine, and can offer you specialized services like acupressure and acupuncture.

> **Hospital Showcase:**
> **University Medical Center, Freiburg, Germany**
> There is an entire department dedicated to naturopathy in this top-quality hospital. They offer some of the most advanced naturopathic therapies, and help patients work through conditions such as tumors, infections, heart disease, psychological trauma and immune system failures. This highly trained group of medical doctors will help you change your life and teach you how to retain permanent health and wellness.

Ayurvedic Medicine

Ayurvedic medicine is an Indian discipline that uses lifestyle changes, natural treatments and a heavy focus on preventative medicine to overcome illness. There is a deeply traditional – even mystic – set of beliefs that accompany this healing art. Ayurvedic practitioners believe that all disease starts in the consciousness of the affected person. When this consciousness is overworked, stressed or pressured, it throws everything out of balance. Using a system of relaxation and meditation, they are able to significantly reduce their patients' risk of getting heart disease. Like naturopathy, Ayurvedic medicine involves a big lifestyle change, grounded in firm principles that have been built up over a period of five thousand years. There is an emphasis on spirituality, physical health and mental tranquility. Though herb-based, Ayurvedic medicine is quite potent and has been documented as a treatment for serious illnesses like cancer, diabetes and AIDS. The word Ayurvedic means life and knowledge. Vedic philosophy is tied to the belief that all people were created from one consciousness. As one of the world's oldest medical disciplines, it has stood the test of time and has helped hundreds of millions of people recover from illness. If you go to India for Ayurvedic treatment, these medical practitioners can remove all of your impurities so you can heal. Here are the three main body types involved with Ayurvedic medicine.

The Vata Type

Ayurvedic practitioners believe that the vata dosha encompasses the powerful elements of both air and ether. Your vata can be disrupted by late nights, extreme sorrow, and terror or overeating. People with this archetype are known to be susceptible to brain, cardiac and skin conditions.

The Pitta Type

As the vata encompasses air and ether, so this archetype encompasses fire and water. The parts of the body most prevalent in this type are the digestive system and hormones. If you have this constitution then you'll have issues with heart disease, tension and digestive conditions. An imbalance for this type could manifest itself in anger, heartburn and compulsive eating.

The Kapha Type

If you are categorized as a kapha archetype, then you rule over the elements of water and earth. If you are imbalanced, this means your immunity will fail and you might experience nausea. A consistently weak kapha means you might contract cancer, obesity or diabetes.

> **Hospital Showcase:**
> **Ayurveda Retreat, India**
> This stunning center doubles as a retreat for medical travelers looking for short- or long-term treatment. With a full range of treatments, including heart disease, diabetes, obesity, epilepsy and arthritis treatments, this top-quality Ayurveda facility is one of the best in the world.

Acupuncture

Acupuncture is the Eastern art of inserting tiny needles into a person's body to achieve a specific reaction. These reactions can be pain relief, calm, stress relief or healing. Acupuncture is one of those ancient branches of medicine that spread across the world because of its great reputation and physical results. There are different forms of acupuncture depending on the country you wish to visit for the treatment. Thailand, Korea, China and Japan each have their own unique way of performing acupuncture procedures. Unlike many of the other alternative medicine practices, acupuncture has been clinically proven to work on a variety of different ailments. Studies have shown that patients with intense back pain, arthritis, headaches and fibromyalgia, and those who need rehabilitation after a stroke, have all received positive results from acupuncture. The only problem is that there are still con men who claim to be qualified and treat people for money, without causing any improvements in their conditions. Be very careful when choosing an acupuncturist; a skilled practitioner can do wonders for your medical problems, while a fake will just relieve you of your money.

There is a philosophy – tied to the traditional use of Chinese acupuncture – that everyone has a life force that flows through them, and that disease arises when that life force becomes disrupted. Acupuncture is a way of realigning that life force, and once again creating a smooth steady flow of it throughout the body.

Chinese Acupuncture

Chinese acupuncture methods are deeply ingrained in their belief system. A practitioner of this method believes that there are specific channels that move through the body, where the chi (or energy) flows. Small, clean stainless steel needles are gently inserted into the skin at strategic places in order to relieve the blockage of chi – and as a result, the body can repair itself.

Japanese Acupuncture

Japanese acupuncture is more specific and touch-oriented. The Japanese practitioner will feel your body for inconsistencies, and then tell you what your problem or condition is. They will then proceed to find the ideal needle location, and will use a small tube to guide little needles to the exact point that needs treatment.

Korean Acupuncture

Korean acupuncture involves a combination of both Japanese and Chinese versions of the medical art. Your acupuncturist will diagnose your symptoms based on your physical condition, and then proceed to insert needles into your hands. They believe that your hand contains pathways to the rest of your body, where channels can then be opened.

Five-Element Acupuncture

This is the oldest form of acupuncture that is still used today. It involves the treatment of all aspects of the person – their body, spirit and mind. Practitioners of this form believe that the elements are directly related to one's emotions, and that these elements must be balanced in order to be healthy.[198] They assess every level of your physical and mental state, and then insert needles where they think they are required.

Auricular Acupuncture

This specialized form of acupuncture treats only the ear. Small needles are placed on specific parts of the outer ear, which is believed to send electrical impulses to the brain and from there to the part of the body that needs to be treated.

Trigger Point Acupuncture

An acupuncturist who uses trigger point therapy hones in on stiff or knotted muscles. They find the exact location from which all of the tightness originates and then probe the spot with thin needles.

> **Hospital Showcase:**
> **ACURA Acupuncture Clinic, Japan**
> One of the best Japanese-style acupuncture clinics in the country, this definitive center offers healing for many injuries, ailments and conditions. Staffed with fully trained acupuncture practitioners, ACURA provides a clean, comfortable and relaxing surrounding where you can enjoy the stimulating treatment in a luxury setting.

Hyperbaric Oxygen Therapy

Hyperbaric Oxygen Therapy involves treating diseases or conditions with pure oxygen, inhaled inside a secure chamber. Oxygen is needed to effectively circulate blood in the body. This kind of therapy improves blood circulation throughout your body, and as a result, provides your cells with a higher level of oxygen than normal. This oxygen is used to help wounds heal faster inside and outside of the body; it also treats burns, bone infections, gangrene infections and damage from radiation therapy. The procedure itself is completely painless; although, after sitting in a pressurized room, you may experience drowsiness and popping ears as they depressurize the area. This kind of therapy is great for people who have very poor circulatory systems or problems with clogged arteries and veins. As a highly proven alternative medicine, this treatment can help you recover from chemotherapy during cancer, and can significantly reduce your risk of having a heart attack or stroke. The entire procedure takes about half an hour to two hours, but you may want to return for repeat treatments until you're feeling better. This means that the minimum stay overseas will be about a week – more if you are having accompanying surgeries and procedures done while you're there. There are several different kinds of oxygen therapy available for the eager patient. The first is hyperbaric oxygen therapy, as we have discussed here. Let's take a look at a few more.

Oxygen Concentrators

An oxygen concentrator works by removing other gases from the air, thus providing a higher concentration of oxygen to the patient. It is a stationary system that can only be found in medical care centers or hospitals. The oxygen concentrator is used most often by patients who need to sleep in high-oxygen atmospheres. This oxygen system is administered via tubes that are placed in the nasal cavity of the patient. This therapy is good for patients with severe respiratory dysfunction, cancer or heart disease.

Compressed Oxygen Cylinders

This kind of oxygen is compressed and stored in a cylinder made out of aluminum. This is the portable solution to oxygen therapy as the oxygen can be moved to your home. The cylinders come in a variety of sizes, and fit onto carts (sold separately) so you always have access to oxygen. You can also get mini compressed oxygen cylinders that fit into a bag worn over your shoulder. The cylinders attach to a breathing or ventilator mask which you place over your mouth and nose, breathing in the oxygen. If they have access to oxygen therapy, people with chronic disease can lead fairly normal lives while having other treatments.

Liquid Oxygen Systems

Liquid oxygen systems can be stationary or portable. Oxygen is cooled and turned into liquid form, then stored in tanks. A patient can get these tanks refilled at the hospital. While this may be the most convenient access to oxygen for the patient, it can be expensive. Why not travel abroad, where you can stay in comfort and where simple health enhancers like this aren't expensive?

Multiplace Chamber

Hyperbaric Oxygen therapy can be done alone or in a multiplace chamber with other people. You are seated in a pressurized room with other patients and administered oxygen through a mask. Medical staff continuously monitors each patient until the time is up. If you are in intensive care and need this treatment, you will be wheeled down in your hospital bed to have it done.

> **Hospital Showcase:**
> **St. Augustine's Hyperbaric Medicine Centre, South Africa**
> This upscale care center offers single and multiplace use of their advanced hyperbaric treatment chambers. The center also has round-the-clock monitoring of patients who need constant attention due to advanced-stage lung disease or an equivalent. As a quality, inexpensive center, St. Augustine's should be your first choice for oxygen treatment.

Biofeedback Therapy

Biofeedback therapy is an effective and revolutionary way of changing one's thoughts patterns in order to achieve physical health. A person is hooked up to a biofeedback machine, and is then able to view what our thoughts and emotions do to our bodies via an external monitor. The biofeedback therapist helps the patient identify what causes his or her stress, and teaches methods for readjusting these stressors so that they don't threaten the patient's digestive system, heart health or mental functioning. The biofeedback machine can read everything from your muscle tension to your sweat production, your temperature and your heart rate. This is an empowering therapy, as it allows patients to control the way they use their internal muscles like the heart. Being aware of how frustrated you are, and what frustration does to your heart, will teach you to slow it down when need be. This gives you greater power over your body and health. This therapy is used to treat such disparate conditions as addiction, epilepsy, incontinence and muscle spasms. When undergoing biofeedback therapy, you will be privy to data from your muscles, brain waves, blood flow, heart rate and respiratory system. Learning how to control the inner workings of your body, and how to change your automatic nervous system into a manual system, is the key to reducing many dangerous symptoms of disease and disorder.

Electromyography (EMG)

An EMG is used to give the patient information about his or her muscle activity. Special sensors or electrodes are placed at specific locations on the patient's skin around the muscle, so that readings can be taken about it. If a patient goes for enough treatment, it often results in their ability to ease muscle tension at will, significantly reducing the amount of stress on the body and preventing spasms, cramps and headaches.

Thermal Biofeedback

Thermal biofeedback is used to provide you with information about your body temperature. This is a great way to learn stress control; you will have your blood flow monitored, and learn when your blood vessels constrict and dilate – thereby causing stress on the body. Eventually, you will be able to detect the signs of stress and to actively increase or decrease your body temperature.

Electroencephalography (EEG)

Also known as neurofeedback, this therapy is used to provide the patient with information about his or her brain wave function. Specialized sensors are attached to the scalp in order to analyze the electrical impulses that the brain is emitting. This treatment results in the patient becoming more aware of brain activity, and in learning how to keep the brain functioning at an optimum frequency. This can help autistic people and those with behavioral problems.

Finger Pulse Measurements

Finger pulse measurements are used to give you information about your heart rate. Your finger goes into a small finger pulse oximeter, which then displays what your current heart rate is on the adjoining machine. Through a series of tests, you will learn to monitor your heart rate and to keep your blood pressure as low as possible.

Respiration Biofeedback

Respiration biofeedback can provide you with information on your breathing cycles. This training system makes you aware of when your breathing becomes rapid or uneven, and can teach you how to prevent problems such as hyperventilation and asthma attacks.

> **Hospital Showcase:**
> **Cyfeed Biofeedback Center, Greece**
> This center is one of the most advanced in the world. Its medical team has more than 25 years of experience in working with biofeedback technology. They are experts, and travel the world giving lectures about the benefits of biofeedback and how these treatments can help people rid themselves of life-threatening problems. Fully equipped for all forms of biofeedback, this center will help you discover exactly how your body works.

Spa Retreats

If health and wellness is connected to your physical and mental state, then it stands to reason that a spa retreat can have enormously beneficial effects on your body – especially if your body is in a diseased or unhealthy condition. Spas have evolved to become more than just nail and massage parlors. These days, you are in for the full experience with a range of healthy procedures that you can do for yourself, and even a private dietician to ensure that you eat well while you're there. Spas are designed to improve your health by stimulating your muscles with massage, giving you hydrotherapy baths and providing specialized supplements with every planned meal. These five-star luxury spas outside of the U.S. have grown in fame, known as popular destinations for medical tourists. They are so affordable and luxurious in certain parts of the world that cancer patients choose to stay there for months, rather than at the hospital down the road. The most common spa treatments include manicures and pedicures, facials, deep cleansing scrubs, body wraps, hot rock massages and reflexology treatment. These lush spa retreats offer their guests classes in everything from Tai Chi to Yoga. There are many specialty spas abroad that cater to the medical tourist. These health spas have full teams of medical physicians, nutritionists and psychologists to cater to your every whim. If you are flying abroad for a fairly small procedure and a nice two-week vacation, then a spa doctor will perform the procedure for you on location. It's just one of the many perks that come with going to a lavish health spa in another country. There are several different types of spa retreats available, so make sure you pick the one that suits your purposes.

Health Spa

The health spa will be your choice if you want to be looked after or pampered by people who want to make you a healthier person. The entire health spa lifestyle is about teaching you, the guest, how to live an extraordinarily healthy life. Here you will enjoy delicate foods made from the freshest, healthiest produce, and a range of relaxing therapeutic treatments will help you unwind and de-stress. The health spa was created specifically to pamper you while educating you on the healthy way to live. When you leave this luxury place, you'll be dying to go back the next chance you get.

Resort Spa

A resort spa is less about helping you maintain a healthy lifestyle and more about making you relax as much as possible. The food here will be richer, and you won't be required to attend health lectures or exercise classes. In fact, it's all about you – giving you a good time. If you need to recover after a hectic accident or a traumatic disease treatment, this is the place where you can take it easy all day long. There will also be sports facilities for the more active traveler as these spas are usually part of a large hotel chain.

Day Spa

If you're abroad for medical treatment and need a day of fun and pampering, why not look for a day spa in the area? From cozy, home-based spas to large, opulent facilities, these spas specialize in all the classics without having to settle in or stay overnight. Enjoy calm, peaceful ambiance with trickling waterfalls and freshly-brewed exotic teas. This is a great place to recover from a stressful cancer treatment or a pre-op checkup before a major surgery. It will steady your nerves and help you to clear your mind for a few hours.

Mineral Springs Spa

Have you ever felt the gentle healing properties of a fresh mineral spring? The world is full of mineral spring spas where you can unwind and experience the glorious properties of hot or cooling springs that will rejuvenate your body and mind. Soak in a geothermal spring and enjoy the healing benefits of the nutrient-rich water, which has been documented as a soothing treatment for a variety of illnesses and conditions.

Medical Spa

This is a superb spa for cosmetic surgery patients, where you can receive quality cosmetic treatments while basking in the glow of a tranquil atmosphere.[199] Medical spas offer everything from laser treatments to botox injections. They might even have an on-staff cosmetic surgeon who will perform your cosmetic surgery on location. These facilities are often immaculate due to the need for hygienic conditions in a medical environment. Imagine going to a spa for two weeks, getting a nose job, then spending the rest of your time in luxury. A medical tourism vacation doesn't get much better than this.

> **Hospital Showcase:**
> **SHA Wellness Clinic, Spain**
> Voted the best spa for medical travelers in 2010, this superb spa is a must-see for any traveler, medical or not. Even the WHO has touted this spa, set in the idyllic Spanish countryside, as a place that can return you to mental, physical and emotional wellness. Everything you need is right here, including treatment facilities for nutrition, psychology, smoking, sleeping and anti-aging.

Testimonial from an Alternative Medicine Patient

Name: AP, New York

Condition: General Chronic Illness
Treatment: Ayurvedic Medicine and Therapy
Hospital: Ayurveda Resort and Health Spa
Medical Travel Agency: Life Smile, India

THIS PATIENT ATTENDED THE WORLD FAMOUS Ayurveda Resort and Health Spa, set in the beautiful Himalayas, for two fulfilling weeks of treatment, relaxation and restoration. After treasured moments of peaceful Yoga classes and meditation in front of the holy river Ganges, and long, relaxing walks in stunning Indian forests on the Himalayan mountains, this patient found tranquility and a chance to recover from illness. Detox was administered through panch karma therapy and traditional Ayurvedic medicines by licensed doctors that eventually cured the patient's long-term illness. Special time was also spent at a gurukul (like a school), where AP observed and learned the teachings of an Indian guru. Life Smile organized the entire trip in three short weeks, then met the patient at the airport and arranged transportation to the spa in the scenic Himalayas. The entire experience was described as spiritual, breathtaking and exactly what the patient was looking for. After experiencing the best physical and mental rehabilitation possible, the patient plans to return to this holy place soon and recommends it to anyone seeking natural holistic treatment for disease and disorder!

Price Chart

Average cost of **DMSO THERAPY** (per course)	U.S.	$2,000–$6,000
	Costa Rica	$300–$1,000
	Mexico	$500–$1,200
	Panama	$400–$1,000
Average cost of **HOMEOPATHIC MEDICINE LIKE ST JOHNS WORT** (per 60 caps)	U.S.	$20
	Australia	$8
	Belize	$4
	Mexico	$6
Average cost of **CHELATION THERAPY** (per treatment)	U.S.	$150–$350
	China	$140–$180
	India	$115–$150
	Mexico	$50–$100
Average cost of **NATUROPATHIC TREATMENT** (per week)	U.S.	$300–$500
	Costa Rica	$80–$150
	India	$40–$100
	Mexico	$30–$100
Average cost of **AYURVEDIC MEDICINE**	U.S.	$100–$350
	India	$20–$50
	Mexico	$30–$70
	South Korea	$30–$100

Average cost of **ACUPUNCTURE**	U.S.	$150–$300
	China	$40–$80
	Japan	$40–$80
	Panama	$20–$60
Average cost of **HYPERBARIC OXYGEN THERAPY (x40)**	U.S.	$6,000–$10,000
	India	$3,000–$6,000
	Mexico	$1600–$2,000
	South Africa	$3,000–$4500
Average cost of **BIOFEEDBACK THERAPY** (per session)	U.S.	$100–$150
	India	$40–$60
	Mexico	$30–$50
Average Cost of **SPA RETREAT STAY** (for two weeks)	U.S.	$3,000–$8,000
	India	$500–$800
	Mexico	$800–$1,200
	Panama	$500–$700

CHAPTER 9

ಐ • ೧೩

EVERYTHING YOU NEED TO KNOW BEFORE YOU GO

Everything You Need to Know Before You Go

☙ • ❧

Traveling overseas for medical care requires planning, preparation and assistance in order to be successful. Without a proper plan in place, you could run out of money, end up in a hospital that isn't what you expected or have serious time delays that ruin your trip. Life is difficult to plan for, and there will always be certain factors beyond your control. The point here is to fully understand, research and formulate the parts of your trip that *are* in your control. Features of your trip like the length of stay could be thrown out of whack by post-surgery medical complications – and there's nothing much you can do to plan for something like that. What you can do is make sure that you research what could go wrong, what additional medical procedures you might need to correct the problem and how long it would take to recover.

> **That's what makes for a successful medical trip— planning for every eventuality before you go**

After you have done all of this research, you can calculate extra time into your trip and take along additional funds in case anything happens. That's what makes for a successful medical trip – planning for every eventuality before you go. This chapter will help you decide exactly what it is you need to do before, during and after your stay at your international hospital. It's a veritable "everything you need to know before you go."

Become a Successful Medical Traveler

There are a ton of medical tourism books and texts that share the same warning: you need to plan months in advance for your trip so that you have everything covered. We disagree completely. Ill health doesn't happen at convenient times in your life, and most people don't have months to spend wading through volumes of medical texts and speaking to dozens of doctors before they go. You need to become a savvy traveler – fast. Aside from elective surgeries than can wait awhile, and some holistic medicine treatments that can be put on hold, every other medical emergency or condition needs treatment as soon as possible. With the economic climate in America being what it is, and now being compounded by the disastrous new healthcare bill, Americans need medical solutions that can be arranged immediately. The entire purpose of this book is to make you aware that you always have an option to fly abroad, even if you are deathly ill or have had multiple surgeries in recent weeks. You can fight back against a failing system that drains your pocket and gives you substandard, limited medical care. The answer is medical tourism, of course – and we're going to show you how to become an expert at getting the medical services you need pronto.

> **You need to become a savvy traveler— fast**

Breaking through the Culture Clash

Every savvy medical traveler knows that there are people who don't "get" medical travel. This is because they have been programmed to believe that America has the best medical care – and that it always will, no matter what happens. They also believe that foreign countries have strange, untested or seedy medical practices that will put your life in danger. Obviously, this is nothing but pure nonsense. Many hospitals abroad are affiliated with U.S. hospital groups, and even more of them are held to higher standards than any hospital in America. There are parts of Europe, for example, where some hospitals are so advanced that even the best American hospitals can't compare. It's all about breaking through these cultural differences and seeing the truth beyond what you've been told to believe. The fact is that if your medical doctor in the U.S. talks you out of medical tourism – you're the one that will suffer. With such a personal decision, you really do need to find out the facts for yourself.

Medical Tourism Safety

Americans tend to believe that foreign countries are teeming with criminals waiting to kidnap, mug or kill them. This is ridiculous, of course. Countries like India, Malaysia, Hungary, South Korea, France and New Zealand have far lower crime rates than the U.S. does. Even in places where the crime rate is higher, there is such a small chance that anything would happen to you that we can say with 99% certainty that you're safe. If you still have concerns about going abroad, then take a travel partner with you. Not only is this a good idea when things go wrong, but it's always smart to have a travel companion whenever you fly overseas. To stay safe in your destination country, just remember to keep a low profile and stay in the decent parts of the city you're in.[200] Keep your money available in traveler's checks or in a bank account that you can access abroad. Being ill or injured can make people feel very vulnerable in other countries, but it doesn't increase your risk of becoming the victim of a crime. There is always a chance of crime reaching you, but the chances are no higher than if you were in

Keep your money available in traveler's checks or in a bank account that you can access abroad

perfect health on vacation in another country. The only thing you have to worry about is getting the best medical services possible.

JCI-approved Hospitals and Other Accreditations

During your search to find the perfect hospital, you will come across hospitals that claim to have accreditations and certifications from medical boards of authority. The safest way to ensure that your experience overseas meets your expectations is to fly to a JCI-approved hospital. The Joint Commission International only awards their accreditation if the hospital in question adheres to certain standards. The presence of this stamp of approval ensures that there is a level of care in the hospital that satisfies a stringent set of rules and practices. A hospital that has this accreditation wants you to know that they have quality standards in place. The entire process is voluntary; any international hospital can apply to be assessed. Also, individual countries have their own regulatory boards and accreditations. Other international and country accreditations include:

1. HA Accreditation – The Thailand Hospital Accreditation
2. ACHSI Accreditation – The Australian Council for Healthcare Standards International
3. The Egyptian Health Care Accreditation Organization
4. MSQH Accreditation – Malaysian Society for Quality in Health
5. The Japan Council for Quality in Healthcare
6. QHA Accreditation – Trent
7. The Irish Health Services Accreditation Board
8. ISQua Accreditation – The International Society for Quality in Healthcare
9. The Council for Health Services Accreditation of Southern Africa

Any one of these accreditations is a good sign that the hospital involved puts its patients first. When you're looking for a hospital, the first stage of elimination should be whether or not it is accredited. There is no reason for a major hospital to go without an accreditation if it has the level of services and medical care that it claims to have. Before you contact your potential hospital about a procedure, make sure that it's accredited by searching for it online.

Finance at the Ready

You're flying overseas for medical treatment – so you can't just pack your handy American Express credit card and get on with it. You need to plan your finances just as carefully as you plan the rest of your trip. After all, you don't want to be stuck in a foreign country, bedridden… and then run out of money. You must organize finances quickly, because your insurance isn't going to cover your trip.

So what are your options? Assuming that you've done your research and asked your international doctor the right questions about money, and received an email or fax detailing all of your costs, you can begin to arrange money for your trip. This all depends on your financial situation.

Scenario #1

You're an average American man who has three nearly maxed-out credit cards and a huge mortgage, and you need urgent treatment for prostate cancer. You have health insurance, but it's so limited that it won't cover any of the costs that you incur on your medical travels. Here are your options:

1. ***A Medical Loan from Your Bank*** – Assuming you're on fairly good terms with your bank, you can discuss your options for taking out a loan that will cover all of your medical expenses during your trip. If you are successful, they will create a tailored plan of repayment over the next few years.
2. ***A Second Mortgage*** – If you have a constant employment history and good credit, you could take out a small second mortgage on

your house to cover your expenses. This can be arranged through your bank or through a private company. Though you will pay higher interest rates on this loan than on your first mortgage, it may be your only option due to the urgent nature of your condition.

3. ***A Loan from a Private Medical Loans Company*** – If you can't get your bank to give you a loan and can't secure a second mortgage, you can try getting a loan through a private company. Most commercial lending companies will view the fact that you have prostate cancer as a medical emergency, and therefore as a viable reason to approve your loan.

4. ***Your International Hospital's Payment Plans*** – Many accredited hospitals abroad now offer their patients flexible payment options so they can tackle large expenses over a period of several months, or even years. Contact the finance office of your hospital and inquire about payment methods they offer to international patients.

Scenario #2

You're a young healthy woman who has never had or needed health insurance. You like to buy things, and this has left you with bad credit scores across the board. You were in a terrible accident and now your face is disfigured. You want to go overseas to have facial reconstructive surgery, but you don't have the money – and private loan companies don't care because they don't view your need as urgent or legitimate.

1. ***Approach a Private Cosmetic Surgery Loan Company*** – You can get financing through a private cosmetic medical loan company, and may get decent repayment options. Because you have bad credit, these loans will have a higher interest rate than others – but at least these companies approve loans based on real need.

2. ***Ask Someone to Co-sign for Your Bank Loan*** – If you still can't get a loan, ask someone close to you like a friend or family member

to co-sign for you so that you can get a bank loan. This means that person will put up assets and guarantee that you will repay the bank or that the other person will shoulder the costs for you if you can't. The point is not to let co-signer pay, but to have a way around being rejected as a result of bad credit.
3. ***Have a Family Member Get a Loan*** – If you are refused at the bank a second time, you'll have to get sneaky. Get someone in your family with good credit and a flawless reputation with the bank to take out a personal loan for you. Deposit the cash into your bank account and you're all set.

Informing Your Local Doctor

Don't make the mistake of thinking that you don't need an American doctor's assistance, because you will – either to obtain records, or for care when you get back from your trip. Make sure that your American doctor has agreed to collaborate with your international doctor on your medical care. It will make your life easier and give you the support base that you'll need when you return home. Plus, having two doctors gives you two ways to find out about your condition and how best to fix it. If your local doctor doesn't like the fact that he or she has to take a backseat to a doctor abroad, then find a new primary doctor. You can't afford to have an uncaring, bitter doctor in your corner when you most need the support.

Planning Your Medical Expedition Abroad

When it comes to planning your trip, speed is of the essence. You want to get the help you need, immediately.[201] Obviously, if you are waiting a few months to go, then you can take your time with this; but for those patients who require urgent medical care, there are several steps to make this work.

STEP 1: BEHOLD, FAST INFORMATION!

If you don't have the luxury of time on your side, there are efficient ways of finding the best doctors at the best hospitals. We do live in the age of information; and though much of that information is misleading, there are credible sources that you can count on for quick, accurate information for your trip.

The Internet

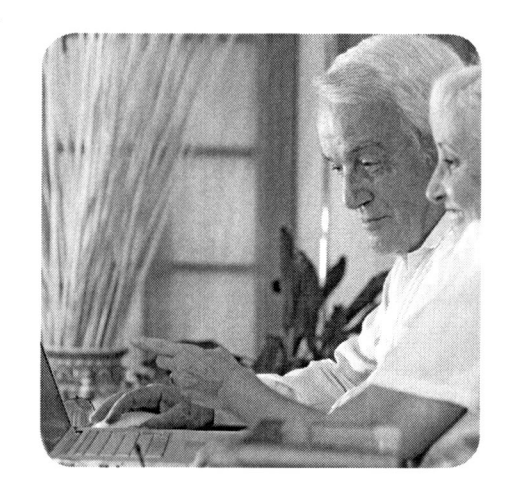

The Internet is a great tool for quickly identifying and contacting hospitals. You'll find that most hospitals have websites with a single email address for contacting general administration. Ask them if you can have the contact details of a doctor who specializes in your condition. Make it clear that you intend to travel to the hospital for the procedure or treatment, but that you need more information from the doctor. Title your email clearly, so that admin staff won't overlook it in their haste to get through requests and answer emails. This is very important. A good title would be "Patient needs more information on your hospital" or "Serious patient from U.S. seeks medical doctor at your hospital." If you title your email properly, then when they browse through their inbox in the middle of a busy day, they will click on your message first. It is part of the administrative department's duty to refer potential medical tourists to the appropriate doctors in their hospital. If you don't receive a reply from them within the next few days, send the same email again three times. Often, emails can be overlooked or lost because of the sheer number of emails that pour into the hospital's admin account daily. Be sure to include your telephone number in your email. You should get a reply email or a phone call from the hospital fairly soon after you send your message. If you don't, then you should scratch that hospital off your list of potential destinations. If they can't even answer a simple email, their service can't be reliable.

There are also some hospital websites that have telephone numbers on them. This is the most direct way of getting answers when searching for the right hospital. If the line is busy, don't give up. Try calling at different times during the day and take time zone differences into account. Your morning could be late night for the staff at the facility, in which case many doctors might be off or the phone might not be answered.

Of course, the Internet is also a great resource for general information about medical procedures and conditions, and for getting extra advice. Some of the best online medical resources are WebMD, MayoClinic, EMedicinehealth and Medicine.Net.

Networking

Thanks to the rise of social media, there are new and exciting ways to get in touch with people online. If you're hitting dead ends with your research and aren't sure which direction to go in, try searching for news articles that contain stories about people with your condition who have had successful surgery or treatment abroad. Once you've found a name, you can run it through the major search engines like Google or Bing. Most people in America have the access to Internet, and millions of them are on social network platforms like Facebook, Twitter and LinkedIn. If you find someone's Facebook page, for example, you can send a message and open a dialogue with a complete stranger about his or her experience abroad. This is a great way to pick up first-hand information from someone who has already been through the experience you're just starting. You can get wonderful insights into treatment, hospital facilities and doctor competency. You might be so impressed with what you learn that you decide to use the very same doctor for your treatment or procedure. One sterling first-hand account of a trip is worth a hundred anonymous text-based testimonials.

Testimonials

To get a better idea about the hospitals and doctors you need, try to locate testimonials on the Internet. These testimonials will often be published on medical tourism websites, but not all of them will be true. Make sure that if you find one particular interesting hospital or doctor, you search for negative testimonials about them as well. Nothing on the Internet is what it seems. If one website feels strongly enough to post thirty positive testimonials about a hospital (trying to sell their package deals), then there will be at least one person who experienced it for real and posted a factual account in opposition to the trumped-up medical tourism site accounts. At any rate, testimonials will give you a good idea about the attention the hospital gets from medical tourism sites. Not all exaggerated testimonials are bad, because the medical tourism websites that sell these package deals make money from those sales. This means they can't be that terrible, or people wouldn't use them.

> **Make sure that you search for negative testimonials as well**

Amazon.com

A word in print is worth a thousand online, as they say. Amazon.com is the quickest way to get researched material and information about hospitals and medical tourism delivered to your door. Delivery is fast and efficient, and one of these texts could happen to have the hospital you end up flying to in it. Just make sure that you choose current, up-to-date books or you'll be getting old, outdated information.

The Three Doctor Rule

To save time and get on the right track fast, use the three doctor rule. If you are investigating hospitals in a certain country, then choose three medical centers to call and speak to three doctors, one at each center. According to the law of averages, speaking to three doctors should give you a good impression of the medical services in that country. From there, you should quickly be able to decide which hospital is the best fit for you. If you choose more than three hospitals, you'll end up speaking to a ton of people and you could lose weeks doing this. The same concept applies when trying to select a doctor at your chosen facility. Try to get quickly to an appropriate doctor by briefly explaining yourself to other staff. Don't waste time by telling them your life story when you know they can't help you themselves. The three doctor rule helps American patients who are pressed for time discover the best hospital and doctor as fast as possible.

STEP 2: MAKING A QUICK GETAWAY

It's time to decide if all of this research is getting you anywhere. If it isn't, then you need to change your strategy and move on to a more efficient solution. That solution is the medical travel agent.

Wouldn't it be great to have insider knowledge on where to go and what to do, over and above everything contained in this book? If you need to make a quick getaway, then you have to contact a great medical travel agent. They are more than your average travel agents. They have excellent connections to overseas medical facilities, doctors and staff. If you're pinched for time, you want one of these professionals in your corner. Medical tourism agencies employ travel agents who specialize in the medical tourism industry. They know how to find you affordable medical care in a hurry – and they will literally plan your trip for you. From start to finish, you will have a complete, structured trip focused on your unique medical needs. They do everything from contacting your hospital to getting hold of your doctor, and they arrange things like checkups, flights, accommodations, transportation and finance. Make sure that the agency you decide to contact is a full-service agency, and not just a glorified travel agency that puts you in contact with their listed hospitals – disregarding your needs in favor of a fat commission. Some of these agencies will even gather your medical documents for you, and many have an agent in the country you are visiting who will greet you and take you through the process. Discuss what package deals you can get with your medical travel agent. There are often discounted packages, and you can get great tour packages after your treatment. Ask about these add-ons.

STEP 3: THE FINER POINTS OF TRAVEL

Either you or your medical travel agent will have to organize all the logistics of travel, so that you get the most for your money *and* the best medical treatment available.

Accommodations

International accommodations aren't difficult to find; in fact, you can get bogged down in the sheer number of options to choose from. In most countries, there are accommodations ranging from five-star luxury resorts to boutique guest houses, from medium-range hotels to cheap self-catering lodges. If you are going for an extended stay, then think about renting an apartment near your medical facility. Keep these four criteria in mind:

1. The cost of accommodations over time
2. The cost of on-site hospital accommodations
3. The transportation costs to and from the hospital
4. Your overall experience

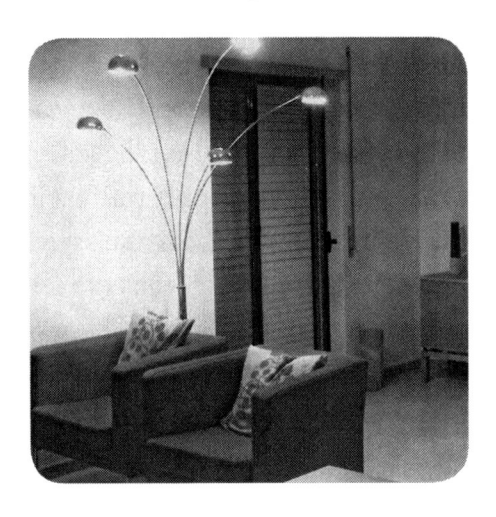

If you are a chronic disease patient, you may require a permanent bed at the hospital. In that case, find out how much it is going to cost your travel companion to stay in the hospital or at hotel accommodations during your treatment. Local travel agents can arrange some good deals for you close to the hospital, and they will know of less expensive accommodation options in the area. If you are recovering from serious surgery or heavy treatment, resort accommodations or recovery centers may be great options for you. Find out where the most comfortable, affordable recovery centers are in the area.

Flights

Flights are expensive. Flights that are booked for immediate departure are even more costly. That's why fewer people go on international vacations every year. But you have to look at this in context. If your medical need is urgent, then it's probably very expensive to treat – which is why you're flying overseas in the first place. In this case, a last-minute flight might cost more, but it still saves you a bucket-load of money in the long run. If you organize your trip through a travel agent, your flight costs will probably be cheaper.

Tours

Let's not forget that medical tourism is half tourism. The vacation portion of your stay can be whatever you want it to be. If you're jetting in for a nose job in India, you can take tours around the country or even hike in the Himalayas. It all depends on your level of health and your interest in the country. Choose from structured or un-structured tours, before your operation or after it. If your medical condition is too unpredictable, then you can always plan on the spot or make fluid plans. A spa resort vacation abroad is a fine option for injured or diseased patients who need a getaway but can't do anything too strenuous. A medical travel agent will know of the best tours to accompany your treatment, and can make all the necessary arrangements for you.

Transportation

Once you land in your destination country, you'll be completely dependent on the public transportation system or on the rental car that you organized beforehand. If you need emergency transportation services from the plane directly to the hospital, this can be arranged through the hospital or via your medical travel agent. If you are renting a vehicle, then research the price of fuel in the country and add it to your list of expenses. You can't predict how much gasoline you will use, but you can estimate. You'd always rather take too much money than too little.

STEP 4: YOUR SAFETY NET

On every trip, there are things that you forget to do that may come back later to haunt you. If you don't create a safety net for yourself, you could run into a lot of trouble. Take these important factors into account:

1. Sometimes things don't go as planned. Doctors get sick or can't do a planned surgery. Always make sure that you know other members

of the medical team involved in your surgery. If anything happens, it will be up to one of them to make you well again.

2. The best doctors in the world are in great demand. If you've chosen an extremely good doctor, that person may not be inclined to help you or have the time to consider your case. These professionals are very busy, all day, every day. If one turns you down, don't give up – he or she may have a colleague who is just as talented and half as busy.
3. The three doctor rule gives you a back-up plan in case you arrive at your researched hospital and things aren't as great as you hoped. Always have another doctor's number on hand – preferably one at a hospital close by. This simple preparation can save you a lot of trauma.
4. Sometimes saving money means settling for a good doctor with a fair reputation instead of a great doctor with a flawless one. If this is what the situation requires, don't despair. You can still get great medical treatment abroad, even if it's on a shoestring budget with no vacation time planned afterwards.

Time Delay Theory

The time delay theory is based on a formula. As long as you use this formula to calculate how much extra time you might have to spend abroad, you will have made the necessary preparations. The formula is: The estimated time for procedure/treatment (+ recovery) + worst-case complication procedure (+ recovery) = estimated worst case scenario stay.

> ***For example:*** tummy tuck = 1 day in the hospital (+ 2 weeks recovery) + infection 2 days in the hospital (+ 2 weeks recovery) = over a month for worst-case scenario.

If you had originally planned to be in the country for only two weeks and then this complication arises, you would be forced to stay unplanned for longer, incurring extra costs and missing work. If you prepared for a full month of travel instead, in order to cover for the worst-case scenario, then you are less likely to miss work or to run out of money.

Finance Calculation Theory
The finance calculation theory is the second part of your safety net system. It is based on your time delay theory, and ensures that you plan financially for any eventuality. The expenses in this case refer to food, accommodations and transportation. The calculation is: estimated procedure cost (+ recovery expenses) + worst-case complication costs (+ recovery expenses) = your basic worst-case scenario cost.

> *For example:* tummy tuck $2,700 (+ recovery $600) + infection $160 (+ recovery $600) = $4,060 amount needed for hospital stay and recovery in the worst-case scenario.

If you hadn't planned for this eventuality and you traveled in India before your tummy tuck, saving only the amount you're meant to pay, you would have been around $1,000 short. Make sure that you always travel prepared for the worst-case scenario – even though the "worst case" will rarely happen to you.

STEP 5: PREPARING YOURSELF

There are a few things that you need to organize from your side – and that will delay your trip if you don't have them on hand, or already complete.

Visas and Passports
To get into a foreign country, you'll need a visa and passport.[202] If you don't have a valid visa/passport, then prepare to wait a while after you

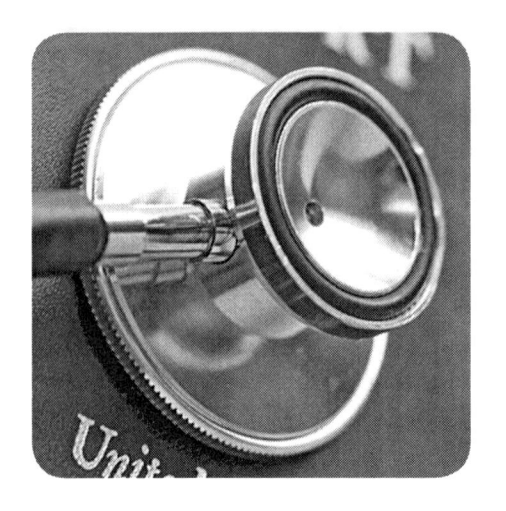

apply to receive one. Renewing your visa/passport costs about $75; the cost is a bit more than that if you have never had one and need it made from scratch. There are ways of getting your passport delivered to you faster than normal but it nearly doubles the price. If you are in a hurry, this might be a viable option. This is a great time to use your medical travel agent. They can get it done for you within one day if you are prepared to pay extra. After all, in America, it's not who you know – it's who you pay.

Travel Insurance

It's always a good idea to take out travel insurance for your trip. It will make it a bit less of a nightmare when your baggage gets stolen, or your plans fall through and you have to move the dates of your trip. Date changes are especially relevant to medical travelers, as you never know when your health might decline and leave you unable to travel. A fair rate for insurance is between 3-5%; when you're choosing an airline, make sure to check out their travel insurance rates as well.

Vaccinations

Requiring vaccination is the CDC's way of ensuring that you don't bring diseases back to America. It can also save you from getting even sicker than you were when you left the country. If you're heading off to Europe, Asia or Australia, then you really don't have to worry about contracting an illness. However, if you're going to India, Africa or the Middle East, these open terrains might present a problem. In this case, all you need to do is have your local doctor give you a shot or two to prevent diseases like malaria, hepatitis A and B, yellow fever and typhoid.

When You Arrive

Arriving at your destination country can be either an exhilarating experience or a significant source of worry for the new medical traveler. If you believe you might have anxiety, it's best to arrange your trip with a medical travel agent who will send someone to meet you at the airport. The agent will also arrange for that person to drive you to your accommodations to get you settled in. If you're traveling with a partner, you can pick up your rental car from the airport or use the local public transportation system. Once you've unpacked, or if you've gone directly to the hospital, you need to get ready for your first experience at the facility.

Meeting Your Doctor

Meeting your doctor for the first time is a big moment for you, because this is the person that you are going to trust with your health for the duration of your stay. He or she will handle your treatment, surgery and pre- and post-operative checkups. If you have more than one doctor, you should try to meet them all as soon as you arrive at the hospital in order to get a better impression of who they are, how they speak to you as a patient and their level of professionalism.

Discussing Treatment Options

Before you are admitted, you should discuss the various treatment options with your doctor. Different doctors have different ideas about the best methods of treatment, so be sure to note what the doctor recommends, then call your doctor at home and get his or her second opinion. This is your opportunity to get an in-depth view into what you are facing, and how you can go about getting healthy. From previous phone calls, you will already know what treatments you are there for; however, it doesn't hurt to exhaust all the options, especially if there is a way to prevent surgery or get a less invasive procedure. Speak with your new doctors about any additional treatments that might increase your success rate or reduce your recovery time. In foreign countries, there are always several natural options that can complement your main treatment. It might be advisable to try one, especially because the healthier you are, the faster your recovery will be.

Handing Over Medical Records

> **Tell him which medications you are on, and which you can't take**

When you meet your new doctors, you should hand them your complete medical records, with all of the tests, histories, allergies and medications that you have had in the past. If you are in the country for something like a knee replacement, your doctors will now be able to look closely at your X-rays, and perhaps run more tests to determine the extent of the damage – then re-diagnose as they see fit. Your medical records are very important because they present a lifetime history of your health, lists of medications that you have been on and any substances that you are allergic to. Even though your new doctors have your records, make sure to tell them directly which medications you are on and which you can't take. Once again, if any new diagnosis is made, check in with your doctor at home.

Poking Around the Hospital

Having a good look around the hospital will tell you a lot about the medical care there. If you are in for the long haul, then pay special attention. When you're walking around, take note of the patients in their rooms and how they are being looked after. Watch doctors go about their daily business. If for any reason you get a bad feeling about the hospital, then you can pull out – and contact your back up doctor in a hospital nearby. You should never stay in a hospital that makes you feel uncomfortable, especially if you can pinpoint a specific reason you feel that way.

Pre-Operative Checks

Once you have returned to the hospital and have been admitted, you will be required to do some pre-operative checks. These checks might include a whole new battery of "conditioning tests," or tests to see how overall fit and healthy you are. You will be screened for common ailments like anemia that may affect your stability on the operating table. As a general rule, stop taking all forms of medication, even if it's natural or prescribed, at least two weeks before surgery. Depending on your level of health, past history and age, you will be asked to complete a questionnaire about your less-than-healthy habits. If you drink or smoke, that's got to go. Sometimes even tea can be a threat, so be sure to list everything you can think of.

Make Copies of Your Test Results

Medical tourism is a round-trip ticket, starting and ending at your local doctor's office. You need to ask your international doctor for copies of all the new medical tests, history, medicine and diagnosis created for you at your overseas facility. This will give your local doctor an update on your health status, including the types of medicines that you were put on, and help him or her continue any treatment when you get back.

Getting the Most Out of Your Stay

This might be a time for correcting whatever health problem you may have; but it's also a time for sightseeing, touring and enjoying the cultural diversity of the country you're in. This is the vacation part of your trip, and it has led to golden memories for the thousands of American medical tourists who have crossed the globe for medical care.

Vacation Time Planning

Depending on the extent of your injuries or treatment, you will have the opportunity to experience your host country for as long as you are there. Even if you only stay in a certain part of the city, you'll still get to enjoy new taste sensations from foreign cuisine, experience a slice of local culture and see how they live as a community on a day-to-day basis. The longer you stay, the more you'll get to see. If you're there for a cosmetic procedure or a quick surgery – even for certain chronic disease treatments – you can branch out and explore the sights and sounds of the country beyond one city. Many medical tourists have had some of their best vacations during their time abroad for medical treatment – and there's no reason why you shouldn't either. Imagine taking a self-guided tour of Japan in your spare time, and seeing world heritage sites, traditional dances – even going to a Japanese rock concert. For most countries, you can download free itineraries off the Internet that highlight the best routes to take to see all the splendor of the country. Or you can take an organized tour (see below) so you can fit in as much as possible before you have to return home. You

> **Many medical tourists have had some of their best vacations during their time abroad for medical treatment**

could also decide to do some sightseeing before your surgery so you can experience the country first and then relax at your destination hospital before heading home. Planning your vacation time is much easier if you know what procedure you are going to have and how long it will take to recover from it. A good vacation is about a week long, but the best are between two and four weeks long because then you really get to see the country.

Tours

If you decide to use a medical travel agent, they will book any tour that catches your eye for you. These tours are usually very specific, and can be booked once in the country or pre-booked before you go. Choose from a variety of the top-rated tours in the country that will take you past some of the tourist hot-spots, where you and your traveling companion can take photos and enjoy the moment. If you don't know how to contact a travel agent in the city you're in, then inquire at your hospital or medical care center. They see a lot of tourist trade and will be able to point you in the right direction. Often, you can get significant discounts if you book through an online travel agency before you go. Once you arrive, you only need to find the starting location for the tour, and off you go.

Things to Pack

Going overseas always presents the problem of what to pack and what to leave behind. The first thing you need to establish is when you are going. Check the dates online and see what season it will be in your destination country. The last thing you want to do is leave America in summer and land a day later in a frigid winter climate. Once you have discovered what the weather is going to be like in your host country, you can pack accordingly. There are a number of other important items that you don't want to leave off your packing list.

Medication and Supplies

Every country has medicine, but it might not be the medicine you're used to.[203] If you are on any prescription medication, take it along with you. Once you're there, you can discuss with your international doctor whether you can keep taking it or if you have to stop for a while. As soon as the medical procedure is over, you can likely resume your medication regimen again. Certain medications pose a risk on the operating table. They may thin your blood, which could cause hemorrhaging, or interact badly with the anesthesia. Always check with your doctor about what medications you can and can't use during your stay. You should also take a basic supply of over-the-counter medication in case you get sick from the food and water, which can cause headaches, diarrhea, vomiting and nausea. Be sure to throw a few emergency painkillers into your bag, along with nausea tablets and diarrhea medication. You don't want to be in severe pain or be violently sick because of strange food. Avoid eating food that is sold in open air markets, and don't drink anything but bottled water on your trip. It's a good idea to steer clear of raw food as well. Contracting food poisoning can be very dangerous just after surgery. Stitches can break, wounds can open and internal injuries can worsen. While you're in the pharmacy, take the opportunity to buy other medical essentials that you might need during your stay. If you're going for a large operation that will require stitches and dressing, then stock up on some of your own so you can keep the wound clean. Cleaning fluids, bandages, gauze, tape and scissors can all come in handy. If you can't get the scissors past security, then make a plan to buy them in your host country before you are admitted into the hospital.

Clothing for a Comfortable Recovery

Think about the procedure that you're going to be having, and pack accordingly. Include comfortable soft fabrics and stretchy pants. These aren't necessary if your surgery is above the neck, but you can imagine how painful jeans would feel if you've just had abdominal surgery. If you're going to be bedridden for a while, include a few pairs of soft, clean pajamas. This might also be the time to invest in a few pairs of pure cotton undergarments. Hospitals don't allow you to wear polyester or nylon on the operating table; if you don't have your own cotton underwear they will give you a pair of theirs, which is not always ideal. A good pair of comfortable slip-on shoes or slippers will also help your recovery along because you won't have to bend awkwardly to lace them up or strap them on.

Your Guide to Recovery

Recovering after a heavy surgical procedure will be the most difficult part of your trip. Depending on the extent of your medical procedure or treatment, you need to plan enough time to recover. Everyone recuperates at their own individual pace, but it's always useful to know how long it takes on average to be travel-ready again. You don't want to end up having to leave early, when you are still in a lot of pain and discomfort. This is the part of your trip when your travel companion will be invaluable to you. You will need plenty of assistance after most surgical procedures, and rest is very important for a successful recovery.

Hospital Stay

When you wake up in the ICU, or have undergone a particularly rough chronic disease treatment, this is when you will be at your most vulnerable. To avoid the risk of infection, relapse and any additional complications that could arise shortly after treatment, you need quality supportive care. Hospitals abroad provide their patients with exceptional round-the-clock care, and monitor their progress until they are able to leave. You need a hospital that will pay special attention to you during this time

> **Hospitals provide their patients with exceptional round-the-clock care until they are able to leave**

so you are left to concentrate on nothing but getting better. Inpatient care in a hospital is the best way for you to recover fully after your surgery. You can also choose to be transported to a recovery center for a few days – or for an extended stay if you need constant care after your procedure. These state-of-the-art outpatient facilities focus solely on your health and well-being, and are there to tend to your every need during this difficult time. These centers are staffed with private doctors, surgeons and nurses, so if anything does happen, action can be taken on premises to save your life or prevent further damage. Your recovery center will keep you clean, and provide you with a list of healthy food choices that are specially prepared for weakened patients. They will also handle your medication regimen for the duration of your stay.

Private Nurses

Both hospitals and recovery centers abroad provide their patients with the option of having a private nurse attend to them during their stay. This is an excellent idea if you are going in for an extensive procedure and will be bedridden for quite a while. These trained health professionals will walk you through each stage of your recovery process, making it their business to keep you on the right track so you don't experience any additional issues that could arise from neglect or bare-minimum treatment. Private nurses can also be hired on a freelance basis to return with you to your hotel and care for you there. This is very beneficial, especially if there are many new medications that you have to take or if the medications have to be administered intravenously. Your nurse will also prepare meals for you, change your surgical dressings and assist you if you need to bathe or use the bathroom.

The Dos and Don'ts after Surgery or Treatment

For every surgical procedure, there will be a list of physical activities that you may not perform if you hope to recover properly. Make sure that when you are recovering in the hospital, you get your doctor or private nurse to create a list of things that you can and can't do, and for how long each of these limiting rules will be in effect. For example, a patient who has just had a face lift must avoid showing any kind of emotion that could affect the face muscles for the first few days. Another patient who has just had spinal surgery may not bend his or her spine or walk around for a few weeks. This can and can't do list will remind you of the rules you have to adhere to during your recovery process. Medications and drowsiness can impair memory function, so it's best to keep them all written down. Follow the doctor's orders to the letter. If you have chosen to recover in a hotel with your travel companion, give your companion the list and make sure that you are forced to follow it. A smoker might be inclined to smoke directly after a big surgery, but this can lead to many complications. Be smart.

Medications

If you were on any medication before going in for the procedure, ask your doctor whether you can start taking it again. Natural supplements, chronic medications, birth control, painkillers and other forms of daily medicine should all be run past your doctor

> **Use this opportunity to discuss with your doctor the safety of mixing certain kinds of medication**

before you decide to use them again. Use this opportunity to discuss with your doctor the safety of mixing certain kinds of medication. You will likely be on antibiotics and a variety of pain medications, so you need to know what will be safe to take and what could potentially be damaging to your body.

Post-Op Checks

After your ordeal, you will need to go for certain post-operative checks so your doctor can monitor your progress and adjust your medication or treatment accordingly. Be sure to mention exactly what you've been experiencing through your recovery. If there has been pain, then mention it. Your doctor might have to give you a higher dosage of pain killers. Post-operative tests will assess whether the operation went as planned, and watch for clots, infections, internal bleeding or other side effects of surgery. A cancer patient who has just had a tumor removed, for example, may be X-rayed to see if the entire mass is gone or if another surgery is needed. Use this time to ask your doctor if you will need any physical therapy so you can make the necessary arrangements when you get home.

New Medical Records

During your post-operative checkups, request all new medical records from your international doctor. You doctor back home will need them to add to your medical history. This includes notes, test results and X-rays – everything your international doctor or nurses did to you while you were at their facility.

Continuity of Care

When you return home, you will still require a certain level of care to make sure that you recover fully. Just because your international doctor has cleared you for travel, it doesn't mean that you can return to drinking and smoking or stop taking your medication. People who do this take much longer to recover, and sometimes it leads to significant complications that mean hospital time. Be vigilant once you're home, and make sure you have someone there who is willing to help.

Returning Home

You have done what you set out to do, and are now on your road to recovery. If you are still in a very fragile state, then hire a private nurse for as long as you need one or keep in close contact with your local doctor. Before you leave for your medical trip abroad, you should make sure that you've made the necessary arrangements for your return home. If you've just had major jaw surgery, for example, you will need to have soft foods on hand. Your recovery might also hinder your movement to the point where you should consider buying a wheelchair or a walking stick to help you move more safely around your house. This is a great time to watch those series that you've never had time to see, or to read that book you've had in your bookcase for three years.

Contacting Your Local Doctor

As soon as you arrive home, you should contact your local doctor to fill him or her in on the trip and to hand over your new medical records. If you can't drop them off yourself, then get someone else to do it. It's important that you fill in your doctor's office as soon as possible so they are up to speed on your medical condition, and can keep prescribing you the medication you need for your recovery. Your local doctor will also support you through the final stages of recovery, and assist with finding you a physical therapist if you need one.

What to Do if the Worst Happens

> **It's important to keep your local emergency services telephone number on hand**

Sometimes, even once you've made it through the dangerous first week of recovery, things can go wrong. Once you are back at home, anything can happen. You could fall and split your wound open, experience terrible pain from an unknown and unforeseen complication or experience a life-threatening reaction to a new medication. If this happens, it's important to have your local emergency services telephone number on hand, and to contact your doctor's office immediately. This is why you filled them in as soon as you got home. If anything happens, they will know what you had done and what medications you were on. If these complications are mild and don't result in hospitalization, then you need to contact your international hospital immediately and tell them about it. If you do end up in the hospital, calling your international doctor is still a good idea once you are stable. If you are recovering from a very large surgery at home, install a panic button or a preprogrammed text message that goes out to your doctor or close family member if you need help and can't talk.

Spreading the Word

Once you have fully recovered and are enjoying the benefits of your amazing surgery abroad, it's time to spread the word about it. Feeling the physical, emotional and financial benefits of an overseas medical trip can change your life. Something like this should never be kept quiet. Imagine the 65-year-old woman who believes that she is wheelchair-bound for the rest of her life because her insurance won't cover her hip replacement surgery. Imagine the child lying in a hospital with cancer, having given up hope of recovery. You need to put the word out that you went through this brave new form of travel – and came out of it healthier, happier and better than you've ever been before. Who knows how many people's lives you could change with something as simple as a heartfelt testimonial online? It's now up to you to get the truth out about the exceptional medical care you received abroad.

Medical Tourism Solves the U.S. Healthcare Crisis

With so many average Americans now at the mercy of a draconian healthcare system, medical tourism will surely rise to help even more people than it did before. As long as there are pristine, world-class hospitals mere hours away from the U.S., there will always be an alternative for you and your family. Use this text as a reference – your guide to the global healthcare market. There are hundreds of exotic locations to visit, each with quality medical care designed for the international medical traveler.

It's time you said no to these new healthcare laws, and moved onto something better for your family – to opportunities that will broaden your global knowledge and help you to live a life of health, wealth and happiness. Isn't that what the American dream is all about? Medical tourism is primed to expand, offering you more choices, higher medical standards and lower costs. The greener pasture is now on the other side of the U.S. border – in Panama, Belize or any of the other fine destinations detailed in this book. Though you will be paying the government insurance rates or the fines for refusing, you can still save money by taking a leap of faith and putting your trust in a top-quality medical facility abroad. In your time of need, there is no better solution than one that goes above and beyond your expectations. If you prepare yourself and your family, you will be able to get quality medical care abroad for the rest of your lives – and enjoy vacations in the sun together – instead of losing your health and your money to a corrupt, greedy system. The time is now. Fight back by doing what is best for you. Explore the world. Become a medical traveler.

CHAPTER 10

❧ • ☙

DESTINATION PROFILING: COUNTRIES, FACILITIES AND TREATMENTS

Destination Profiling: Countries, Facilities and Treatments

Choosing where in the world you would like to go for medical services is always a challenge, especially if you are in dire need of medical attention. Making the right decision will have long-term consequences on your health, so it's best to explore your options thoroughly before setting out on your medical journey. In this section, we break down the countries you should consider traveling to, some of the individual facilities that these countries offer and which would be most appropriate for your specific medical concern. It's a veritable three-step guide to discovering your dream medical destination. If you follow the advice given here, you are bound to find a destination, hospital and treatment plan that will get you back on the fast track to good health.

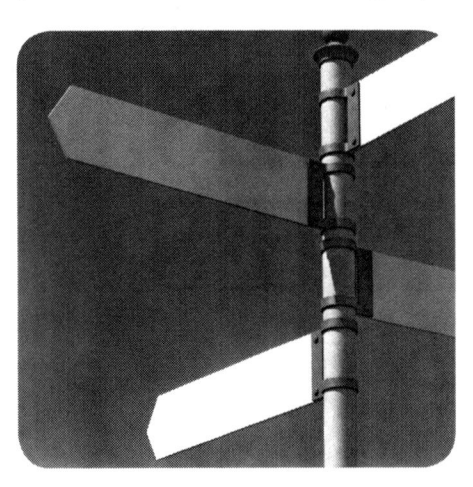

Where Do I Go for My Specific Medical Concern?

The bottom line for any successful medical trip is finding the best hospital for your medical concern. After all, when you take away the beautiful travel destinations, the appealing climates and the wonderful sights, you want to be left with top-class medical care in a top-class medical facility. It's difficult to narrow down which countries are best at each field of medicine; and truth be told, you'll probably be able to find excellent care for your condition in any country. But if you want to know which of them has the best reputation for your medical condition, then this is the section to read. It might broaden your ideas about where you should go.

SPOTLIGHT ON PANAMA: ORTHOPEDICS

Panama is most often visited for its excellent orthopedics centers, but they are also great at treating any age-related illness or condition. Because of the growing trend of Americans choosing to move to Panama for retirement, the country's hospitals have become particularly skilled in the areas of broken bones, bone-related diseases and surgeries.

SPOTLIGHT ON DUBAI: DENTAL CARE

Dubai has an excellent and affordable healthcare system, but they excel most in the area of dental care and surgery. With thousands of Americans traveling each year to Dubai for a better smile, stronger teeth and healthier gums, this is the ideal location for someone seeking low-cost implants, bridges or gum treatments.

SPOTLIGHT ON SOUTH AFRICA: COSMETIC SURGERY

South Africa is the best location for a nice quiet cosmetic procedure while on an African safari. With top-notch cosmetic surgery centers and some of the finest tour/surgery packages in the world, this country sees a lot of Americans who want to keep their surgeries private – and recover in style.

SPOTLIGHT ON SINGAPORE: NEUROSURGERY

Singapore has incredible standards of healthcare, and nowhere is this more prominent than in neurosurgery. For such a complex specialty, this country excels at dealing with matters of brain disease and surgery. You'll find some of the world's best neurosurgical departments in the 13 private hospitals here.

SPOTLIGHT ON SAUDI ARABIA: DIABETES

Saudi Arabia has recently experienced a massive increase in the number of diabetic medical travelers. As a result, its treatment of this chronic disease has become very sophisticated, with research and revolutionary treatments being administered here that can't be found anywhere else in the world.

SPOTLIGHT ON NEW ZEALAND: PEDIATRICS

New Zealand has emerged as a great place for pediatric surgeries, where they deal with all branches of medicine as they relate to children. If you're looking for caring doctors who can help your sick child, then contact a specialist hospital in this country for higher success rates.

SPOTLIGHT ON INDIA: CARDIOLOGY

India is by far the best country to travel to for matters of the heart. With the latest medical technology and exemplary service to international patients, you couldn't be in safer hands for heart surgery, pacemaker implants, valve replacements or other heart disease treatments. They also have unbeatable prices for some of these extreme surgeries.

SPOTLIGHT ON MEXICO: EMERGENCY SURGERY

Mexico shares a border with America, and as a result, they see a lot of medical travelers who need emergency surgeries. These surgeries include everything from heart surgery and neurosurgery, to gastrectomies and tumor removal. You'll find Mexican hospitals with excellent facilities, fully prepared for a range of emergency conditions.

SPOTLIGHT ON THAILAND: ALTERNATIVE MEDICINE

Thailand is best known for their long history of effective alternative medicine. Here you'll find ancient herbal treatments for a number of chronic diseases, as well as acupuncture and a wide variety of other complementary medicines to help you recover from almost any illness.

SPOTLIGHT ON PHILIPPINES: WEIGHT LOSS SURGERY

The Philippines has a booming medical tourism trade, with an ever-increasing demand for bariatric surgery and other weight loss surgeries. Marrying quality medical care to affordable prices, this country is the best place to achieve a thinner, healthier you – especially when weight loss is going to correct other dire health problems.

SPOTLIGHT ON SOUTH KOREA: SPINAL DISORDERS

South Korea remains one of the most technologically advanced countries in the world; in particular, they have great medical treatments and surgeries for spinal disorders and disease. If your problem is in the central nervous system, you want to travel to South Korea to get the best, most accurate treatment of spinal injuries and conditions – and treatment with the highest rate of success.

SPOTLIGHT ON EUROPE: STEM CELL TREATMENT

In countries like Germany, France and even Hungary, you can find exceptional and experimental stem cell treatment that may help cure you when everything else has failed. For the best option when all others have run out, find a hospital in Europe for stem cell therapy.

SPOTLIGHT ON MALAYSIA: REPRODUCTIVE HEALTH

Malaysia offers the struggling family an opportunity to secure the finest fertility treatment in the world from one of their accredited medical centers. This country does it all – IVF, ICSI and IUI – and will help to make your dream of starting a family come true. For expert advice on fertility matters across the board, contact a hospital in Malaysia.

SPOTLIGHT ON COSTA RICA: ONCOLOGY

Costa Rica provides excellent medical facilities and treatments for patients suffering from cancer. The greatest benefit of all is that this country offers some of the most affordable long-term treatment to patients in the final stages of the disease. If you want a great live-in treatment destination, this is it.

SPOTLIGHT ON BELIZE: EYE SURGERY

Belize has world-class ophthalmology treatments to help you see clearer than you ever have before. For normal eye surgery and LASIK eye surgery, find a hospital or outpatient center to attend to your eyesight professionally and affordably in this country.

The Top Four Destinations for Fast, Excellent Medical Care

Panama, Belize, Mexico and Costa Rica are all very close to the U.S., and are ideal locations for fast medical travel. If you need great medical services, and you need them as soon as possible, these four locations boast some of the finest hospitals and medical staff in the world. There are no better countries for immediate medical care on our doorstep and each of these excellent locations can meet your medical needs, whatever they may be.

TOP DESTINATION #1: PANAMA

Panama is situated in Central America at the southernmost point, and connects the landmasses of North and South America. With Costa Rica to the north and Columbia to the south, this dynamic country has one of the fastest-growing economies in South America.

Language: Spanish/English
Air Travel Time: 4 – 5 hrs
JCI-accredited Hospitals: 1
Currency: Balboa/Dollar
Top Three Specialties: Orthopedics, Cosmetic Surgery, Oncology

Contact for Travel Packages:
http://www.panama-health.com/
http://www.panamamedicaltourism.com/
http://www.agelesswonders-pma.com/
http://www.abpanama.com/panama-medical-tourism/panama-spas.php

Contact for Hospitals:
www.hospitalpuntapacifica.com/
www.hospitalsanfernando.com/
www.hospitalnacional.com/
www.centromedicopaitilla.com/

Sights to See:
1. The Beaches of Panama Islands
2. The Panama Canal
3. San Lorenzo Fort
4. Boquette, a small mountain village

Panama Medical Care

As a medical tourism destination, this is one of the best, with comprehensive medical services and friendly, supportive medical staff. Panama is home to a number of world-class medical institutions, but there is only one JCI-approved hospital in the entire country. Hospital Punta Pacifica leads the way in the thriving metropolis of Panama City, pioneering advances in a number of complex medical disciplines that are in demand around the world. Often touted as the best location for medical services in Latin America, this bright and colorful country is also a big tourist destination, attracting Americans every year with its tropical climate and many surrounding islands. It is also situated relatively close to the U.S., so Americans can travel with ease between the two countries for next to nothing. If you need an international destination that offers quality healthcare, low prices and a great atmosphere, then Panama is the next stop on your medical tourism journey.

Top Hospital #1: Hospital Punta Pacifica

Location: Punta Pacifica Avenue, Paitilla, Panama City
Contact Details: (Tel) 011 507 204 8000 (Fax) 011 507 204 8010
Email Address: info@hpp.com.pa
Description: A modern, up-market hospital in the heart of Panama City that is affiliated with Johns Hopkins International, and holds JCI accreditation. With patient-centered service and over 350 doctors on staff, this hospital offers seven floors of 52 private rooms, recovery rooms and suites. They have a wide variety of specialty departments, including cardiology, neurology, gastroenterology, nefrology, dermatology, plastic surgery and hematology. They also assist their patients with an alternative medicine department, a psychiatric center and advanced cancer treatments.

Clinica Hospital San Fernando

Location: Via Espana Final, Panama City
Contact Details: (Tel) 011 507 305 6399 (Fax) 011 507 305 7000
Email Address: elewis@hospitalsanfernando.com, tmendez@hospitalsanfernando.com

Description: A well-rounded and established hospital with over 500 doctors on staff and 159 patient beds. This private hospital is affiliated with Pana-Health Corporation, which brings medical tourists to the hospital from all over the world. This fine medical institution offers patients services that include cardiology, cosmetic surgery, cancer treatment, orthopedic surgery, fertility treatment, laser eye surgery and pediatrics. There are also a number of other treatments available, so inquire for further information. Situated close to the Panama City Airport, this is a convenient hospital for patients in dire need.

Hospital Nacional
Location: Avenue Cuba, 38th and 39th Street, Panama City
Contact Details: (Tel) 011 507 207 8100 (Fax) 011 507 207 8337
Email Address: mercadeo@hospitalnacional.com
Description: From humble beginnings comes this advanced medical care center, with 160 doctors on staff and 33 rooms for you to choose from, as well as a selection of special private rooms upon request. This hospital has the best gynecological staff in Panama. Other medical services include pediatrics, excellent diagnostics equipment, cardiology, gastroenterology, stem cell therapy and physical rehabilitation. For your convenience, there is also an on-site pharmacy and doctors who speak a variety of languages. For a quiet, supportive hospital stay, this is one of Panama City's great hospitals.

Centro Medico Paitilla
Location: Avenue Balboa y Calle, 53 Panama City
Contact Details: (Tel) 011 507 265 8891 (Fax) 011 507 265 8862
Email Address: aclientes@cmpaitilla.com
Description: As an up-to-date medical center with 166 beds to keep occupied, this hospital in Panama City employs over 250 trained and

certified staff members. They have long been known for successful heart surgeries, and it is still one of their most requested surgeries. Their medical services include cardiac surgery, oncology, neurology and general surgery. Like Punta Pacifica, they have an alternative medicine department and a psychology center. As one of Panama's four leading hospitals, Centro Medico Paitilla will help you sort out your medical problems at almost 30% less than you would have paid in the U.S.

TOP DESTINATION #2: BELIZE

Belize is situated to the south of Mexico, and is one of the only English-speaking Central American countries. This is because, unlike its neighbors who were owned by Spain in the colonial period, Belize was occupied by the British. This led to an interesting amalgamation of the local dialect and English, which has now become a language called Kriol. As a truly breathtaking country with a lot to offer the medical tourist, Belize could be exactly what you need to kick your addiction, fix your illness or raise your quality of life.

Language: Kriol/English
Air Travel Time: 3 – 4 hrs
JCI-accredited Hospitals: 0
Currency: Belize Dollar
Top Three Specialties: Eye Surgery, Gastroenterology, Addiction Treatment

Contact for Travel Packages:

http://www.revahealth.com/dentists/belize/belize/belizedental

Contact for Hospitals:

http://www.health.gov.bz/www/index.php/regions/central-health-region-articles/karl-heusner-memorial-hospital

http://www.belizemedical.com/
http://www.12steptreatmentcentres.com/Centres/New_River_Cove_44565.asp

Sights to See:
1. Mayan Temples
2. The Five Sisters Falls
3. Baboon Sanctuary
4. The Cayes (Islands)

Belize Medical Care

Belize was once a backwater nation with terrible medical care and nearly no tourist trade. These days, the Ministry of Health keeps a close eye on the hospitals, ensuring that they are up to standard and that they are edging nearer to world-class medical services. Belize City is the medical hub of the country, with the best trauma services, surgeries and disease treatments all located within city limits. Economically, Belize has a lot to prove to the international community. As time passes and the business, tourism and medical sectors expand, one day we'll see Belize on par with countries like Mexico and Panama. In the meantime, if you need simple procedures done, then stop down to Belize for adequate medical care and nearly insignificant bills that won't hurt your pocket at all.

Top Hospital #1: Karl Heusner Memorial Hospital
Location: Princess Margaret Drive, Belize City, Belize
Contact Details: (Tel) 501 2231 548 (Tel2) 501 2233081
Email Address: N/A
Description: This is Belize's biggest and most popular hospital, with 115 beds and full facilities, drawing locals and people from beyond the Belizean border to its doors. The most shocking part of receiving

treatment at this hospital is receiving the bill. It's so ridiculously cheap that you could save up to 90% on medical care if you choose to fly to Belize for treatment. Granted, the center isn't as evolved as others in surrounding countries – but the doctors are competent and passionate, and they work to make sure everyone gets the best treatment possible.

Belize Medical Associates

Location: Belize City, Belize

Contact Details: Fill in a contact form on their website

Description: This private hospital started out as a clinic, and has now morphed into one of the largest medical facilities in Belize. Affiliated with the Baptist Health System of South Florida, this hospital boasts an on-site pharmacy, room for 25 patients and advanced laboratory facilities. There are also modern radiology services and two specialty units – neurology and cardiology. With highly trained medical staff dedicated to your health and wellbeing, their operating rooms have state-of-the-art machinery to facilitate any surgical procedure. This means that you get the benefit of the best surgery – in a quiet, tropical country. Recovery is the best part of this experience, because you get to relax in a humble village or a lush beachfront resort.

New River Cove

Location: Belize, Central America

Contact Details: None available

Email Address: kadam@newrivercove.com

Description: New River Cove is a secluded drug and alcohol rehabilitation center for people struggling with addiction. Built to look more like a tropical cabana than a treatment center, this beautiful building is surrounded by greenery and effectively removes the patient from the temptation of taking drugs or alcohol. Said to have been inspired by the

Mayan people, this center caters to the needs of men and women who require intensive counseling, detox facilities and psychological treatment. They use a twelve-step program much like ones used in the U.S. The compassionate staff members are supportive, understanding and trained to deal with the ravages of addiction. Set in the lush jungles of a green paradise, New River Cove offers hope to those who have lost it, and the treatment to help them reclaim their lives. The program includes family counseling, meditation, education, relapse prevention, fitness, horse riding, acupressure and one-on-one therapy.

TOP DESTINATION #3: MEXICO

Mexico shares its northern border with the U.S. Many Americans move to Mexico in search of a more temperate climate – but recently droves of them have been flooding in for medical services. Mexico remains one of the cheapest options when looking for medical treatment abroad.

Language: Spanish/English
Air Travel Time: 2 – 4 hrs
JCI-accredited Hospitals: 9
Currency: Mexican Peso
Top Three Specialties: Emergency Surgery, Cosmetic Surgery, Dental Surgery

Contact for Travel Packages:
http://www.discovermedicaltourism.com/mexico/
http://www.newmedicalhorizons.com/

Contact for Hospitals:
http://www.amerimed-hospitals.com/
http://www.christusmuguerza.com.mx/

Sights to See:
1. Ancient Mayan Ruins at Chichen Itza
2. Tijuana Nightlife
3. Templo Mayor, Aztec Temple
4. San Angel

Mexico Medical Care

Mexico should be one of your first choices if you are strapped for cash and looking for a nearby place to get your surgery done. Mexico has excellent medical care centers and they are continually being improved. There has never been a better time to start your medical tourism journey in Mexico.

Top Hospital #1: AmeriMed American Hospital
Location: Cabo San Lucas, Mexico
Contact Details: (Tel) 52 624 105 8500
Email Address: N/A
Description: This hospital is still fairly new but in the short time it's been around, it's built up a great reputation. With JCI accreditation and emergency surgery facilities, this is the perfect hospital to flee to if you've been in an accident. Each room has a private bathroom, and you can sign up for a private nurse to make you well again.

Christus Muguerza Alta Especialidad Hospital
Location: Nuevo Leon, Mexico
Contact Details: (Tel) 011 52 81 8399 3400 (Fax) 011 52 81 8174 3484
Email Address: internationalpatients@christusmuguerza.com.mx
Description: This JCI-accredited hospital was the first to garner a higher quality medical reputation from the international community. It is part of a hospital group so there is more than enough funding going

into the 200-bed hospital, which makes it both up-market and exclusive. Specializing in vascular surgery, general surgery and ophthalmology – this hospital is one of Mexico's best, with a professional staff to prove it. If you're looking for a tiny medical bill and a whole lot of renewed health, then this is your dream destination.

Angel's Touch Dental Clinic
Location: Los Cabos, Mexico
Contact Details: (Tel) +52 624 142 6192 (Fax) +52 624 142 2459
Email Address: angelsdental@gmail.com
Description: This highly sought-after dental clinic feels more like a day resort when you walk in the front doors. Of course, once you get inside, it's all down to business – with talented dentists and the latest dental equipment filling every room. There are five dentists on staff, each with his or her personal specialty. The clinic handles surgeries and routine procedures with finesse and grace – which is probably the reason that nearly all of their clients are from outside of Mexico. Fly here to get everything from endodontic treatments to full maxillofacial reconstruction surgery.

TOP DESTINATION #4: COSTA RICA

Costa Rica is situated in Central America, with Panama and Nicaragua as its neighbors. A fair potion of it also runs along the Caribbean ocean. When it comes to medical tourism, this country lands itself in the top five, every time. With medical services that can make even the most modern U.S. hospitals blush, Costa Rica is a bustling haven for American medical travelers. Year after year, it proves to be so popular that many Americans have even moved there after treatment. One thing is certain – as long as Costa Rica is just around the corner from the U.S., Americans will always have the opportunity to the get the best medical care in the world.

Language: Spanish/English
Air Travel Time: 4 – 5 hrs
JCI-accredited Hospitals: 3
Currency: Colon
Top Three Specialties: Oncology, Weight Loss Surgery, Dental Surgery

Contact for Travel Packages:
http://costaricanmedicaltours.com/medical-tours-packages.html
http://www.placidway.com/country/9/Costa-Rica-Medical-Tourism
http://www.medicaltourismofcostarica.com/

Contact for Hospitals:
http://www.hospitalcima.com/
http://www.hospitallacatolica.com/site.php?lang=eng
http://www.clinicabiblica.com/esp/index.php

Sights to See:
1. Monteverde Cloud Forest Biological Reserve
2. Parque Nacional Manuel Antonio
3. Parque Nacional Volcán Arenal
4. Puerto Viejo de Talamanca Village

Costa Rica Medical Care

Costa Rica has long been the dream medical tourism destination for Americans. Not only do they have a first-world infrastructure, but their medical services are phenomenal and draw thousands to the country every year. If their medical services are cheap, their prescriptions are even cheaper, saving you as much as 80% on certain medications. There is no reason to go anywhere else when Costa Rica is an option.

Top Hospital #1: CIMA Hospital

Location: 500 metros oeste del Peaje a Snata Ana Escazu, Costa Rica
Contact Details: (Tel) 011 506 208 1068 (Fax) 011 506 208 1107
Email Address: cima@hospitalcima.com
Description: If you think you've seen a modern hospital, wait until you visit the pristine grounds of this one in Costa Rica. With 62 beds in the hospital, and over 500 doctors ready to help you at any given time, there is nothing but 24-hour top-quality care for the medical traveler. Specializing in over 60 different medical disciplines, these doctors are at the top of their fields. Most people venture to this hospital for orthopedics and cosmetic surgery; it's also excellent for laparoscopic surgery, general surgery, cosmetic surgery and cardiac care. Their slogan pretty much sums up this effortless and affordable experience: "Your Safest Medical Care, Close to Home."

Hospital Hotel La Catolica

Location: Guadalupe, Goicoechea, San José, Costa Rica
Contact Details: (Tel) 506 2246 3000 (Fax) 506 2246 3176
Email Address: callcenter@hospitallacatolica.com, servicioalcliente@hospitallacatolica.com
Description: This JCI-accredited hospital has taken a revolutionary step and combined the immaculate service of a hotel with a hospital – ensuring that every individual patient admitted here gets the five-star treatment. From the outside, it looks more like a luxury resort. Best of all, it gives patients and their families an opportunity to stay together on the same premises. With a host of highly qualified medical staff and the most cutting-edge medical equipment money can buy, you couldn't be safer than in a hospital of this caliber. Situated 45 minutes away from the International Juan Santa Maria Airport, it may be possible to fly to this location in an emergency situation.

Hospital Clinica Biblica

Location: 1st and 2nd Street, 14th and 16th Avenues, Costa Rica

Contact Details: (Tel) 506 2522 1000 (Fax) 506 2258 7184

Email Address: info@clinicabiblica.com

Description: This is one of the oldest hospitals in Costa Rica, but because it's been updated every few years it's also one of the most modern. A very large portion of this hospital's patient base is international; as such, they strive to make your stay here perfect. With over 200 specialists on hand and an international department to help you organize your stay, you'll be in good hands. There isn't an illness, disease or surgery they aren't prepared for, with excellent disease treatment facilities and surgery specializations that include cardiology, ophthalmology, hernia repair, cosmetic and gall bladder surgery, to name just a few.

Other Worthy Destinations for Global Medical Travel

Dubai

Dubai sits on the Arabian Peninsula, with the Persian Gulf to the south of this busy emirate. It is part of the United Arab Emirates, and is one of the most popular tourist destinations in the UAE. Americans have been known to travel to this bustling trade center to buy the most amazing products for next to nothing. The same is true for their medical treatment.

Language: Arabic/English

Air Travel Time: 14 – 15 hrs

JCI-accredited Hospitals: 2+

Currency: Dirham

Top Three Specialties: Endocrinology, Urology, Obstetrics

Contact for Travel Packages:
http://www.placidway.com/search/UAE,,/search.html

Contact for Hospitals:
http://www.ehl.ae/WH/
http://www.ehl.ae/TheCityHospital/
http://www.belhoulspeciality.com/home.aspx
http://www.ahdubai.com/main/index.aspx

Sights to See:
1. Dubai Museum (once a historical fort)
2. The Grand Mosque
3. Jumeirah archeological site
4. Gold Souk, Dubai's own gold shopping Mecca

Dubai Medical Care

Dubai has always been known for its inexpensive trade items, and now you can get medical services at that same reduced cost. As a developing country, and after realizing its potential in the tourism market, Dubai has crossed over to first-world standards of medical care. With 20 solid medical care centers dotted around the country, you can take your pick of which works best for you. An element of the medical culture in Dubai is the private house call that a doctor pays to his patient after the patient has left the hospital. This is considered to be a very important part of patient care, and is practiced at most hospitals in the region.

Welcare Hospital
Location: Dubai, UAE
Contact Details: (Tel) 971 4282 7788 (Fax) 971 4282 8226
Email Address: info@welcarehospital.com

Description: A confidential and attractive hospital in Dubai with a 12-bed emergency unit, dedicated medical staff and specialized equipment for chronic disease patients. This hospital is equipped to handle complete diagnostic testing, and is particularly proud of their kidney disease department. With hotel-like accommodations and five-star service, your recovery will feel more like a vacation in this excellent medical care center. They make a point of acquiring the latest technology as it is invented so you can receive all the benefits of modern medical care as it progresses. Welcare also won the prestigious Dubai Quality Appreciation Award, as well as an ISO certification in 2000. Though they are not yet JCIaccredited, it's only a matter of time before they achieve it.

The City Hospital
Location: Dubai Healthcare City, Dubai, UAE
Contact Details: (Tel) 971 4435 9999 / 800 THECITY (Fax) 971 4435 9900
Email Address: info@thecityhospital.com
Description: A modern architectural delight, this hospital has room for 210 admitted patients, and sticks closely to their patient-centered credo. The equipment in their hospital is not only the best available, but if anything better ever comes out they'll grab it for their facility as soon as possible. This hospital looks more like a hotel than a clinical place of healing. Its testing centers have warm wood paneling on the walls, accented with rich gold floors and cheery sculptures scattered around. If you're looking for a top-quality medical center that knows how to be a home away from home, then you might want to consider the City Hospital in Dubai. The luxury perks include an indoor heated swimming pool, saunas and a full gym onsite. They are best known for helping patients recover after trauma, and nursing them back to health using rehabilitative equipment and positive reinforcement.

Belhoul Specialty Hospital

Location: Dubai, UAE

Contact Details: +971 4 2733333 +971 4 2733332

Email Address: bsh@belhoulspeciality.com

Description: This fully equipped hospital concentrates on making your time there the best that is can possibly be. With a full resident staff on hand and a number of international doctors that fly in for specific surgeries, you'll get the best of what you need. Belhoul is a family-centered hospital with a number of specialty medical services available. These include cardiology, neurology, laparoscopic surgeries, dentistry, psychiatry and cosmetic surgery. It's a virtual one-stop medical healthcare center. There is also a nutrition center, a medical shop, lab services and rehabilitation facilities. Each specialty is treated individually, with teams of doctors ready to help you overcome your medical condition, whatever it may be.

The American Hospital, Dubai

Location: OudMetha Road, Dubai, UAE

Contact Details: (Tel) 971 4336 7777 (Fax) 971 4336 5176

Email Address: mktg@ahdubai.com

Description: The name gives you some indication of the quality of services available at this 143-bed surgical hospital. Fully accredited by the JCI, they work tirelessly to ensure that every part of your medical experience is as pleasant as possible. With stunning grounds surrounded by palm trees and manicured lawns, this hospital towers above many of the smaller ones in the region. It's the old American standard of medical care transferred into a luxurious location, giving its patients better care at lower costs. With a top-quality heart center, cancer treatment center and diabetes center as well as great orthopedics programs, neurology departments and pediatric care, this hospital should pop up first on your radar if you're flying into Dubai for medical care.

South Africa

South Africa is situated at Africa's southernmost point. As a multicultural nation, South Africa has consolidated its medical care and enticed strong corporate interests to invest heavily in its medical industry. With some of the best travel/surgery package deals in the world, South Africa is waiting.

Language: English/Afrikaans/African Languages
Air Travel Time: 18 – 20 hrs
JCI-accredited Hospitals: 0
Currency: Rands
Top Three Specialties: Cosmetic Surgery, Heart Surgery, Addiction Treatment

Contact for Travel Packages:
http://www.surgeon-and-safari.co.za/
http://www.surgicalbliss.com/medical-tourism-packages/
http://surgicalattractions.co.za/

Contact for Hospitals:
http://www.mediclinic.co.za/hospitals/Pages/about.aspx?h=2
http://www.olivedaleclinic.co.za/profile.asp
http://www.netcare.co.za/live/content.php?Item_ID=250

Sights to See:
1. Table Mountain, Cape Town
2. Safaris
3. Garden Route
4. Gold Reef City

Cape Town Medi-Clinic
Location: Stellenbosch, South Africa

Contact Details: (Tel) 021 809 6500 (Fax) 021 809 6756
Email Address: Contact form on website
Description: This hospital is known throughout the whole of Africa as a quiet, worthy place to get the best medical care in the country. Situated close to Cape Town Airport, this hospital boasts an excellent orthopedic unit and emergency center with topnotch facilities and fully trained medical staff who are up for the challenge.

Netcare Olivedale Hospital
Location: Johannesburg, South Africa
Contact Details: (Tel) 011 27 11 777 2000 (Fax) 011 27 11 462 8382
Email Address: wilmarie@olivedale.netcare.co.za
Description: This large and established hospital is part of the Netcare Group and has private hospitals all over South Africa. With an excellent emergency department and a 24/7 rape crisis center, this is a leading hospital in South Africa's biggest city. The hospital itself comes equipped with 263 beds and 11 operating theaters, each with state-of-the-art facilities. Known best for its excellent cardiothoracic surgeons and a multitude of other world class specialists, Olivedale also has the best in diagnostic testing equipment at its disposal. For a light, friendly and modern hospital visit, this should be high on your list of quality medical care centers.

Christiaan Barnard Memorial Hospital
Location: Cape Town, South Africa
Contact Details: (Tel) 011 27 21 480 6111 (Fax) 011 27 21 424 0826
Email Address: info@netcare.co.za
Description: This hospital is a monument to South African medical innovation and was named after cardiac pioneer Christiaan Barnard, the doctor who performed the world's first heart transplant. All forms of

cardiac treatment can be found here along with excellent general surgery, pediatrics, orthopedics, urology treatments and emergency surgery. Christiaan Barnard Memorial Hospital attracts the nation's best surgeons, and is also owned and operated by the Netcare Group. If you need heart disease treatment and surgery, then this is the hospital to visit.

Singapore

Singapore is situated in Southeast Asia, and is an island close to the Malay Peninsula. As an already thriving tourist nation with one of the highest tourist densities and expatriate communities in the world, Singapore makes a point of always being brilliant at whatever it does.

Language: Malay/English/Mandarin
Air Travel Time: 19 – 20 hrs
JCI-accredited Hospitals: 16
Currency: Singapore Dollar
Top Three Specialties: Neurosurgery, Cardiac Surgery, General Surgery

Contact for Travel Packages:
http://www.medicalsingapore.com/
http://www.discovermedicaltourism.com/singapore/

Contact for Hospitals:
http://www.ttsh.com.sg/
http://www.cgh.com.sg/
http://www.nccs.com.sg/

Sights to See:
1. Singapore Zoo
2. The Merlion
3. The Singapore Flyer
4. Buddha Tooth Relic Temple

Tan Tock Seng Hospital

Location: 11 Jalan Tan Tock Seng, Singapore
Contact Details: (Tel) 6256 6011 (Fax) 6256 6252
Email Address: contact@ttsh.com.sg
Description: This large hospital in Singapore was designed to help combat disease and to rehabilitate people who have been injured from accidents. There are 1,200 beds and the medical departments in the hospital have won many awards. JCI accredited and ISO certified. Most hospitals do not come as highly regarded as Tan Tock Seng.

Changi General Hospital

Location: Simei Street 3, Singapore
Contact Details: (Tel) 011 65 6850 3388 (Fax) 011 65 6782 1353
Email Address: international@cgh.com.sg
Description: Changi General Hospital is a JCI-accredited medical care center that embraces modern technological advancement and uses it daily to cure their patients of a variety of life-threatening conditions. Known for its special treatment of sports injuries, gastroenterology and conditions that affect only men, this hospital has emerged as one of Singapore's finest. With nine stories and 790 beds, this building is home to a score of expert doctors waiting for your arrival. There are also 22 specialist centers dedicated to patient care housed in this hospital.

National Cancer Center Singapore

Location: Hospital Drive, Singapore
Contact Details: (Tel) 011 65 6236 9433 (Fax) 011 65 6536 0611
Email Address: foreign_patients@nccs.com.sg
Description: For cancer treatment and recovery, there is no better place in Singapore than the National Cancer Center. This center assists patients at any stage of the illness and has support facilities for families.

They also use holistic medicine to complement the modern treatments that are provided here, so you get an all-round boost in health while coping with your disease. With the largest collection of expert oncologists in Singapore, your chance of recovery will improve significantly if you fly to this hospital for treatment. The center has also won numerous awards over the years for their contribution to fighting this chronic disease.

Saudi Arabia

Saudi Arabia is situated in the mysterious Middle East. Close to Iraq and the UAE, this country has a monarchy that understands how important it is for a country to enjoy an energetic medical tourist trade. In the process of improving medical facilities in the country, they have attracted more Americans to it.

Language: Arabic/English
Air Travel Time: 15 – 18 hrs
JCI-accredited Hospitals: 33
Currency: Riyal
Top Three Specialties: Diabetes Treatment, Dentistry, Heart Surgery

Contact for Hospitals:
http://bportal.kfshrc.edu.sa/wps/portal/bportal
http://www.almanahospital.com.sa/en/index.aspx
http://www.sghgroup.com/main-en.html

Sights to See:
1. Al Musmak Castle
2. City of Old Diriyah
3. Al Masjid Al Haram, the biggest mosque in the world
4. Black Stone

King Faisal Specialist Hospital and Research Center

Location: Riyadh, Kingdom of Saudi Arabia

Contact Details: (Tel) 966 1 464 7272 (Fax) 966 1 441 4839

Email Address: kfshwebmaster@kfshrc.edu.sa

Description: This extraordinary hospital is the best in South Arabia. It has over 894 beds with some of the brightest doctors in the kingdom working to cure cancer, heart disease and other chronic illnesses. Specializing in liver dysfunction, neuroscience, orthopedic surgery and cardiac surgery, this fine institution also trains future doctors for work in the hospital.

Almana General Hospital

Location: Dammam, Saudi Arabia

Contact Details: (Tel) +966 3893 7000 (Fax) +966 3898 0694

Description: This JCI-accredited hospital is part of a large hospital chain called the Almana General Hospital Group. As a highly respected hospital in the region with advances in medical specialties like nuclear medicine, fertility treatment and care for mentally ill patients, Almana General leads the way with quality medical care in Saudi Arabia. You can also get all the main branches of medical specialization here like cardiology, neurology and even dentistry. This particular hospital has over 200 beds, and is dedicated to providing healthcare for international patients at affordable prices.

Saudi German Hospital

Location: Jeddah, Saudi Arabia

Contact Details: (Tel) +966 (2) 6829000 (Fax) +966 (2) 6835874

Email Address: webmaster@sghgroup.com

Description: The Saudi German Hospital in Jeddah is one of a group of hospitals owned by the Saudi German Hospitals Group. With multi-

DESTINATION PROFILING: COUNTRIES, FACILITIES AND TREATMENTS

functional facilities and world-class doctors to tend to your every need, this medical care center is the largest in the region. Travel to this hospital for exceptional cardiac surgeons, general surgeons, and neurosurgeons, or for their great psychiatric department. All in all, a neatly-run quality hospital with a JCI accreditation.

New Zealand

New Zealand is a small country just off the Southeast coast of Australia. It is completely surrounded by water, and has a lively medical tourism industry because of the high quality standards of practice the facilities have put into effect there.

Language: English/Maori
Air Travel Time: 19 – 20 hrs
JCI-accredited Hospitals: 0
Currency: New Zealand Dollar
Top Three Specialties: Pediatrics, General Surgery, Urology

Contact for Travel Packages:
http://www.medtral.com/

Contact for Hospitals:
http://www.starship.org.nz/
http://www.mercyascot.co.nz/

Sights to See:
1. New Zealand National Maritime Museum
2. Tamaki Maori Village
3. Hobbiton, set of *Lord of the Rings*
4. International Antarctic Center

Starship Children's Health Service

Location: Auckland, New Zealand

Contact Details: (Tel) 649 3072800

Email Address: ssfis@adhb.govt.nz

Description: This hospital offers the international family a chance to get quality medical care from a great pediatric center. Starship is a teaching center as well, and provides surgical, medical and psychiatric services for the young child. This hospital with 194 beds is dedicated solely to children and looks kind of like a starship, which is how is it got its name.

Ascot Hospital

Location: Auckland, New Zealand

Contact Details: (Tel) 09 520 9500 (Fax) 09 520 9508

Email Address: You can send a message direct from their website

Description: This double-story hospital is affiliated with MercyAscot and acts as its partner facility. As a small but powerful hospital with 88 beds, this care center also has room for 12 state-of-the-art operating theaters. They specialize in same-day surgeries and most of the main medical specialties as well. If you're looking for a private, cozy and comfortable hospital in New Zealand, this is the one to choose.

Mercy Hospital

Location: Auckland, New Zealand

Contact Details: (Tel) 09 623 5700 (Fax) 09 623 5702

Email Address: You can send a message direct from their website

Description: Mercy Hospital is also part of the MercyAscot Group and is New Zealand's largest surgical hospital. This hospital has 155 beds with seven full operating theaters in the building. As a hospital best known for its intensive care unit and excellent surgical staff, Mercy Hospital is a great medical tourism destination if you need bariatric surgery, plastic surgery, vascular surgery or gynecology. Offering patient-centered care and advanced medical facilities, this is a safe destination for the medical traveler looking for medical treatment.

India

India is situated in Southeast Asia and is an enormously large country. It has a busy economy with a vibrant array of people living in both the cities and in the rural areas. Over the past few years, Indian doctors have been the ones making the most headway with medical discoveries and as such, the tourism trade is booming.

Language: Hindi/English
Air Travel Time: 15 – 19 hrs
JCI-accredited Hospitals: 16
Currency: Rupee
Top Three Specialties: Cardiology, Transplant Surgery, Neurosurgery

Contact for Travel Packages:
http://www.medicaltourismindia.com/india-medical-packages/index.html
http://www.indian-medical-tourism.com/
http://www.medicaltourisminindia.net/

Contact for Hospitals:
http://www.krishnaheart.org/
http://www.apollohospdelhi.com/index.html
http://www.hiranandanihospital.org/

Sights to See:
1. The Red Fort
2. The Amber Palace
3. Crawford Market
4. The Port City of Kochi

Krishna Heart and Super Specialty Institute

Location: Ghuma, Ahmedabad, India

Contact Details: (Tel) 910 2717 230877 81 (Fax) 91 02717 230876

Email Address: info@krishnaheart.org

Description: This is an advanced and technological medical center for the treatment of heart diseases. With the latest in diagnostic testing facilities, this ISO-certified institute is a haven for international patients suffering from cardiac dysfunction. Their specialties include arterial bypass surgery, transplant surgery and angioplasties.

Indraprastha Apollo Hospital

Location: Delhi, India

Contact Details: (Tel) 011 91 11 2692 5858 (Fax) 011 91 11 2682 5709

Email Address: helpdesk_delhi@apollohospitals.com

Description: This hospital sees more international traffic than most American hospitals, and holds a JCI accreditation and financial backing from the largest hospital group in Asia. Providing 560 beds for the international traveler and offering a wide range of medical services, it's no wonder this is one of the most popular hospitals in India. There are 14 operating rooms, each used over the years to perform many successful transplant surgeries – a specialty of the hospital. Indraprastha Apollo is also exceptionally good at cardiac and orthopedic surgeries, with a tiny 1% failure rate.

Dr. LH Hiranandani Hospital Powai

Location: Mumbai, India

Contact Details: (Tel) +91 22 25763300/33 (Fax) +91 22 25763311/44

Email Address: wecare@hiranandanihospital.org

Description: Because this is a new hospital in India only recently opened in 2004, it was specifically designed with international patients

DESTINATION PROFILING: COUNTRIES, FACILITIES AND TREATMENTS

in mind. As a result, everything is top quality, easy and effortless – from arranging your stay there to getting hold of educated professionals to help you find what you need. With 130 beds at their disposal, there will always be place for you. This is an exceptional hospital for chronic disease patients who need to save money by traveling. This hospital offers several packages to treat disease with modern medical advances and surgery. Stay in luxury at this modern hospital.

Thailand

Thailand is situated near Malaysia and Cambodia in Southeast Asia. It has one of the world's business powerhouses in the capital city of Bangkok. It attracts businessmen and tourists alike and as such, the medical trade has evolved and improved over time.

Language: Thai/English
Air Travel Time: 18 – 20 hrs
JCI-accredited Hospitals: 11
Currency: Baht
Top Three Specialties: Alternative Medicine, Oncology, Orthopedics

Contact for Travel Packages:
http://www.phuket-health-travel.com/
http://www.discovermedicaltourism.com/thailand/

Contact for Hospitals:
http://www.bnhhospital.com/en/contact.aspx?idCD=12
http://www.thaisuperiorart.com/

Sights to See:
1. City of Bangkok
2. Phuket Island

3. Doi Suthep Temple
4. Phra Buddha Chinnarat

Thailand Medical Care

In 2008, over a million medical travelers from around the world went to Thailand for medical care. According to the report, most of them loved the experience and saved a ton of money in medical costs. This should give you a decent insight into the medical tourism trade in Thailand. It's on the rise.

BNH Hospital

Location: Silom Bangkok, Thailand
Contact Details: (Tel) 662 686 2700 (Fax) 662 632 0577 79
Email Address: info@bnhhospital.com
Description: This JCI- and ISO-accredited hospital has 100 beds and the option to have your own private room. With a 440-strong staff of medical practitioners, this hospital is one of the best in the city. Great for medical specialties that include physical rehabilitation, nutrition and cardiology, this hospital is bound to get you back into good shape once your surgery is done.

Superior A.R.T, Fertility Clinic

Location: Bangkok, Thailand
Contact Details: (Tel) 660 2 255 4848 (Fax) 66 02 255 8455
Email Address: services@thaisuperiorart.com
Description: This is one of South East Asia's jewels in the infertility field. Through dedicated research, testing and balancing procedures, this clinic manages to get women pregnant when it was previously impossible. ISO certified and specializing in IVF, this clinic also does a range of other fertility treatments, testing each one until the woman gets pregnant.

Philippines

The Philippines is a Southeast Asian country known for its rich history, incredible landscapes and stunning modern epicenters. As a growing power in the medical tourism industry, this island-laden state has some of the best medical facilities in the East.

Language: Filipino/English
Air Travel Time: 18 – 20 hrs
JCI-accredited Hospitals: 3
Currency: Peso
Top Three Specialties: Weight Loss Surgery, Vascular Surgery, Cardiology

Contact for Travel Packages:
http://www.medicaltourismphilippines.rxpinoy.com/v2/tours-wowvid.php
http://www.philmedtourism.com/default/why-the-philippines/sports-packages

Contact for Hospitals:
http://www.stluke.com.ph/
http://www.rxpinoy.com/metropolitanmedicalcenter/index.php?page=vmap.php
http://themedicalcity.com/Site/MedicalCity/Home.aspx?SS=886

Sights to See:
1. San Agustin Church
2. Malacanang Palace
3. Corregidor Island
4. Jumalon Musuem

Philippines Medical Care
There are some who say that medical care in the Philippines is still

developing, and it is – in the rural areas. In the cities, you can expect to find the best of the best, with tall hospitals filled with talented doctors from all over the region. If the Philippines is your dream vacation destination, then you won't be disappointed at the level of care you get here. The majority of doctors in the Philippines study in America, so you get the benefit of a great education at a less expensive location.

St. Luke's Medical Center
Location: Quezon City, Philippines
Contact Details: (Tel) 632 723 0101 (Fax) 632 723 1199
Email Address: info@stluke.com.ph
Description: St. Luke's is one of the oldest and most established names in the medical field. This particular St. Luke's is the most respected hospital in the entire country. It should come as no surprise that their expertise, technology and surgical success rate cannot be rivaled anywhere else in the Philippines. This institution is JCI accredited and offers patients the chance to stay in one of their 650 beds. There are over 1,700 trained medical professionals ready to make your stay as comfortable as possible. The hospital specializes in aesthetics, cardiology, cosmetic surgery and dental care.

The Metropolitan Medical Center
Location: Manila, Philippines
Contact Details: (Tel) 63 2 254 1111
Email Address: Contact form on website
Description: This esteemed hospital has been around for more than 37 years, and in that time it has seen a lot of growth and expansion. The hospital includes recent additions like a 27-story tower and brand new, state-of-the-art medical technology. With over 300 qualified doctors staffing the hospital, you won't have to worry about lack of experience or

quality control. This hospital also offers package deals that include kidney transplants, bariatric surgeries and modern procedure like laparoscopic non-invasive surgeries.

The Medical City
Location: Metro Manila, Philippines
Contact Details: (Tel) 632 635 6789 (Tel2) 632 631 86 26
Email Address: mail@medicalcity.com.ph
Description: As the name suggests, this is a massive hospital, but it doesn't compromise on quality because of its size. The building looks like a hotel from a distance and, once you get inside, that feeling lingers. With 1,000 highly qualified medical staff and 800 rooms in the hospital, it really is a city. Along with this super force of doctors comes the allied health professionals, and this hospital has over 2,000 of them. Look forward to advances in cancer treatment, cardiology, neurology and regenerative medicines.

South Korea

South Korea is situated between China, Japan and North Korea in the East. With a long, proud history and many modern innovations coming out of this country in the digital age, it has a lot to offer the medical traveler.
Language: Korean/English
Air Travel Time: 14 – 18 hrs
JCI-accredited Hospitals: 5
Currency: Won
Top Three Specialties: Spinal Disorders, Oncology, Ophthalmology

Contact for Travel Packages:
http://www.healthbase.com/
http://www.placidway.com/package-search/South%20Korea,/search.html

Contact for Hospitals:
http://eng.amc.seoul.kr/lang/MedicalServiceController.do?forward=/jsp/en/Service/Intrntnl/Intrntnl.jsp&state=viewpg

http://www.cmcseoul.or.kr/global/eng/front

Sights to See:
1. Lotte World
2. Namsan Park
3. Gyeongbokgung Palace
4. Jogyesa Temple

South Korea Medical Care
Medical care in South Korea used to be quite antiquated but has caught up in a big way over the last decade, thanks to the combined effort of area universities and private companies. The South Korean government is also excited about this new form of industry and has sanctioned a number of 'healthcare towns' to be built in the country. With medical complexes on the rise and more American tourists set to travel abroad for medical care, Korea may have the edge with their new healthcare-cluster idea. Only time will tell how many of these towns will be built and how popular they will be with overseas patients.

ASAN Medical Center International Clinic
Location: Songpa-Gu, Seoul, South Korea
Contact Details: (Tel) 822 3010 5001 (Fax) 822 3010 5004
Email Address: int@amc.seoul.kr
Description: This unique center in South Korea was specifically built due to the influx of medical tourists. The Asian Medical Center opened this clinic and within a few years, numbers began to climb and tourists started flocking to the institution. With many different centers making up

the whole, there are a large variety of centers to choose from. Whether you need treatment for Alzheimer's disease, diabetes or cell therapy, there's a center here that can help you.

Seoul St. Mary's Hospital
Location: Seoul, South Korea
Contact Details: (Tel) 822 2258 5745 (Fax) 822 2258 5752
Email Address: ihcc@catholic.ac.kr
Description: One of the largest Korean hospitals available, St. Mary's welcomes every opportunity to provide excellent medical care for the international patient. The hospital has 1,200 beds and enough medical staff to keep each one of their patients happy. With a self-proclaimed cutting-edge infrastructure, St. Mary's specializes in family medicine, urology, obstetrics, infectious disease and a gigantic range of other medical disciplines.

Europe

Europe is one of the smallest continents, bordered by several different oceans and seas. Despite its size, most of the world's innovation comes from the countries on this continent. The following provides a brief introduction to the continent, highlighting the main institutions that stand out among the several European countries.

Language: Many/English
Air Travel Time: 8 – 10 hrs
JCI-accredited Hospitals: 90+
Currency: Euro
Top Three Specialties: Stem Cell Treatment, Transplant Surgery, Laparoscopic Surgery

Contact for Travel Packages:
http://www.en.zz-l.de/dental-tourism-germany.html

http://www.debsonmedicaltourism.com/
http://www.worldeyelasik.com/medical-tourism-packages.html

Contact for Hospitals:
http://www.drk-kliniken-berlin.de/
http://www.arsmedica.hu/eng/
http://www.anadolumedicalcenter.com/

Sights to See:
1. Eiffel Tower, France
2. Roman Architecture, Italy
3. Neuschwanstein Castle, Bavaria
4. Archeological Museums, Greece

Europe Medical Care

It goes without saying that a continent like Europe would house some of the most advanced medical facilities in the world. Even in a place like Europe, the American medical traveler can find low-cost, quality healthcare. The continent focuses on safety and guaranteed service, and you can secure medical procedures that you can't get anywhere else. Stem cell treatments, hyperthermia cancer treatments and spinal disk replacement surgery are all available if you know where to look. Countries like Hungary, Germany, Turkey, Poland and Spain all fall under this banner.

DRK Kliniken Berlin
Location: Berlin, Germany
Contact Details: (Tel) 493 03035 5210 (Tel2) 493 03035 5211
Email Address: N/A
Description: This is not a single hospital but rather a group of hospitals that fall under one name. Situated in some of the most striking and

picturesque parts of Berlin, these medical care centers are all JCI accredited. With a combined 1,325 beds and over 450 qualified medical specialists working here, it's no wonder this group has such a sterling international reputation. DRK Kliniken includes pain specialists and has earned the 'Pain Free' certification from the German Association for Qualified Pain Therapy. This means that the staff works hard to ensure that no clients are ever in pain, even if they are suffering through the worst kinds of treatments. Cancer treatment is a particular specialty, as are cardiology, neurology and fertility treatments.

Ars Medica Laser Clinic, Hungary
Location: Budapest, Hungary
Contact Details: (Tel) 361 266 7766 (Fax) 361 235 0661
Email Address: arsmedica@arsmedica.hu
Description: This medical clinic is world-renowned for their one-day laser treatments that solve a variety of problems for the medical traveler. The clinic is ISO certified and has a full staff of 12 qualified doctors and surgeons. They treat their patients with respect and as individuals so that you leave as happy as you arrived. This clinic specializes in laser and cosmetic surgery, gynecology, dentistry and ear, nose and throat medicine. As a Hungarian clinic that keeps releasing success stories, these are the guys to talk to if you need a one-day surgical procedure.

Anadolu Medical Center, Turkey
Location: Istanbul, Turkey
Contact Details: (Tel) 90 262 678 53 89 (Fax) 90 262 654 00 53
Email Address: int.patients@anadolusaglik.org
Description: This prestigious hospital is JCI and ISO accredited, and is a partner of John Hopkins International in America. The building itself was built next to the sea, so each hospital room has a view. There are 209

of these private rooms, each watched closely by one of the 230 doctors that are permanently employed at the medical care center. The great thing about this hospital is that family members can stay on premises with the ailing patient. As an emporium of the best medical specialties in the world, this hospital offers a range of surgical disciplines, diagnostic testing, women's health services, cardiac care and oncology. They are also a very forward-thinking establishment, providing departments for nutrition, sports, genetics and microbiology.

Malaysia

Malaysia is a large area of land encompassing various Southeast Asian states. Some of these states include Kuala Lumpur, Johor, Penang, Sarawak and Malacca. Malaysia is land of incredible diversity and amazing plant and animal life. It has endless rolling hills with tree canopies that stretch for miles, and open bodies of water that create tiny islands close to the shorelines.

Language: Malay/English
Air Travel Time: 19 – 21 hrs
JCI-accredited Hospitals: 6
Currency: Ringgit
Top Three Specialties: Reproductive Health, Cosmetic Surgery, Stem Cell Therapy

Contact for Travel Packages:
http://www.wellnessvisit.com/
http://www.urekascapade.com/
http://www.placidway.com/search/Malaysia,,/search.html

Contact for Hospitals:
http://www.princecourt.com/default.asp
http://www.gleneagles-penang.com/

http://healthcare.simedarby.com/Sime_Darby_Medical_Centre_Subang_Jaya.aspx

Sights to See:
1. Merdeka Square
2. Lake Gardens
3. Batu Caves
4. Bako National Park

Malaysia Medical Care

The medical care in Malaysia has always been good, but over the last decade we have seen a sudden boost in the main city centers as the government seeks to expand medical services to include foreign tourism. These days, Malaysia maintains a balance between traditional medicine and modern medicine, incorporating the two to the benefit of the international patient. Medical travelers know that many of Malaysia's medical professionals studied in other top medical countries.

Prince Court Medical Center
Location: 39, Jalan Kia Peng, 50450 Kuala Lumpur, Malaysia
Contact Details: (Tel) 603 2160 0000 (Fax) 603 2160 0010
Email Address: N/A
Description: This JCI-accredited hospital is a private institution found in Kuala Lumpur that specializes in areas of medical care like burn treatment, cosmetic surgery, cardiology, pediatrics and a host of other comprehensive medical disciplines like breast and endocrine surgery, general surgery, nephrology and oncology. This stylish hospital gives you the opportunity to choose either a private single room or a secure suite. As the new favorite medical travel destination, Prince Court leads the way in the eclectic city of Kuala Lumpur.

Gleneagles Medical Center, Penang

Location: 1 Jalan Pangkor, Penang, Malaysia

Contact Details: (Tel) 011 604 2276 111 (Fax) 011 604 2262 994

Email Address: pr@gmcpenang.com.my

Description: Gleneagles prides itself on being one of Malaysia's most up-to-date medical facilities. With a full range of choice, this hospital provides its patients with group rooms or with private quarters for extra privacy and security. They specialize in cardiothoracic surgery, orthopedic surgery and pediatrics. The hospital requires a deposit upon admission and will accept credit card payments or payments by check. As a leading medical service provider in Malaysia, this is one hospital you want to consider if you are looking for services in the area.

Sime Darby Medical Centre Subang Jaya

Location: Sdn. Bhd, 1 Jalan SS 12/1A Subang Jaya

Contact Details: (Tel) 011 603 5639 1466 (Fax) 011 603 5639 1675

Email Address: Contact form on the website

Description: This medical care center is part of one of Malaysia's biggest conglomerate companies, Sime Darby. The hospital itself has 393 beds and ten centers that practice the latest and most advanced medicine. Specialties include cardiology, clinical psychology, radiotherapy, hematology and nuclear medicine. The hospital is also close to many luxury hotels, shopping areas and restaurants.

℘•ℜ

Medical Glossary

Abdominal Aortic Aneurysm. A ballooning or widening of the main artery (the aorta) as it courses down through the abdomen.

Abscess. A localized collection of pus in any body part, resulting from invasion of a pyogenic bacterium, or other pathogen.

ACE inhibitors. A group of pharmaceuticals which lower the blood pressure by inhibiting the formation of angiotensin 11.

Acupuncture. The practice of inserting needles into the body to reduce pain or induce anesthesia.

Addiction. A chronic relapsing condition characterized by a compulsion to seek out drugs, food, gambling, sex or alcohol, and by chemical changes in the brain.

Adjunctive Therapy. A treatment used together with the primary treatment. Its purpose is to assist or boost the primary treatment.

Adult Stem Cell Treatment. A natural repair mechanism for many tissues of the body. Such treatment has cured many illnesses and disease by healing damaged tissues and cells in the body.

AIDS. The advanced stage of HIV infection. Symptoms and signs of AIDS include pneumonia.

Allergodes. A homeopathic preparation created from an allergen.

Allogenic Stem Cell Transplant. A procedure in which a patient receives stem cells from a donor. Allogeneic transplants are preferred in certain cases, such as in the treatment of leukemia.

Alport Syndrome. A hereditary condition characterized by kidney disease, sensorineural deafness and eye defects.

Alternative Medicine. Healing arts not taught in traditional Western medical schools, which promote alternatives to conventional medicine.

Alzheimer's Disease. A progressive neurologic disease of the brain that leads to dementia and the irreversible loss of neurons.

Amputation. The removal of a body extremity by trauma or surgery.

Anesthesia. A state of total unconsciousness resulting from general anesthetic drugs.

Anesthesiologist. A physician trained in anesthesia and peri-operative medicine.

Antiangiogenesis Therapy. The administration of one of two types of drugs in a new class of medicines that restores health by controlling blood vessel growth.

Antineoplastons. Chemicals derived from phenylacetate salts, phenylacetate, glutamine and isoglutamine, which are purported to combat or prevent cancer.

Anxiety Disorders. A blanket term covering several different forms of abnormal and pathological fear and anxiety.

Aortic Aneurism. A general term for any swelling (dilation or aneurysm) of the aorta, usually signifying an underlying weakness in the wall of the aorta at that location.

Aortic Valve Replacement. A cardiac surgical procedure in which a patient's failing aortic valve is substituted with a healthy valve.

Appendectomy. The surgical removal of the vermiform appendix.

Appendicitis. Inflammation of the appendix. It is thought that appendicitis begins when the opening from the appendix into the cecum becomes blocked.

Arthritis. Inflammation of one or more joints, which results in pain, swelling, stiffness and limited movement. There are over 100 different types of arthritis.

Asthma. A common chronic inflammatory disease of the airways, characterized by airflow obstruction and bronchospasm.

Astigmatism. An optical defect in which vision is blurred due to the inability of the eye to create a sharp focused image on the retina.

Atherosclerosis. A disease in which plaque builds up inside the arteries.

MEDICAL GLOSSARY

Atrial Fibrillation. An irregular and often rapid heart rhythm. This arrhythmia results from abnormal electrical impulses in the heart, and can be continuous or intermittent.

Autoimmune Disease. A disorder in which the body's immune system reacts against some of its own tissue and produces antibodies to attack itself.

Autologous Stem Cell Transplants. Stem cell transplants that utilize cells from the recipient's own body.

Ayurvedic Medicine. A system of traditional medicine native to the Indian subcontinent, practiced in other parts of the world as a form of alternative medicine. "Ayurveda" means "the science of life."

Bariatric Surgery. A type of procedure performed on patients who are dangerously obese for the purpose of losing weight.

Bariatrics. The branch of medicine that deals with the causes, prevention and treatment of obesity.

Beta Blockers. Medicines used to treat high blood pressure, congestive heart failure, abnormal heart rhythms and chest pain.

Biofeedback Therapy. A technique that trains patients to improve their health by controlling bodily processes. Biofeedback is an effective therapy for many conditions, but is primarily used to treat high blood pressure, tension headache, migraine headache, chronic pain and urinary incontinence.

Biological Therapies. A class of treatments that use biological agents to alter the body's immune system. These therapies are used to treat cancer and other illnesses.

Biopsy. The removal and examination of a sample of tissue from a living body for diagnostic purposes.

Blepharoplasty. The surgical modification of the eyelid.

Bone Marrow Transplant. A technique in which bone marrow is transplanted from one individual to another, or removed from and replaced into the same individual.

Botanical Medicine. An alternative health care option that utilizes compounds prepared from plants to treat various types of illnesses. Also known as phytotherapy.

Brain Hemorrhage. Bleeding within the brain. Also known as cerebral hemorrhage or intracerebral hemorrhage.

Breast Augmentation. A procedure which enlarges one or both breasts by installing plastic or saline implants.

Breast Cancer. Cancer originating from breast tissue, most commonly from the inner lining of milk ducts or the lobules that supply the ducts with milk.

Bronchoscopy. A procedure in which a hollow, flexible tube called a bronchoscope is inserted into the airways through the nose or mouth to provide a view of the tracheobronchial tree.

Cancer. Any malignant growth or tumor caused by abnormal and uncontrolled cell division. It may spread to other parts of the body through the lymphatic system or the blood stream.

Cardiologist. A medical doctor with special training in finding, treating and preventing diseases of the heart and blood vessels.

Cardiology. A medical specialty dealing with disorders of the heart.

Cardiomyopathy. The functional deterioration of the myocardium (heart muscle) for any reason. The term means "heart muscle disease."

Cardiothoracic Surgeon. A medical doctor who performs surgery on the heart or related blood vessels accessed through the chest (or thorax).

Cardiovascular Disease. A term used to describe a variety of heart diseases, illnesses and events that impact the heart and circulatory system, including high blood pressure and coronary artery disease.

Cataract. A clouding of the lens within the eye, causing blurred vision.

Catheter. A tube that can be inserted into a body cavity, duct or vessel. Catheters allow drainage, injection of fluids or access by surgical instruments. Catheterization is the process of inserting a catheter.

MEDICAL GLOSSARY

Chelation Therapy. The administration of chelating agents to remove heavy metals from the body.

Chemotherapy. The treatment of disease through the use of chemicals, generally by killing micro-organisms or cancerous cells.

Cerebral Palsy. A condition that affects muscle control.

Cholecystectomy. The surgical removal of the gall bladder. It is the most common method for treating symptomatic gallstones.

Cholecystitis. Inflammation of the gall bladder.

Cholesterol. HDL ("good") cholesterol is a substance found in your body that is needed to produce hormones, vitamin D and bile, and is also important for protecting the structure of cells and nerves. Having a high level of "bad" cholesterol (LDL) puts you at risk of cardiovascular disease.

Chrohn's Disease. An inflammatory disease that may affect any part of the gastrointestinal tract, causing a wide variety of symptoms.

Chronic Bronchitis. A form of bronchitis characterized by excess production of sputum, leading to a chronic cough and obstruction of air flow.

Chronic Disease. A specific disease that has lasted for longer than 3 months, and can't be cured outright.

Chronic Renal Insufficiency. The progressive loss of renal function over a period of months or years.

Chronic Respiratory Illness. A disease of long duration and slow progression, affecting the respiratory system. Symptoms may be continual or intermittent, but the patient usually has the condition for life.

Colon Cancer. A malignant tumor of the colon; early symptom is bloody stools.

Comatose. Related to or associated with a coma, as in "comatose breathing" or a "comatose state."

Congenital Abnormalities. A type of congenital disorder, primarily structural in nature, which is present at birth. Also called a "birth defect."

Congenital Heart Disease. A problem with the structure of the heart that is present at birth.

Coronary Artery Disease. A condition in which plaque builds up inside the coronary arteries.

Coronary Bypass. Open-heart surgery in which the rib cage is opened and a section of a blood vessel is grafted from the aorta to the coronary artery, to bypass the blocked section of the coronary artery and improve blood supply to the heart.

Coronary Disease. The failure of adequate coronary circulation to supply the cardiac muscle and surrounding tissue.

Cosmetic Surgery. Surgery intended to reverse or hide the effects of aging, or to improve appearance.

CNS Infection. A bacterial attack on the central nervous system, which is comprised of the brain, spinal cord and associated membranes. May result in abscesses or empyemas.

CT Scan. Also known as CAT or computerized axial tomography scan. An imaging test that provides a three-dimensional image of the brain, used to spot irregularities.

Curative Surgery. Removes a cancerous tumor or growth from the body. Surgeons use curative surgery when the tumor is localized to a specific area of the body.

Cyst. A closed sac with a distinct membrane. It may contain air, fluids or semi-solid material. A cyst may go away on its own or may have to be removed surgically.

Cystic Duct. The short duct that joins the gall bladder to the common bile duct. It is of variable length, and usually lies next to the cystic artery.

Defibrillator Implant. A cardiac medical procedure for regulating abnormal heart rhythm.

Dental Bridge. A technique used to bridge the gap between missing teeth; it is essentially a fixed partial denture.

Dental Veneer. A thin layer of restorative porcelain that is placed over the surface of a tooth to improve the aesthetics of the tooth and protect it.

MEDICAL GLOSSARY

Dentures. A prosthetic device that is supported by surrounding soft and hard tissues of the oral cavity and replaces missing teeth. They may be either fixed or partial.

Depression. A mental state signified by a sense of inadequacy and a desire to avoid activity.

Diabetes Mellitus. A chronic condition characterized by high levels of sugar (glucose) in the blood.

Diabetes Type 2. A chronic lifelong disease marked by high levels of sugar (glucose) in the blood. It is the most common form of diabetes.

Diagnostic Surgery. A procedure used to determine whether or not cells are cancerous. Tissue samples are removed for testing.

Dialysis. A process in which blood is cleansed or filtered by a dialysis machine when the kidneys are not working properly.

DMSO (Dimethylsulfoxide) Therapy. A popular form of therapy for professional athletes that can be topically applied to reduce pain and inflammation, or used broadly for relief of joint pain, muscular pain and connective tissue damage. It is also commonly used in veterinary medicine.

Drug and Alcohol Abuse. When an individual has no control over the use of drugs or alcohol.

EDTA Endrate. A chelating agent capable of removing heavy metal like lead or mercury from the blood.

Elective Surgery. Surgery that is subject to choice, whether made by the patient or doctor.

Electroconvulsive Therapy. A procedure used to treat patients with depression, in which an electric current is passed through the brain to produce controlled seizures.

Electroencephalography (EEG). A test in which electrodes are placed on the scalp, recording spontaneous electrical activity over a short period of time.

Electromyography (EMG). A technique used to evaluate and record the electrical activity produced by the skeletal muscles.

Emphysema. A long-term progressive disease of the lungs that destroys the tissue necessary to support the physical shape of the lungs, causing shortness of breath.

Endodontic Surgery. Root canals, retreatments and related procedures.

Endoluminal Grafts. A new technique for aneurysms, and an innovative development in treating abdominal aortic aneurysms and other arterial disease.

Endometrial Cancer. One of several types of malignancy which arise from the endometrium (lining of the uterus) and the most common gynecologic cancer.

Energy Therapies. A collective term which refers to a variety of alternative and complementary treatments which are based on the use, modification or manipulation of energy fields.

Epilepsy. A neurological disorder characterized by recurrent unprovoked seizures.

Excimer Laser. A form of ultraviolet laser, also called an exciplex laser, commonly used in eye surgery.

Extracorporeal Shock Wave Lithotripsy. A non-invasive treatment of kidney stones and stones in the gall bladder or liver.

Fallopian Tubes. Part of the reproductive system that transports the egg from the ovary to the uterus (womb).

Fracture. A break in bone or cartilage caused by trauma.

Frozen Embryo Transfer. A fertility procedure, in which embryos are frozen, then thawed and placed in the uterus.

Gallstones. Crystalline formations that form in the body by accretion or concretion of normal or abnormal bile components.

Gamma Knife Technique. A form of radiation therapy in which gamma rays are aimed at a focal point, such as a brain tumor, in order to stop its growth.

Gamete Intrafallopian Transfer (GIFT). A fertility treatment in which the eggs are removed from the ovaries and mixed with the man's sperm, then placed in one of the fallopian tubes. Used in conjunction with fertility drugs.

Gastrectomy. A surgery which removes part or all of the stomach, used in cases of stomach cancer, gastric ulcers or polyps.

Gastric Bypass Surgery. A surgery used to treat morbid obesity. It makes the stomach smaller and allows food to bypass part of the small intestine so the patient feels full more quickly.

Gastric Ulcer. A raw, eroded area in the lining of the stomach. Also known as a stomach ulcer.

Gastroenterologist. A physician who specializes in the diagnosis and treatment of diseases in the digestive tract.

Gynecology. A branch of medicine that deals with the study and treatment of the female reproductive system.

Heart Attack. A traumatic event which normally occurs when the blood supply to an area of heart muscle is blocked by a clot in a coronary artery. Also known as a myocardial infarction.

Heart Disease. An umbrella term for a variety of diseases affecting the heart.

Heart Failure. A long-term treatable condition in which the heart can't pump enough blood throughout the body.

Heart-Lung Machine. A device used in open heart surgery to support the body while the heart is stopped during the surgical procedure.

Heart Valve Disease. A condition in which one or more of the valves in the heart does not work as it should.

Hematologic Cancer. Cancers of the blood or bone marrow, such as leukemia and lymphoma.

Hematologist. A physician who specializes in treating conditions involving the blood.

Hemodialysis. The most common method used to treat advanced and permanent kidney failure.

Hemorrhoidectomy. A surgical procedure for hemorrhoid removal when the hemorrhoids have not responded to conservative treatments.

Hepatitus A. An infectious disease of the liver caused by the hepatitis A virus. It does not cause permanent damage to the liver.

Hepatitus B. An infectious disease of the liver caused by the hepatitis B virus, causing inflammation, vomiting and jaundice.

Hernia Repair Surgery. A surgery to correct a hernia; that is, when the large blood vessel that supplies blood to the abdomen, pelvis, and legs becomes abnormally large or balloons outward.

High Blood Pressure. A serious condition that can lead to coronary heart disease, heart failure, stroke, kidney failure and other health problems.

Hodgkin's Lymphoma. A common type of lymphoma, which is a cancer that originates in the lymphatic system.

Homeopathy. A form of treatment that uses small doses of natural substances to stimulate the immune system in the body, encouraging it to bring about healing.

Hyperbaric Oxygen Therapy. The medical use of oxygen in condensed form.

Hyperglycemia. Higher than normal levels of sugar in the blood. It occurs when the body has too little insulin or is unable to use insulin properly.

Hyperthermia. Occurs when the body produces or absorbs more heat than it can dissipate. Also know as heatstroke.

Hypertrophic Pyloric Stenosis. A narrowing of the opening from the stomach to the intestines. It is common in children, and causes severe vomiting in the first few months of life.

Hysterectomy. A surgical procedure in which the uterus (or a part of it) is removed.

Immunization. The process by which an individual's immune system becomes fortified against an agent through injection of a vaccine.

Immuno-Augmentative Therapy. A cancer therapy that involves injecting blood proteins from healthy donors into a patient.

Immunosuppressive Drugs. Drugs that suppress or inhibit the activity of the immune system.

Impulse Control Disorders. A specific group of impulsive psychiatric behaviors such as kleptomania, skin picking or compulsive gambling, in which an individual cannot refrain from performing harmful actions.

Inguinal Hernia Repair. The repair of a protrusion of abdominal cavity contents through the inguinal canal.

Intervention Therapy. A process that brings families together in times of addiction crisis. The dependent family member is generally put into an inpatient program.

Intracytoplasmic Sperm Injection. The direct injection of sperm into eggs obtained from in vitro fertilization.

In Vitro Fertilization. The fertility treatment in which egg cells are fertilized by sperm outside the womb.

Ionized Water. Drinking water that has undergone a process known as ionization, which splits the acid and alkaline content and gives the water health benefits.

Irritable Bowel Syndrome. A condition affecting the colon, or large bowel. It causes abdominal pain and chronic diarrhea or constipation.

Issels Whole Body Immunotherapy. A holistic approach to treating cancer, restoring natural immunities and resistance while also managing the symptoms.

Jaw Bone Grafting. When there is insufficient bone mass in the mouth, a bone graft from the hip or tibia is the easiest way of filling in a hole in the jaw bone or it can be obtained from a tissue bank.

Kidney Disease. A progressive loss of renal function over a period of time.

Kidney Reflux. A condition in which one or both valves in the ureters fail to work properly, causing urinary tract infections.

Knee Transplant. The removal of a damaged knee and replacement with a mechanical implant that mimics the movement of a natural knee.

L-Arginine. An amino acid that is used to make nitric oxide, which reduces blood vessel stiffness, increases blood flow and improves blood vessel function.

Laceration. A tear or cut in skin, tissue or muscle. They can be deep or shallow. Treatment varies depending on the injury.

Laparoscopic Surgery. A surgical technique in which small incisions are made in the abdomen and a laparoscope is used. Also called minimally invasive surgery or keyhole surgery.

Laser (Lasik) Eye Surgery. Laser treatment to correct certain vision problems, eliminating the need for glasses.

Laser Lithotripsy. A surgical procedure used to remove stones from the urinary tract (kidney, ureter, bladder or urethra).

Lipoplasty. A procedure that uses high frequency sound waves to liquefy fat beneath the skin's surface then suck it out.

Liposuction. A procedure in which excess fat is removed from a targeted area with a vacuum, reshaping the body.

Liquid Oxygen Systems. Portable liquid oxygen systems for patients who need supplemental oxygen; can be used at home or on the road.

Lung Cancer. A disease of uncontrolled cell growth in the tissue of the lung.

Lung Transplant. A surgical procedure in which the patient's lungs are partially or totally removed and replaced by lungs from a donor.

Lung Volume Reduction Surgery. Surgery used to improve the quality of life for certain COPD (chronic obstructive pulmonary disease) and emphysema patients by removing the part of the lung that is badly damaged, allowing the relatively good lung to expand and function better.

Lupus. An autoimmune disease in which the immune system loses the ability to differentiate foreign substances (antigens) from its own cells and tissues. The body makes antibodies which are directed towards itself; causing inflammation, injury to tissues, pain and life-threatening problems.

Lymphatic System. The system which protects the body against antigens (viruses, bacteria, etc.). It contains immune cells called lymphocytes.

Macrobiotic Nutrition. A low fat, high fiber diet that is predominantly vegetarian, with an emphasis on whole grains and vegetables. It is rich in phytoestrogens from soy products. "Macrobiotic" means "long life."

Magnetic Resonance Imaging (MRI). A diagnostic tool that produces a detailed image of the interior of a body. It aids in the diagnosis of diseases and conditions.

Malaria. A mosquito-borne infectious disease, which brings on high temperatures, shaking chills and anemia.

Mastectomy. The surgical removal of one or both breasts.

Menopause. The transition phase in a women's life when her ovaries stop producing eggs and her body produces less estrogen and progesterone.

Mental Illness. A disease or condition affecting the brain that influences the way a person thinks, feels and behaves.

Microkeratome. A highly precise surgical instrument with an oscillating blade, designed for creating the corneal flap in Lasik surgery.

Mood Disorder. A condition which leads to a person experiencing emotional highs and lows of greater intensity and for longer periods than most people experience. They can also lead to reckless behavior and suicide if not treated.

Multiplace Chamber. A form of Hyperbaric Oxygen Treatment in which more than one person can be treated at a time in a highly pressurized room.

Multiple Sclerosis. A neurological condition that affects the ability of nerve cells in the brain and spinal cord to communicate with each other, and often leads to cognitive and physical disability.

Naturopathic Obstetrics. Alternative obstetrics which promote natural prenatal care, natural childbirth and non-use of anesthesia, and less invasive interventions in birthing and postnatal care are carried out.

Naturopathy. An alternative medical system which focuses on natural remedies and the body's ability to maintain and heal itself.
Nephropathy. Damage or disease to the kidney.
Neurology. Medical specialty dealing with disorders of the nervous system.
Neurosurgeon. A physician trained in surgery of the brain and other parts of the nervous system.
Neurosurgery. Surgery that involves the nervous system (brain, spinal cord or peripheral nerves).
Nosodes. A homeopathic remedy prepared from a pathological specimen. It is an oral vaccine given to immunize the body against a specific disease.
Obesity. An excess proportion of total body fat. A person is considered obese when his or her weight is 20% or more above normal weight.
Oncologist. A medical doctor who specializes in the treatment of cancer.
Oophorectomy. The surgical removal of an ovary or ovaries.
Ophthalmologist. A medical doctor who specializes in medical and surgical eye problems.
Orthopedic surgery. A branch of surgery that deals with conditions involving the musculoskeletal system.
Osteoporosis. A disease of the bones that leads to an increased risk of fracture.
Ovarian Cancer. A cancerous growth which begins in the ovaries.
Ovary Transplant. A drastic method of restoring female fertility.
Oxygen Concentrators. A device used to provide oxygen to a patient at substantially higher concentrations than available in ambient air.
Pacemaker. A medical device that uses electrical impulses, delivered by electrodes contacting the heart muscles, to regulate the beating of the heart.
Parkinson's Disease. A degenerative disorder of the central nervous system that impairs the sufferer's motor skills, speech and other functions.
Pediatrician. A medical practitioner who specializes in pediatrics.

MEDICAL GLOSSARY

Pediatrics. The branch of medicine that deals with the medical care of infants, children and adolescents.

Peptic Ulcer. An ulcer in an area of the gastrointestinal tract that is usually acidic.

Pericarditis. An inflammation of the pericardium.

Pericardium. A double-walled sac that contains the heart and the roots of the great vessels.

Peritoneal Dialysis. A treatment for patients with severe chronic kidney failure.

Personality Disorders. Atypical behavioral patterns, usually involving several areas of the personality.

Photodynamic Therapy. A treatment that combines a light source and a photosensitizing agent (a drug that is activated by light) to destroy cancer.

Physical Medicine. A form of rehabilitative medicine implemented to achieve better physical health through practices like physical therapies, medications and other non-invasive methods.

Physical Therapy. One form of treatment for people who have functional problems resulting from conditions or injuries. The physical therapist evaluates and diagnoses movement dysfunction, and uses physical interventions to treat patients.

Physiotherapy. A profession that uses physical methods, such as massage and manipulation, to promote healing and wellbeing.

Pickwickian Syndrome. The combination of hyperventilation, red skin and drowsiness, caused by obesity.

Plastic Surgery. Aesthetic surgery which alters appearance. It includes reconstructive surgery, hand surgery, microsurgery and the treatment of burns.

Polychrest. A term used in homeopathy to mean a remedy that has many uses.

Polycystic Kidney Disease. A cystic genetic disorder of the kidneys.

Prediabetes. The condition when a person's blood glucose levels are higher than normal, but not high enough for a diagnosis of diabetes.

Pregestational Diabetes. Diabetes (Type 1 or 2) that existed when a woman became pregnant. Without glucose control in early pregnancy, the risks of miscarriage and congenital abnormalities are increased.

Presbyopia. A condition in which the eye exhibits a progressively diminished ability to focus on near objects.

Preventative Surgery. Surgery used to remove tissue that does not contain cancerous cells but that may develop into a malignant tumor.

Prosthetic. An artificial replacement for a body part, either internal or external.

Prostate Cancer. A form of cancer that develops in the prostate, a gland in the male reproductive system.

Proton Therapy. A type of particle therapy which uses a beam of protons to irradiate diseased tissue; most often used in the treatment of cancer.

Psychiatric Treatment. The medical specialty devoted to the treatment of mental disorders – affective, behavioral, cognitive and perceptual.

Psychiatrist. A physician who specializes in psychiatry and is certified in treating mental disorders.

Psychotic Disorders. Mental disorders in which the personality is severely disorganized and a person's contact with reality is impaired.

Pulmonary Arterial Hypertension. A disease of the arteries connecting the lungs to the heart (the pulmonary arteries) causing shortness of breath, chest tightness, fatigue and limited exercise capacity.

Pyloromyotomy. A surgical procedure in which an incision is made in the longitudinal and circular muscles of the pylorus. It is used to treat hypertrophic pyloric stenosis.

Radiation. Energy that travels in the form of waves or high-speed particles. Man-made radiation is used in X-rays and cancer treatment.

Radiation Therapy. The medical use of ionizing radiation, used as a part of cancer treatment to control malignant cells.

Radiologists. Medical doctors trained to diagnose disease and injury with the use of internal imaging devices such as MRI and CT scanners.

Reconstructive Surgery. The use of surgery to restore the form and function of the body.

Renal Acidosis. A medical condition involving an accumulation of acid in the body, due to the failure of the kidneys to appropriately acidify the urine.

Revici Therapy. A nontoxic chemotherapy for the treatment of cancer, using lipids, lipid-based substances and essential elements to correct an underlying imbalance.

Rhinoplasty. A surgical procedure used to improve the function (reconstructive surgery) or the appearance (cosmetic surgery) of the nose.

Sarcodes. Homeopathic medicines obtained from healthy endocrine or ductless glands, or normal secretions of living organs, human and nonhuman. The secretions are mostly hormones.

Sclerotherapy. A procedure used to treat blood vessel malformations, and those of the lymphatic system. A medicine is injected into the vessels, causing them to shrink.

Sleep Apnea. A sleep disorder characterized by pauses in breathing during sleep.

Spinal Disease. Any pathology which affects the spinal column, spinal cord or spinal nerves which are contained therein.

Spinal Fusion. A surgical technique used to attach two or more vertebrae.

Splenectomy. A surgery to remove a diseased or damaged spleen.

Staging Surgery. Surgery used to determine the location and the extent of a disease, usually cancer.

Stem Cell Therapy. A type of genetic medicine that introduces new cells into damaged tissue in order to treat a disease or injury.

Stent. An artificial tube inserted into a natural passage/conduit in the body to prevent or counteract a disease-induced, localized flow constriction.

Stroke. The rapidly developing loss of brain function(s) due to a disturbance in the blood supply to the brain.

Syngeneic Stem Cell Transplant. A procedure in which a patient receives blood-forming stem cells (cells from which all blood cells develop) donated by his or her healthy identical twin.

Thermal Biofeedback. The monitoring of skin temperature as an index of blood flow changes.

Ureteropyeloscopy. A method of minimally invasive surgery. A technique that permits access to the internal organs without the use of a customary large incision.

Vaccination. The administration of antigenic material (a vaccine) to produce immunity to a disease.

Valvuloplasty. A procedure in which a small balloon is inserted and inflated to stretch and open a narrowed (stenosed) heart valve.

Vascular Surgeon. A surgeon who deals with special surgery in which diseases of the vascular system, or arteries and veins, are managed by medical therapy, minimally-invasive catheter procedures and surgical reconstruction.

Wellness. The active process of becoming aware of and making choices toward a more successful existence.

Wheatgrass Therapy. An alternative cancer treatment using wheatgrass.

X-Ray. A form of electromagnetic radiation, similar to light but with a shorter wavelength, which can penetrate solids; used for imaging solid structures inside the body.

Yellow Fever. An acute viral hemorrhagic disease, transmitted by the bite of female mosquitoes.

Resources for the Medical Traveler

All Medical Tourism

www.allmedicaltourism.com

This has become a trusted resource for medical tourism and surgery abroad, where you will find standardized information on prices and high quality health care from different countries around the world.

eMedicineHealth

www.emedicinehealth.com

This consumer health information site contains health and medical articles written by physicians for patients and consumers.

Global Medical Service Inc.

www.globalsurgerycenter.com

If you're looking for affordable cosmetic or weight loss surgery outside of the U.S., these industry professionals will simplify the process and provide you with high quality medical services performed by some of the best surgeons in the world.

Healism

www.healism.com

This is a very informative and interactive website run by highly trained professionals. It will answer your questions and address your concerns, helping you find out what the best options are for you as a medical traveler.

Healthbase

www.healthbase.com

This is an award-winning medical tourism company and a great resource if you're looking for alternative health care abroad. They will arrange first-class services abroad for you.

Health Travel Guides

www.healthtravelguides.com

A good travel company and resource, facilitating high-quality affordable care for the medical tourist.

Life Smile India

www.lifesmileindia.com

This is one of the best resources on the Internet, managed by highly experienced medical and life sciences professionals. They deliver high-quality services to the medical traveler, using sophisticated technology and an experienced team of professionals.

Mayo Clinic

www.mayoclinic.org/international

This is the first and biggest non-profit group practice in the world, where specialty doctors work together to care for patients. It's also one of the best resources on the Internet if you want to find out more about your condition.

Med Retreat

www.medretreat.com

If you're looking for a trusted medical tourism company that will simplify and take care of all your healthcare needs, Med Retreat offer various medical travel programs for American patients. You will receive successful and safe medical procedures at world-class healthcare facilities, at a fraction of the cost in the U.S.

Med Terms
www.medterms.com

This is a great medical dictionary, and serves as a medical reference for MedicineNet.com. It breaks down medical language into easy-to-understand terms.

MedicineNet.com
www.medicinenet.com

This is a nationally recognized online healthcare publishing company that offers insight into medicine, Internet technology and business. The content is produced by a network of seventy board-certified physicians, bringing you the latest in healthcare.

Medical Tourism
http://medicaltourism.com

This website is full of reliable information that will give you a better understanding of medical tourism, costs and countries, and can connect you with medical tourism companies that fit your requirements.

Medical Tourism Companies
www.medicaltourismcompanies.net

This site outlines and reviews medical tourism companies and procedures and is a great reference website for the medical traveler, helping you make an informed decision.

Medical Tourism Corporation
www.medicaltourismco.com

This is an international medical travel company, based in Texas, that will help to get you the best medical care abroad.

Medical Travel

http://medicaltravel.pl

This website offers world class treatment services at excellent prices. They also guarantee patient safety, and offer high quality technology with professional care and experienced doctors. Great if you need dentistry or cosmetic procedures.

MedlinePlus

http://medlineplus.gov/

This is a comprehensive medical resource produced by the National Library of Medicine, the world's largest medical library. You will find information on diseases, conditions, wellness, new treatments, and medical videos and illustrations.

Placidway

www.placidway.com

This is a helpful website offering the medical tourist a variety of high-quality destinations at affordable prices. Packages and free quotes are also available.

Surgeon and Safari

www.surgeon-and-safari.co.za

If you are looking for private health care, first-world infrastructure and personalized after care, this is an excellent medical retreat and facilitation service in South Africa with world class surgeons. Lorraine Melvill will be there to help and assist you with every detail of your surgery and stay.

WebMD

www.webmd.com

This is an informative health website that provides quality health information and up-to-date news on health issues. This is a credible and trustworthy source for medical information.

WorldMedAssist

www.worldmedassist.com

This is a leading medical tourism company, offering affordable options for high-quality treatments, tailor-made to your unique situation. It is also contracted to many of the JCI-accredited hospitals.

Endnotes

Notes on Chapter One

1. Dorgan, Byron, *The Patient Protection and Affordable Care Act,* http://dpc.senate.gov/dpcdoc-sen_health_care_bill.cfm (2009).
2. Rasmussen Reports, *Health Care Reform,* http://www.rasmussenreports.com/public_content/politics/current_events/healthcare/september_2009/health_care_reform (March 2010).
3. Tobin, Maryann, *Obama's Health Care Bill Will Save Money, Control Insurance Companies and Make History,* http://www.examiner.com/x-33986-Political-Spin-Examiner~y2010m3d19-Obamas-health-care-bill-will-save-money-control-insurance-companies-and-make-history, (March 2010).
4. Murdock, Patrick, *The Evolution of Health Care Control,* http://www.campaignforliberty.com/article.php?view=567, (January 2010).
5. Feldstein, Martin, *Obamacare is All About Rationing,* http://online.wsj.com/article/SB10001424052970204683204574358233780260914.html (August 2009).
6. Lane, Moe, *Obamacare to Overwhelm Emergency Rooms,* http://www.redstate.com/moe_lane/2010/05/17/obamacare-to-overwhelm-emergency-rooms/ (May 2010).
7. Coburn, Tom, *The Stimulus Package is More Debt We Don't Need,* Wall Street Journal, http://online.wsj.com/article/SB123371083449746103.html (February 2009).
8. Tawney, Stephen, *Private Insurance Company Shuts Down Due to Obamacare,* The American Pundit, http://amerpundit.com/2010/06/08/private-insurance-company-shuts-down-due-to-obamacare/ (June 2010).

9. Crouse, Janice, *Obamacare is Tyranny, Not Legislation*, American Thinker, http://www.americanthinker.com/2010/03/obamacare_is_tyranny_not_legis.html (March 2010).
10. Cheplick, Thomas, *Obamacare Expected to increase Loss of Doctor Owned Practices*, Health Care News, http://www.heartland.org/healthpolicy-news.org/article/27508/Obamacare_Expected_to_Increase_Loss_of_DoctorOwned_Practices.html (June 2010).
11. Binder, Jeffrey, *Specialists Under Fire: Health Care Reform Takes Aim at the Most Highly-Trained Physicians*, http://www.biomet.com/corporate/ceoBlog/postDetail.cfm?postID=39 (August 2009).
12. Kristian, Bonnie, *Obamacare Will Implicitly Tax the Middle Class*, Young Americans For Liberty, http://www.yaliberty.org/posts/obamacare-will-implicitly-tax-the-middle-class (April 2010).
13. Goldberg, John, *The Reality of Obamacare*, Los Angeles Times, http://articles.latimes.com/2010/mar/23/opinion/la-oe-goldberg23-2010mar23 (March 2010).
14. Portnoy, Howard, *Is More Government Control the Answer to the Problem of Childhood Obesity?* The Examiner, http://www.examiner.com/examiner/x-34929-Manhattan-Conservative-Examiner~y2010m5d12-Is-more-government-intervention-the-answer-to-the-problem-of-childhood-obesity (May 2010).
15. Aron, Judy, *The Obamacare Vaccination Squad*, http://yedies.blogspot.com/2009/07/obamacare-vaccination-squad.html (July 2009).
16. Richards, Hank, *Help Wanted Doctors: Fast-forward, Five Years into Obamacare*, The Examiner, http://www.examiner.com/x-43399-Huntsville-Conservative-Examiner~y2010m4d30-Help-Wanted--Doctors-Obamacare-fastforward-five-years?cid=exrss-Huntsville-Conservative-Examiner (April 2010).
17. Pinkerton, James, *Why Obamacare Will Fail and the Media Will Fail to Notice Its Flaws*, FOXNews.com, http://www.foxnews.com/

opinion/2009/09/08/james-pinkerton-obama-health-care-media/ (September 2009).
18. Limbaugh, David, *Obamacare Equals Socialism on Steroids*, Newsmax, http://www.newsmax.com/Limbaugh/Obama-Obamacare-healthcare-public/2010/05/13/id/358958 (May 2010).
19. Moosa, EJ, *How to Destroy the Private Sector via Health Care Reform*, http://www.nolanchart.com/article7530.html (March 2010).
20. Kelly, Brian, *Obamacare is Full Government Control*, http://www.briankellyforcongress.com/index.php?option=com_content&view=article&id=98&Itemid=83 (March 2010).
21. JDT, *Obamacare Bans New Doctor Owned Hospitals*, http://speaknowamerica.org/2010/04/12/obamacare-bans-new-doctor-owned-hospitals.aspx (April 2010).
22. Merits, GJ, *For Obamacare's Impact Look to Canada and Great Britain*, http://www.wolvesofliberty.com/2010/06/02/for-obamacares-impact-look-to-canada-and-great-britain/ (June 2010).
23. Pear, Robert, *Coverage for Sick Children? Check the Fine Print*, NYTimes, http://www.nytimes.com/2010/03/29/health/policy/29health.html (March 2010).
24. Pundit, Allah, *Great News: CBO Says Obamacare Will Cost $115 Billion More than Thought*, http://hotair.com/archives/2010/05/11/great-news-cbo-says-obamacare-will-cost-115-billion-more-than-thought/ (May 2010).
25. Nix, Kathryn, *CBO: Obamacare Unlikely to Reduce Spending on Healthcare*, http://fixhealthcarepolicy.com/in-the-news/cbo-obamacare-unlikely-to-reduce-spending-on-health-care/ (July 2010).
26. Little, Richard, *The Obamacare Acceptance Strategy*, http://www.americanthinker.com/2010/03/the_obamacare_acceptance_strat.html (March 2010).
27. Editorial, *Obamacare Would Hurt Small Business*, Washington

Examiner, http://www.washingtonexaminer.com/opinion/Obamacare-would-hurt-small-business-7954840-50488667.html (July 2009).

28. Ruberry, John, *Obamacare Already Hurting Small Business*, http://marathonpundit.blogspot.com/2010/03/obamacare-already-hurting-small.html (March 2010).

29. Malkin, Michelle, *Inside the Monstrous Obamacare Bureaucracy*, http://townhall.com/columnists/MichelleMalkin/2009/07/17/inside_the_monstrous_obamacare_bureaucracy/page/full (July 2009).

30. Morris, Dick, *Obamacare: Taxes for Everyone*, http://thehill.com/opinion/columnists/dick-morris/59853-obamacare-taxes-for-everyone (September 2009).

31. Gottlieb, Scott, *You're Losing Your Plan: Obamacare's True Face Emerges*, New York Post, http://www.nypost.com/p/news/opinion/opedcolumnists/you_re_losing_your_plan_O2H1EFmYlHSoQmqp48uDHI (June 2010).

32. Tanner, Michael, *Perils of Obamacare: Three Big Lies*, http://www.cato.org/pub_display.php?pub_id=10367 (July 2009).

33. Klein, Joseph, *Much Less Access to Decent Health Care under Obamacare*, http://www.newsrealblog.com/2010/03/18/less-access-to-decent-health-care-under-obamacare/ (March 2010).

34. Calle, Brian, *Keep the Heart of Innovation Pumping*, http://www.ocregister.com/opinion/-249916--.html (May 2010).

35. White, Tom, *UK Woman Punished for Paying Private Doctor – an Obamacare Preview*, http://www.varight.com/health/uk-woman-punished-for-paying-for-private-doctor-an-obamacare-preview/ (April 2010).

36. Ackerman, Todd, *Texas Doctors Opting out of Medicare at Alarming Rate*, Houston Chronicle, http://www.chron.com/disp/story.mpl/metropolitan/7009807.html (May 2010).

37. Bloom, Stephen, *A Dangerous Cure: Seven Obamacare Health Myths*,

http://www.crosswalk.com/news/commentary/11606388/ (July 2009).

38. Staff Contribution, *What Lies Beneath*, http://spectator.org/archives/2010/04/26/what-lies-beneath (April 2010).

39. Wall Street Journal, *The War on Specialists*, http://online.wsj.com/article/SB10001424052748704471504574443472658898710.html (October 2009).

40. Limbaugh, Rush, *Shazam! Obamacare Will Mean Lost Insurance, Won't Cut Deficit*, http://www.rushlimbaugh.com/home/daily/site_050710/content/01125109.guest.html (May 2010).

41. Morris, Dick, *High Price of Obamacare*, http://thehill.com/opinion/columnists/dick-morris/62893-high-price-of-obamacare (October 2009).

42. Orient, Dr. Jane, *Obamacare: Embattled Doctors and Patients*, http://www.thenewamerican.com/index.php/usnews/health-care/3405-obamacare-embattled-doctors-a-patients (April 2010).

43. Nix, Kathryn, *Obamacare Increases Unemployment, Insurance Premiums, Deficit and Debt*, http://fixhealthcarepolicy.com/in-the-news/obamacare-increases-unemployment-insurance-premiums-deficit-and-debt/ (March 2010).

44. *AT&T to Take $1 Bln Charge on Health-Care Bill*, http://www.marketwatch.com/story/att-to-take-1-bln-charge-on-health-care-bill-2010-03-26-1411190 (March 2010).

45. Suderman, Peter, *Employers Expect Costs to Rise under Obamacare*, http://reason.com/blog/2010/06/01/employers-expect-costs-to-rise (June 2010).

46. Weckesser, Bill, *Obamacare: Rack and Ruin for Small Business*, http://www.americanthinker.com/blog/2010/03/obamacare_rack_and_ruin_for_sm.html (March 2010).

47. Domenech, Ben, *Exempted from Obamacare: Senior Staff Who Wrote the Bill*, http://newledger.com/2010/03/exempted-from-obamacare-senior-staff-who-wrote-the-bill/ (March 2010).

48. Skorburg, John, *Obamacare Tanning Salon Tax Kicks In, Violates President's Pledge*, http://www.heartland.org/healthpolicy-news.org/article/27820/Obamacare_Tanning_Salon_Tax_Kicks_In_Violates_Presidents_Pledge.html (June 2010).
49. Cannon, Michael, *Dear Pool People: Please Remain Poor. Sincerely, Obamacare*, http://www.cato-at-liberty.org/2010/01/13/dear-poor-people-please-remain-poor-sincerely-obamacare/ (January 2010).
50. Fuller, C, *Obamacare's Economic Dominoes*, http://www.americanthinker.com/2010/04/obamacares_economic_dominoes.html (April 2010).
51. *Jail and/or $25K Fine for Refusing Obamacare*, World Finance News, http://ceogroups.net/2010/05/jail-andor-25k-fine-for-refusing-obamacare/ (May 2010).
52. Watson, Paul, *ADL Calls for Major Law Enforcement Operation to Deal with Obamacare Critics*, http://www.prisonplanet.com/adl-calls-for-major-law-enforcement-operation-to-deal-with-obamacare-critics.html (April 2010).
53. Watson, Joseph, *Under Obamacare Prepare to Wait 18 Months to See a Doctor*, http://www.infowars.com/under-obamacare-prepare-to-wait-18-months-to-see-a-doctor/ (December 2009).
54. Carroll, Conn, *Obama Knows Obamacare Increases Government Control, Right?* http://blog.heritage.org/2010/02/10/obama-knows-obamacare-increases-government-control-right/ (February 2010).
55. Barone, Michael, *With Absolute Power, Team Obama Grows Stupid*, Washington Examiner, http://www.washingtonexaminer.com/politics/With-absolute-power_-Team-Obama-grows-stupid-83945567.html (February 2010).
56. Carney, Tim, *AP: Big Pharma Hits the Jackpot with Obamacare*, http://www.washingtonexaminer.com/opinion/blogs/beltway-confidential/AP-Pharma-hits-the-jackpot-with-ObamaCare-89412682.html (March 2010).

57. Berlau, John, *Obamacare Equals Huge Tax Hike on OTC Drugs*, http://www.heartland.org/full/26629/ObamaCare_Equals_Huge_Tax_Hike_on_OTC_Drugs.html (December 2009).
58. Nimmo, Kurt, *Obamacare: It's about Enriching the Bankers and Wall Street*, http://www.infowars.com/obamacare-its-about-enriching-bankers-and-wall-street/ (March 2010).
59. Rall, Ted, *Obamacare! Bill a Bailout for Insurers, Disastrous for Americans*, http://www.boiseweekly.com/boise/obamacare/Content?oid=1532522 (March 2010).
60. Ralston, Richard, *Obamacare Contorts the Constitution*, http://www.ocregister.com/articles/government-250369-insurance-constitution.html (May 2010).
61. Lendman, Stephen, *Obamacare: A Health Care Rationing Scheme to Enrich Insurers, Drug Companies and Large Hospital Chains*, http://www.globalresearch.ca/index.php?context=va&aid=14444 (July 2009).
62. Smithwick, Benjamin, *The Fight to Repeal Obamacare*, http://www.humanevents.com/article.php?id=37698 (May 2010).
63. Schlafly, Phyllis, *Obamacare Versus Freedom*, http://townhall.com/columnists/PhyllisSchlafly/2010/03/23/obamacare_versus_freedom (2010).
64. Paul, Ron, *We Need Free-Market Healthcare, Not Obamacare*, http://www.ronpaul.com/2010-03-22/we-need-free-market-healthcare-not-obamacare/ (March 2010).
65. Fazio, Ryan, *Why Obamacare is Bad For Young Adults Part 2*, http://www.chron.org/2010/06/why-obamacare-is-bad-for-young-adults-part-ii/ (June 2010).
66. O'Hara, Shefali, *Obamacare and your Family –the Good, the Bad and the Ugly*, http://www.examiner.com/x-4365-Austin-Marriage-Examiner~y2010m3d24-Obamacare-and-your-Family--the-Good-

the-Bad-and-the-Ugly (March 2010).

67. Steve, *Doctor Discusses Problems with Obamacare, Liberty Central*, http://www.libertycentral.org/doctor-discusses-problems-with-obamacare-2010-06 (June 2010).
68. *Obamacare's Worst Tax Hike, Wall Street Journal*, http://online.wsj.com/article/SB10001424052748704131404575117623860083574.html?mod=djemEd%20itorialPage_h (March 2010).
69. John, *Stupak vs. Waxman: Obamacare Uses Tax Money to Pay for Abortions*, http://www.verumserum.com/?p=12925 (March 2010).
70. Cotter, Dianna, *Why is Obamacare Unconstitutional?* The Examiner, http://www.examiner.com/x-7715-Portland-Civil-Rights-Examiner~y2010m4d7-Why-is-Obamacare-unconstitutional (April 2010).
71. Carney, Timothy, *Student Loans get the Obamacare Treatment*, Washington Examiner, http://www.washingtonexaminer.com/opinion/columns/Student-loans-get-the-Obamacare-treatment-88460757.html (March 2010).
72. Jeffrey, Terence, *Sen. Hatch Questions Constitutionality of Obamacare*, http://www.cnsnews.com/news/article/56447 (November 2009).
73. Hennenfent, Dr. Bradley, *Obamacare Will Kill Future Patients Compared to What Could Be*, http://bradmd.blogspot.com/2010/03/obamacare-will-kill-future-patients.html (March 2010).

Notes on Chapter Two

74. *If Obamacare is Bad, Why is Stock in Big Health Insurance Companies Going Up?* http://urbanelephants.com/index.php/component/content/article/64/2425-if-obamacare-is-bad-why-is-stock-in-big-health-insurance-companies-going-up.html (March 2010).
75. Bernard, Stephen, *Health Stocks Rise after Passage of Health Care Reform Bill*, http://www.huffingtonpost.com/2010/03/22/health-stocks-rise-after_n_508256.html (March 2010).

76. Moncrief, Anita, *Obama, ACORN and Stealth Socialism*, http://hotair.com/archives/2010/05/29/obama-acorn-and-stealth-socialism-dire-domestic-threat/ (May 2010).
77. Zahn, Drew, *Obamacare Hospitals Killed: 60, with 200 on Life Support*, http://www.wnd.com/index.php?fa=PAGE.printable&pageId=153941 (May 2010).
78. *Side Effects: Physician-Owned Hospitals Face New Regulations, Limits on Growth*, http://fixhealthcarepolicy.com/tag/doctor-shortage/ (May 2010).
79. *Big Pharma Sells Out*, http://online.wsj.com/article/SB10001424052748704782304574541841256040358.html (November 2009).
80. Dollard, Pat, *Obamacare Hidden Provision Shocker*, http://www.sodahead.com/united-states/obamacare-hidden-provision-shocker/blog-287321/ (March 2010).
81. Lonely Conservative, *Obamacare Will Force Small Businesses to Issue Millions of Extra 1099s*, http://lonelyconservative.com/2010/05/obamacare-will-force-small-businesses-to-issue-millions-of-extra-1099s/ (May 2010).
82. Scatigna, Lou, *Obamacare Prescription: Emergency Health Army*, http://www.thefinancialphysician.com/blog/?p=2495 (March 2010).
83. *Ready Reserve Corps (Private Army) in Obamacare Bill*, http://www.dailypaul.com/node/130157 (March 2010).
84. Watson, Bruce, *With Obamacare, Calorie Counters Find a Strange Ally: Fast Food Restaurants*, http://www.dailyfinance.com/story/company-news/with-obama-care-calorie-counters-find-a-strange-ally-fast-food/19413142/ (March 2010).
85. Smith, Wesley, *Obamacare: Taxing Cosmetic Surgery*, http://www.firstthings.com/blogs/secondhandsmoke/2009/11/19/obamacare-taxing-cosmetic-surgery/ (November 2009).
86. *Obamacare Tax Targets Women Business Owners*, http://www.

cosmopolitanconservative.com/2010/03/24/obamacare-tax-targets-women-business-owners/ (March 2010).

87. Wolverton, Joe, *Obamacare and Taxes: Promises Broken*, http://www.thenewamerican.com/index.php/usnews/health-care/3295-obamacare-and-taxes-promises-broken (April 2010).

88. Domenech, Ben, *Will Obamacare Create Two Americas?* http://www.cbsnews.com/stories/2010/03/15/opinion/main6300344.shtml (March 2010).

89. *Obama Today on Obamacare: Most Lies in a Presidential Speech in American History*, http://www.redstate.com/ahffgeoff/2010/03/19/obama-today-on-obamacare-most-lies-in-a-presidential-speech-in-american-history/ (March 2010).

90. *$222 Billion, Ho Hum*, http://online.wsj.com/article/SB10001424052748703652104574652563562216036.html (January 2010).

91. Pethokoukis, James, *How Obamacare is Killing Free Trade*, http://blogs.reuters.com/james-pethokoukis/2010/03/10/how-obamacare-is-killing-free-trade/ (March 2010).

92. Graham, John, *Critical Condition: Let the Gaming Begin: How the Sick Will Suffer under Obamacare*, http://www.nationalreview.com/critical-condition/47303/let-gaming-begin-how-sick-will-suffer-under-obamacare/john-r-graham (April 2010).

93. Murrin, David, *Obamacare Sign of U.S. Empire Decline, Economic Expert Says*, http://illinoisreview.typepad.com/illinoisreview/2010/03/obamacare-sign-of-us-empire-decline-economic-expert-says.html (March 2010).

Notes on Chapter Three

94. *Specter of Doctor Shortage Looms over Obamacare*, http://www.newsmax.com/Headline/doctor-shortage-healthcare-reform/2010/03/28/id/354034 (March 2010).

95. Carroll, Conn, *Morning Bell: Obamacare's Effect on Seniors*, http://blog.heritage.org/2009/07/28/morning-bell-obamacares-effect-on-seniors/ (July 2009).
96. Stossel, John, *A Glimpse of the Obamacare Future*, http://stossel.blogs.foxbusiness.com/2010/07/01/a-glimpse-of-the-obamacare-future/ (July 2010).
97. National Institute of Mental Health, *Suicide in the U.S. Statistics and Prevention*, http://www.nimh.nih.gov/health/publications/suicide-in-the-us-statistics-and-prevention/index.shtml (2009).
98. Editorial, *Obamacare Meets the Reality of Nationalized Health Care: Rationing and Long Lines*, http://www.washingtonexaminer.com/opinion/Obamacare-meets-the-reality-of--48764587.html (June 2009).
99. Morris, Dick and Eileen McGann, *Here Comes Health Care Rationing*, http://www.dickmorris.com/blog/2009/06/06/here-comes-health-care-rationing/ (June 2010).
100. *Obamacare: Doctors Refusing New Medicare Patients Because of Low Government Reimbursement Setting New High*, http://theblogprof.blogspot.com/2010/06/obamacare-doctors-refusing-new-medicare.html (June 2010).
101. Pipes, Sally, *Mass Health Meltdown is Your Future*, http://www.nypost.com/p/news/opinion/opedcolumnists/mass_health_meltdown_is_your_future_qA65Dx77kppzP5lHJN23pN (May 2010).
102. Vidal, Gabriel, *Why Obamacare Can't Work: The Calculation Argument*, http://mises.org/daily/3543 (July 2009).
103. Reed, John, *Obama's You've Had a Good Life Now Drop Dead Plan: Preventative Medicine*, http://www.johntreed.com/Obamapreventive.html (2010).
104. Benchener, Matt, *Obamacare's Impact on Obesity, Liberty and Cost*, http://thebulletin.us/articles/2009/08/10/commentary/op-eds/doc4a8064c80fd5f937691673.txt (August 2009).

ENDNOTES

105. Jones, Susan, *Fighting Obesity is at the Heart of Obama's Plan to Provide Better and Lower Cost Healthcare*, http://www.cnsnews.com/public/content/article.aspx?RsrcID=51675 (July 2009).
106. Price, Josh, *The Freedoms Lost to Obamacare*, http://theconservativebeacon.net/2010/03/23/the-freedoms-lost-to-obamacare/ (March 2010).
107. Unrah, Bob, *Obamacare's Control Plan? Behavior Modification*, http://www.wnd.com/?pageId=167317 (June 2010).
108. Costa, Robert, *House GOP: Obamacare's IRS Connection*, http://www.nationalreview.com/critical-condition/47375/house-gop-obamacares-irs-connection/robert-costa (March 2010).
109. Best, Dr. Steve, *Neo-McCarthyism, the Patriot Act and the New Surveillance Culture*, http://www.animalliberationfront.com/ALFront/AgainstALF/PatriotAct.htm (2008).
110. *Gallup: Majority Don't Want Obama Re-elected*, http://www.newsmax.com/InsideCover/gallup-obama-reelection-independents/2010/06/18/id/362442?s=al&promo_code=A1BA-1 (June 2010).
111. Pipes, Sally, *Obamacare Wins: Now the Pain Begins*, http://www.nypost.com/p/news/opinion/opedcolumnists/obamacare_wins_TeY4JN6V6eJk9ALVwmPYbK (March 2010).
112. Connolly, Michael, *Obamacare – It's Not about Healthcare*, http://www.sodahead.com/united-states/obamacare---its-not-about-healthcare--/blog-160329/ (September 2009).
113. Tanner, Michael, *Lessons from the Fall of Romneycare*, http://www.cato.org/pubs/policy_report/v30n1/cpr30n1-1.html (February 2008).
114. *Side Effects: Obamacare Fueling Higher Insurance Costs*, http://blog.heritage.org/2010/04/05/side-effects-obamacare-fueling-higher-insurance-costs/ (April 2010).
115. Mills, Stephanie, *Obamacare: College Kids Will Get Hit Hard*, http://www.vutorch.com/?p=458 (September 2009).
116. Capretta, James, *Obamacare: Impact on Future Generations*,

http://www.heritage.org/Research/Reports/2010/06/Obamacare-Impact-on-Future-Generations (June 2010).

117. Cross, Melissa, *Death, Taxes and Two Trillion Lies*, http://www.americanthinker.com/2009/10/death_taxes_and_two_trillion_1.html (October 2009).

118. Goodman, John, *Medical Tourism –A Solution for Healthcare*, http://medicaltourismmag.com/issue-article/solution.html (July 2010).

119. Sehgal, Neka, *U.S. Healthcare System Ranks Worst in Global Survey*, http://www.themoneytimes.com/featured/20100624/us-health-care-system-ranks-worst-global-survey-id-10118512.html (June 2010).

120. Herrick, Devon, *Medical Tourism: Global Competition in Health Care*, http://www.ncpa.org/pub/st304?pg=6 (November 2007).

121. Paulson, Matthew, *Medical Tourism: Getting Healthcare Overseas to Save Money*, http://www.associatedcontent.com/article/382701/medical_tourism_getting_healthcare.html?cat=5 (September 2007).

122. Parker-Pope, Tara, *Medical Bills Cause Most Bankruptcies*, http://well.blogs.nytimes.com/2009/06/04/medical-bills-cause-most-bankruptcies/ (June 2009).

123. *Cosmetic Surgery Tourism Briefing Paper*, http://www.plasticsurgery.org/Media/Briefing_Papers/Cosmetic_Surgery_Tourism.html (June 2009).

124. Flaherty, Matt, *Millions of Americans Look Outside U.S. for Drugs Desire for Low Prices Often Outweighs Obeying Law*, http://www.opioids.com/offshorepharmacy/overseas.html (2003).

125. Khoury, Christopher, *Americans Consider Crossing Borders for Medical Care*, http://www.gallup.com/poll/118423/americans-consider-crossing-borders-medical-care.aspx (May 2009).

126. *Puerto Vallarta Mexico Gastric Bypass Surgery*, http://www.medicaltourismco.com/weight-loss/puerto-vallarta-gastric-bypass-surgery-testimonial.php (2010).

Notes on Chapter Four

127. *Medical Tourism*, http://www.medic8.com/medical-tourism/index.html (2009).
128. Pilling, Jennifer, *Why Many Americans are Electing to Travel Abroad for Healthcare*, http://www.rt-image.com/1016Tourism (2006).
129. *Cosmetic Surgery Insurance*, http://www.professional-and-liability.com/cosmetic-surgery-insurance.html (2008).
130. *Health Plans Refuse Coverage for Laser Eye Surgery*, http://www.insure.com/articles/healthinsurance/laser-eye-surgery.html (March 2008).
131. CPR Staff, *Obamacare's Mounting Tax Burden Punishes Families, Small Business*, http://www.cprights.org/2010/06/obamacares-mounting-tax-burden-punishes-families-small-business.php (June 2010).
132. *Air Ambulance Services*, http://www.airambulance.net/ (2010).
133. *Guide to Diagnostic Tests*, Harvard Health Publications, http://www.health.harvard.edu/diagnostic-tests/?URL=/diagnostic-tests/back-x-rays.htm (2010).
134. *Different Types of Air Ambulances*, Air Ambulance Services, http://air-ambulance-resources.com/types-of-air-ambulances.php (2010).
135. *Chronic Disease Prevention and Health Promotion*, http://www.cdc.gov/chronicdisease/index.htm (2009).
136. Van Dusen, Allison, *America's Most Expensive Medical Conditions*, http://www.forbes.com/2008/02/06/health-diseases-expensive-forbeslife-cx_avd_0206health.html (February 2008).
137. *More than 50% of Americans Have a Chronic Health Condition!* http://weightoftheevidence.blogspot.com/2008/06/more-than-50-of-americans-have-chronic.html (June 2008).
138. *Diabetes*, E-medicine Health, http://www.emedicinehealth.com/diabetes/article_em.htm (2010).
139. *Complementary and Alternative Medicine*, http://www.nlm.nih.gov/medlineplus/complementaryandalternativemedicine.html (2010).

140. Jaroff, Leon, *Wasting Big Bucks on Alternative Medicine*, http://www.time.com/time/columnist/jaroff/article/0,9565,237613,00.html (May 2002).
141. *The History of Acupuncture*, http://www.americanacupuncture.com/history.htm (2007).
142. Dharmananda, Dr. Subhuti, *Countering the Side Effects of Modern Medical Therapies with Chinese Herbs*, http://www.itmonline.org/arts/sidefx.htm (September 1998).
143. *Medical Spa Treatment Abroad*, http://www.placidway.com/search/,Medical%20Spa%20Treatment,/search.html (2010).
144. Gahlinger, Dr. Paul, *Part 1 What Your Doctor Doesn't Know About Medical Tourism*, The Medical Tourism Travel Guide, 10-13 (2008).
145. *Is Medical Tourism Dangerous?* http://www.healism.com/blogs/the_stanley_rubenti_medical_tourism_blog/is_medical_tourism_dangerous?/ (2010).
146. Allen, Arthur, *Europe is Killing off Hospital Infections. Why isn't the United States Following Suit?* http://www.slate.com/id/2152118 (October 2006).
147. *Medical Tourism*, http://www.medtourismreview.com/ (2010).
148. *Hospitals*, https://www.healthbase.com/hb/pages/hospitals.jsp (2007).
149. Perry, Mark, *Medical Tourism: Comparable to How Competition Changed the U.S. Auto Industry*, http://www.britannica.com/blogs/2009/02/medical-tourism-comparable-to-how-competition-changed-the-us-auto-industry/ (February 2009).

Notes on Chapter Five

150. *Having Surgery? What You Need to Know*, http://www.ahrq.gov/consumer/surgery/surgery.htm (2008).
151. *Breast Augmentation and Breast Implant Info*, http://www.breastaugmentation.com/ (2010).

ENDNOTES

152. *Facelift Surgery – Rejuvenate Your Appearance*, http://www.your plasticsurgeryguide.com/face-lift/ (June 2010).
153. *What is Liposuction?* http://www.liposuction.com/ (2010).
154. *Nose Surgery (Rhinoplasty)*, http://www.docshop.com/education/cosmetic/face/rhinoplasty/ (2008).
155. *Endodontic Surgery: Save the Tooth*, http://endodonticsurgery.net/ (2010).
156. *Tooth Extraction*, http://www.mynewsmile.com/dental/tooth_extraction.htm (2010).
157. *Dental Bridges*, http://www.docshop.com/education/dental/general-dentistry/bridges/ (2008).
158. *Teeth Whitening and Cosmetic Dentistry*, http://dentistry.about.com/od/cosmeticdentistry/Teeth_Whitening_and_Cosmetic_Dentistry.htm (2010).
159. Soni, Dr. Mukesh, *Porcelain Veneers for Smile Makeovers*, http://www.cosmeticdentistryguide.co.uk/veneers.html (2008).
160. *Gum Disease*, http://hcd2.bupa.co.uk/fact_sheets/html/gum_disease.html (June 2009).
161. *Hip Replacement*, http://www.nlm.nih.gov/medlineplus/hipreplacement.html (April 2010).
162. *Hysterectomy*, http://www.nyhealth.gov/community/adults/women/hysterectomy/ (January 2010).
163. *IVF*, http://www.sharedjourney.com/ivf.html (2010).
164. *Frozen Embryo Transfer, FET Cycles after IVF*, http://www.advancedfertility.com/fet-cycle.htm (2010).
165. GIFT (Gamete Intra-Fallopian Transfer), http://www.infertile.com/infertility-treatments/gift.htm (2010)
166. *Laser Eye Surgery*, http://www.aboutlasereyesurgery.com/ (July 2010).

Notes on Chapter Six

167. *General Surgery Articles*, http://emedicine.medscape.com/general_surgery (2010).

168. Timpone, Dr. Peter, *Emergency Gastrectomy in the Surgical Treatment of Perforated Peptic Ulcer*, http://www3.interscience.wiley.com/journal/120171195/abstract?CRETRY=1&SRETRY=0 (June 2008).

169. *Gallbladder Removal*, http://www.healthsquare.com/mc/fgmc6007.htm (2010).

170. *Appendectomy*, http://www.nlm.nih.gov/medlineplus/ency/article/002921.htm (2009).

171. *Inguinal Hernia*, http://digestive.niddk.nih.gov/ddiseases/pubs/inguinalhernia/ (2008).

172. Lee, Dr. James, *Mastectomy*, http://www.nlm.nih.gov/medlineplus/ency/article/002919.htm (2009).

173. *Internal Hemorrhoids*, http://hemorrhoidstreatment.us/internal-hemorrhoids/ (2010).

174. *Brain Tumor: Understanding Your Disease*, http://www.medhelp.org/lib/Brainqi.htm (1995).

175. *Orthopaedic Surgery Articles*, http://emedicine.medscape.com/orthopedic_surgery (2010).

176. Robinson, Richard, *Spinal Fusion*, http://www.surgeryencyclopedia.com/Pa-St/Spinal-Fusion.html (2010).

177. *Heart Surgery*, http://www.nlm.nih.gov/medlineplus/heartsurgery.html (June 2010).

178. *What is a Pediatric Surgeon?* http://www.pediatricsurgerymd.org/What_is_a_Pediatric_Surgeon_.htm (2010).

179. *Testimonial for Angioplasty in Mexico – Sue Nagy*, http://www.worldmedassist.com/testimonials/angioplasty-in-mexico-sue-nagy/ (2010).

180. *Conchetta Procopio Testimonial,* http://www.medtogo.com/conchetta-procopio-testimonial.html (2009).

Notes on Chapter Seven

181. *Cancer Types,* http://www.cancer.net/patient/Cancer+Types (2010).
182. *Cancer Surgery,* http://www.lef.org/protocols/prtcl-026.shtml (2010).
183. *Surgery for Kidney Stones,* http://kidney-stones.emedtv.com/kidney-stones/surgery-for-kidney-stones.html (2010).
184. Berns, Dr. Jeffrey, *Patient Information: Dialysis or Kidney Transplantation – Which is Right for me?* http://www.uptodate.com/patients/content/topic.do?topicKey=~MSMtBwVDqkDVzS (April 2009).
185. Bousquet, J., R. Dahl and N. Khaltaev, *Global Alliance Against Chronic Respiratory Diseases,* http://erj.ersjournals.com/cgi/content/full/29/2/233 (2007).
186. *Lung Disease,* http://www.nlm.nih.gov/medlineplus/ency/article/000066.htm (2008).
187. Meyer, Maria M., Paula Derr and Mary Gilmartin, *Surgical Options for Chronic Lung Disease,* http://www.caring.com/articles/lung-disease-surgery (2010).
188. *Obesity Medications,* http://www.cchs.net/health/health-info/docs/2400/2468.asp?index=9475 (2010).
189. *The Stem Cell Controversy,* http://www.wilsoncenter.org/index.cfm?event_id=161696&fuseaction=topics.event_summary&topic_id=116811 (January 2006).
190. *The Numbers Count: Mental Disorders in America,* http://www.nimh.nih.gov/health/publications/the-numbers-count-mental-disorders-in-america/index.shtml (2010).
191. Doebbeling, Dr. Caroline, *Treatment of Mental Illness,* http://www.merck.com/mmhe/sec07/ch098/ch098d.html (May 2007).
192. *Addiction and Health,* http://www.nida.nih.gov/scienceofaddiction/

health.html (September 2008).

[193.] *Centers for Disease Control and Prevention*, http://www.cdc.gov/healthyliving/ (2010).

Notes on Chapter Eight

[194.] Guthrie, Michael, *Alternative Cancer Treatments*, http://www.alternative-cancer-treatments.com/ (May 2006).

[195.] *Hyperthermia*, American Cancer Society, http://www.cancer.org/Treatment/TreatmentsandSideEffects/TreatmentTypes/hyperthermia (2007).

[196.] *What is Homeopathy?* http://www.homeopathy-soh.org/about-homeopathy/what-is-homeopathy/ (2000).

[197.] *Chelation Therapy for Heart Disease*, http://www.mayoclinic.com/health/chelation-therapy/MY00159 (April 2010).

[198.] Fadhley, Christine, *What is Five Element Acupuncture? A Primer*, http://chinese-medicine.suite101.com/article.cfm/five_element_acupuncture (June 2008).

[199.] Beil, Laura, *Doctors Cashing in on Cosmetic Work, Saying it Keeps Practices Afloat*, http://www.medicalspasociety.com/viewpress.cfm?ID=34 (September 2006).

Notes on Chapter Nine

[200.] *Tips for Travelling Abroad*, http://travel.state.gov/travel/tips/tips_1232.html (2010).

[201.] Gasparoni, Lourdes, *Planning Your Medical Trip Abroad*, http://www.medicaltourismmag.com/issue-detail.php?item=101&issue=5 (February 2008).

[202.] *Online Passport*, Travisa When Your Need it Fast, http://www.travisa.com/passporc.htm (2010).

203. Smith, Elizabeth, *Medical Pack for Travellers*, http://traveltips.usatoday.com/medical-pack-travelers-12525.html (2010).

References

"The Patient Protection and Affordable Care Act." *Wikipedia, the Free Encyclopedia.* Web. 21 May 2010. <http://en.wikipedia.org/wiki/Obamacare Patient Protection and Affordable Care Act>, <http://dpc.senate.gov/dpcdoc-sen_health_care_bill.cfm.>

Andrews, Tim. "What IS Obamacare?" *Americans for Tax Reform.* 22 July 2009. *Americans for Tax Reform.* Web. 21 May 2010. <http://www.atr.org/obamacare-a3568# What IS Obamacare?>

Norris, Chuck. "Reasons Why Obamacare is Bad Medicine" July 2009. 2010 Human Events. Web. 21 May 2010.

<http://www.humanevents.com/article.php?id=32894 6 Reasons Obama-Care Is Bad Medicine.>

Goldberg, Jonah. "Obama and the Democratic Leadership Have Nationalized Healthcare by Proxy." 23 March 2010. *Los Angeles Times.* Web. 21 May 2010. <http://articles.latimes.com/2010/mar/23/opinion/la-oe-goldberg23-2010mar23 The reality of Obamacare.>

Starr, Penny. "The Federal Fat Police: Bill Would Require Government to Track Body Mass of American Children." *CNSNews.com.* 13 May 2010. 1998-2010 Cybercast News Service. Web. 21 May 2010. <http://www.cnsnews.com/news/article/65781The Federal Fat Police: Bill Would Require Government to Track Body Mass of American Children.>

Democratic National Committee. "Health Reform" *BarackObama.com.* Web. 21 May 2010. <http://my.barackobama.com/page/content/benefits ofreform?source=issues Health Reform.>

Bluey, Rob. "Obamacare has a Poison Pill for Doctor-Owned Hospitals." May 4 2010. *The Washington Examiner.* The Examiner. Web.

REFERENCES

21 May 2010. <http://www.washingtonexaminer.com/opinion/columns/OpEd-Contributor/Obamacare-has-a-poison-pill-for-doctor-owned-hospitals-92705029.html.>

HughS. "More Surprises From ObamaCare: Preexisting Conditions Not Immediately Covered." 29 March 2010. *Wizbang.* Web. 21 May 2010. <http://wizbangblog.com/content/2010/03/29/more-surpises-from-obamacare-preexisting-conditions-not-immediately-covered.php.>

Ponnuru, Ramesh. "The Fatal Flaw of Obamacare." 17 August 2009. *Time Magazine.* Web. 21 May 2010. <http://www.time.com/time/magazine/article/0,9171,1914973,00.html The Fatal Flaw of Obamacare.>

Sherk, James. "Unions Using Obamacare to Punish Small Business." 6 January 2010. *The Foundry.* 21 May 2010. <http://blog.heritage.org/2010/01/06/unions-using-obamacare-to-punish-small-business/.>

"Socialized Medicine." Merriam-Webster Online. 24 May 2010 *Merriam-Webster Online Dictionary. 2010.* Web. May 2010. <http://www.merriam-webster.com/dictionary/socialized medicine>

Brewton, E. Thomas. "Obamacare: Quintessential Socialism." 22 September 2009. *Intellectual Conservative.* Web. 22 May 2010. <http://www.intellectualconservative.com/2009/09/22/obamacare-quintessential-socialism-2/ Obamacare: Quintessential Socialism.>

Tanner, D. Michael. "Perils of Obamacare: The Three Big Lies." *New York Post* 20 July 2009. *CATO Institute.* Web. 22 May 2010. <http://www.cato.org/pub_display.php?pub_id=10367.>

Huston, Warner Todd. "Obamacare Will Kill Medical Technology" 3 May 2010. *Big Government.* Web. 22 May 2010. <http://biggovernment.com/wthuston/2010/05/03/obamacare-will-kill-medical-technology/Obamacare Will Kill Medical Technology.>

"More Obamacare Lies." 18 May 2010. *Uncoverage.Net.* Web. 22 May 2010. <http://www.uncoverage.net/2010/05/more-obamacare-lies/>

Hoft, Jim. "Obama Finally Admits You Can Kiss Your Doctor Good-Bye Under Obamacare (Video)." 3 February 2010. *First Things.* <http://gatewaypundit.firstthings.com/2010/02/obama-finally-admits-you-can-kiss-your-doctor-good-bye-under-obamacare-video/>

Wolf, Milton. "ObamaCare: Turning your family doctor into your health care denier." 1 March 2010. *The Wolf Files.* Web 22 May 2010. <http://wolffiles.blogspot.com/2010/03/obamacare-turning-your-family-doctor.html>

Cooper, Robert. "Obamacare Will Ruin Medical System and Dems Knew It!" 28 April 2010. *Desert Conservative.* Web. 22 May 2010. <http://www.desertconservative.com/2010/04/28/obamacare-will-ruin-medical-system-and-dems-knew-it/>

Morrissey, Ed. "CBO: Obamacare Will Cost $1T, Still Leaves 30 Million Uninsured." 16 June 2009. *Hotair.com.* Web. 22 May 2010. <http://hotair.com/archives/2009/06/16/cbo-obamacare-will-cost-1t-still-leaves-30-million-uninsured/>

James, Dr. N. Kristin. "How Obamacare Will Instantly Destroy The Private Health Care Industry and Lead to Socialized Medicine." 16 March 2010. *Amnation.com.* Web. 22 May 2010. <http://www.amnation.com/vfr/archives/015975.html>

Weckesser, Bill. "Obamacare: Rack and ruin for small business." 26 March 2010. *AmericanThinker.com. Web. 23 May 2010.* <http://www.americanthinker.com/blog/2010/03/obamacare_rack_and_ruin_for_sm.html>

Wells, Jane. "Business Owner on Healthcare: I'm Confused." 24 March 2010. Funny Business with Jane Wells CNBC first in business worldwide. *CNBC.com.* Web. 23 May 2010. <http://www.cnbc.com/id/36023914/Business_Owner_on_Health_Care_I_m_Confused>

Bowers, Brenda. "18 New Taxes Slipped into Obamacare Bill." 16 April 2009. An Opinionated Older Lady on Lessons Learned. *Brendabowers.wordpress.com.* Web. 23 May 2010. <http://brendabowers.wordpress.

REFERENCES

com/2010/04/16/18-new-taxes-slipped-into-obamacare-bill/ And So I Go: Yesterday, Today and Tomorrow 18 new taxes slipped into Obamacare bill>

Schenker, Mark. "Charles Krauthammer: Obamacare to Result in National Sales Tax on Americans; Public Option Already Here." 24 March 2010. *Associated Content. Web. 23 May 2010.* <http://www.associatedcontent.com/article/2820580/charles_krauthammer_obamacare_to_result.html?cat=75>

"Obamacare Taxes the Poor at 100 Percent." 5 May 2010. *Politi Fi.* Web. 23 May 2010. <http://politifi.com/news/Obamacare-taxes-the-poor-at-100-percent-850021.htmlObamacare taxes the poor at 100 percent>

Steven. "Saying No To Obamacare? Pay $1900 or Go to Jail" 26 September 2009. *The Daily Caller.* Web. 23 May 2010. <http://www.sodahead.com/united-states/saying-no-to-obamacare-pay-1900-or-go-to-jail/question-644125/Saying no to Obamacare? Pay $1900 or go to jail.>

Doctor Biobrain. "Obamacare Ruins Market-Based Rationing." 12 September 2009. *Biobrain.blogspot.com.* Web 24 May 2010. <http://biobrain.blogspot.com/2009/09/obamacare-ruins-market-based-rationing.html>

Domenech, Ben. "Exempted From Obamacare: Senior Staff Who Wrote the Bill." 22 March 2010. *The New Ledger.* Web. 24 May 2010. <http://newledger.com/2010/03/exempted-from-obamacare-senior-staff-who-wrote-the-bill/>

Elmendorf, W. Douglas. "Congressional Budget Office." 16 June 2009. *U.S. Congress, Washington DC.* Web. 24 May 2010. <http://www.cbo.gov/ftpdocs/103xx/doc10311/06-16-ConradLetter.htm>

Condon, Stephanie. "Health Care Bill brings Debate Over Importing Drugs." 11 December 2009. *CBSNews.* Web 24 May 2010. <http://www.cbsnews.com/8301-503544_162-5967799-503544.html>

"Democrats Using Drug Company Money to Push Obamacare?" 17 March

2010. *Christian Coalition of America*. Web. 24 May 2010. <http://www.cc.org/blog/democrats_using_drug_company_money_push_obamacare>

"Obamacare Will Benefit Wall Street, Insurance Corporations & Pharmaceutical Companies." 21 March 2010. *Buffalorange*. Web. 24 May 2010. <http://www.buffalorange.com/showthread.php?175728-Obamacare-Will-Benefit-Wall-Street-Insurance-Corporations-amp-Pharmaceutical-Companies&p=2684687>

Nimmo, Kurt. "Obamacare: It's About Enriching Bankers and Wall Street." 20 March 2010. *Infowars.com*. Web. 24 May 2010. <http://www.infowars.com/obamacare-its-about-enriching-bankers-and-wall-street/>

Nimmo, Kurt. "Americans Fear Totalitarian Obamacare Will Result in Violence." 31 March 2010. *PrisonPlanet.com*. Web. 24 May 2010. <http://www.prisonplanet.com/americans-fear-totalitarian-obamacare-will-result-in-violence.html>

Hogberg, David. "20 Ways Obamacare Will Take Away Our Freedoms." 25 March 2010. *Investors.com*. Web. 24 May 2010. <http://www.investors.com/NewsAndAnalysis/Article.aspx?id=528137 20 Ways Obamacare Will Take Away Our Freedoms.>

Jeffrey, P. Terence. "Sen. Hatch Questions Constitutionality of Obamacare: If Feds Can Force Us to Buy Health Insurance Then There's Literally Nothing the Federal Government Can't Force Us to Do." 26 November 2009. *CNSNews*. Web. 24 May 2010. <http://www.cnsnews.com/news/article/56447.>

Lendman, Stephen. "Obamacare: A Health Care Rationing Scheme to Enrich Insurers, Drug Companies and Large Hospital Chains." 20 July 2009. *Global Research*. Web. 24 May 2010. <http://www.globalresearch.ca/index.php?context=va&aid=14444.>

"ObamaCare Includes Provision To Takeover Student Loan Program." 12 March 2010. *The Traditional Values Coalition*. Web. 24 May 2010.

REFERENCES

<http://www.traditionalvalues.org/read/3866/obamacare-includes-provision-to-takeover-student-loan-program/>

Weiler, Jonathan. "Health Care Reform and Corruption." 1 October 2009. *The Huffington Post*. Web. 25 May 2010. <http://www.huffingtonpost.com/jonathan-weiler/health-care-reform-and-co_b_306386.html>

Andrew. "Healthcare Reform Eve: A Pork Fest of Corporate Welfare." 20 March 2010. *Swifteconomics.com*. Web. 25 May 2010. <http://www.swifteconomics.com/2010/03/20/healthcare-reform-eve-corporate-welfare-run-amok/>

Young, Jeffrey. "Big Pharma's Top Lobbyist Said What?" 6 March 2010. *The Hill*. Web. 25 May 2010. <http://www.theatlantic.com/business/archive/2009/03/big-pharmas-top-lobbyist-said-what/1284/>

Paul, Ron. "Obamacare Could Bankrupt America." 3 August 2009. *RonPaul.com*. Web. 25 May 2010. <http://www.ronpaul.com/2009-08-03/obamacare-could-bankrupt-america/>

Morgan, Nancy. "Is Obama Trying to Bankrupt America?" 2 March 2010. *Rightbias.com*. Web. 25 May 2010. <http://rightbias.com/news/022810econ.aspx>

Zahn, Drew. "Obamacare Hospitals Killed: 60, With 200 On Life Support." 17 May 2010. *WorldNetDaily*. Web. 25 May 2010. <http://www.wnd.com/?pageId=153941>

Hennenfent, Dr. Bradley. "Obamacare Will Kill Future Patients Compared to What Could Be. Please Stop Obamacare." 16 March 2010. BradMD. Web. 26 May 2010. <http://bradmd.blogspot.com/2010/03/obamacare-will-kill-future-patients.html>

Kouri, Jim. "Obamacare: Death and Misery on the Horizon?" 20 April 2010. *Law Enforcement Examiner*. Web. 26 May 2010. <http://www.examiner.com/x-2684-Law-Enforcement-Examiner~y2010m4d20-ObamaCare-Death-and-misery-on-the-horizon>

Adams, Mike. "Health Care Reform Bill Dooms America to Pharma-Dominated Sickness and Suffering." 22 March 2010. *DProgram.net*. Web. 26 May 2010. <http://dprogram.net/2010/03/22/health-care-reform-bill-dooms-america-to-pharma-dominated-sickness-and-suffering-mike-adams/>

Merrie, Marie. "Obamacare Hidden Provision Shocker (Deduct $150-$240 A Month From Your Paycheck)" 27 March 2010. *Merriemarie.Amplify.com*. Web. 26 May 2010. <http://merriemarie.amplify.com/2010/03/27/3956/>

Favish, J. Allen. "Racial Preferences in the Democrats' Health Care Bill." 21 July 2009. *AmericanThinker.com*. Web. 26 May 2010. <http://www.americanthinker.com/2009/07/racial_preferences_in_the_demo_1.html>

DeMause, Neil. "Health Care Law's Massive, Hidden Tax Charge." 5 May 2010. *CNNMoney*. Web. 26 May 2010. <http://money.cnn.com/2010/05/05/smallbusiness/1099_health_care_tax_change/index.htm>

CNN, "Stealth IRS Changes Mean Millions of New Tax Forms." 21 May 2010. *Wibw.com*. Web. 26 May 2010. <http://www.wibw.com/nationalnews/headlines/94611384.html>

Portnoy, Howard. "Obama's Civilian Army." 4 April 2010. *Hotair.com*. Web. 26 May 2010. <http://hotair.com/greenroom/archives/2010/04/04/obamas-civilian-army/>

"Obamacare Prescription: 'Emergency Health Army'" 25 March 2010. *WorldNetDaily*. Web. 26 May 2010. <http://www.wnd.com/?pageId=132001>

"Costly Marriage Penalty in Proposed Health Care Bill Draws Criticism." 8 January 2010. *CatholicNewsAgency.com*. Web. 26 May 2010. <http://www.catholicnewsagency.com/news/costly_marriage_penalty_in_proposed_health_care_bill_draws_criticism/>

Trobee, Kim. "Marriage Penalty Hidden in Health Care Reform." 12 October 2009. *Citizenlink.com*. Web. 26 May 2010. <http://www.citizenlink.org/content/A000011651.cfm>

REFERENCES

Drummond, Katie. "Hidden Health Care Clause: Menu Labels Go National." 2010. *AOL Inc.* Web. 26 May 2010. <http://www.aolnews.com/healthcare/article/health-care-bill-mandates-nutritional-labels-on-chain-restaurant-menus/19409727>

Gold, Grace. "Is The Health Care Bill's Cosmetic Surgery Tax Sexist?" 8 December 2009. Stylist.com. Web. 26 May 2010. <http://www.stylelist.com/2009/12/08/is-the-health-care-bills-cosmetic-surgery-tax-sexist/>

O'Callaghan, Tiffany. "Bo-tax: A Levy on Nips and Tucks?" 30 November 2009. *Wellness.blogs.time.com.* Web. 26 May 2010. <http://wellness.blogs.time.com/2009/11/30/bo-tax-a-levy-on-nips-and-tucks/>

Morrison, Pat. "Healthcare Reform Fun Facts: The 10% Tan Tax." 23 March 2010. *LATimes.com.* Web. 26 May 2010. <http://opinion.latimes.com/opinionla/2010/03/health-care-reform-fun-facts-the-ten-percent-tan-tax.html>

Berger, Judson. "Plan to Restrict Health Accounts Will Hurt The Disabled, Critics Warn." 25 November 2009. FoxNews. Web. 26 May 2010. <http://www.foxnews.com/politics/2009/11/25/plan-restrict-health-accounts-hurt-disabled-critics-warn/>

Cheplick, Thomas. "President's Plan Limits Flexible Spending Accounts." 24 March 2010. *The Heartland Institute.* Web. 26 May 2010. <http://www.savemyflexplan.org/media_news/10-03-24_heartland.html>

Goldstein, Jacob. "What The Senate Health Bill Says About Breast Feeding." 30 November 2009. *WSJ Blogs.* Web. 26 May 2010. <http://blogs.wsj.com/health/2009/11/30/what-the-senate-health-care-bill-says-about-breast-feeding/?utm_source=feedburner&utm_medium=feed&utm_campaign=Feed:+wsj/health/feed+(WSJ.com:+Health+Blog)>

Klein, Philip. "Why Obamacare Would Fail." 19 March 2010. Spectator. Web 26 May 2010. <http://spectator.org/archives/2010/03/19/why-obamacare-would-fail>

Pinkerton, P. James. "Why Obamacare Will Fail and The Media Will Fail to Notice its Flaws." 8 September 2010. *FoxNews*. Web. 26 May 2010. <http://www.foxnews.com/opinion/2009/09/08/james-pinkerton-obama-health-care-media/>

Pillay, Srinivasan. "Is Health Care Reform Possible Without Caring For The Providers?" 28 July 2009. *Huffington Post*. Web. 26 May 2010. <http://www.huffingtonpost.com/srinivasan-pillay/is-health-care-reform-pos_b_245089.html>

Troy, Tevi. "Medical Brain Drain." 11 March 2010. *National Review*. Web. 26 May 2010. <http://www.nationalreview.com/critical-condition/47441/medical-brain-drain/tevi-troy Medical Brain Drain?

Little, Ilene. "U.S. Brain-Drain of Physicians: What's Driving Our Physicians to Practice Abroad?" 20 December 2009. *Traveling4Health.com*. Web. 26 May 2010. <http://blogs.traveling4health.com/resources-medical/us-brain-drain-of-physicians-whats-driving-our-physicians-to-practice-abroad/>

Fodeman, D. Jason. "Obamacare's Doctorless World." 4 April 2010. *Washington Times*. Web. 26 May 2010. <http://www.washingtontimes.com/news/2010/apr/04/obamacares-doctorless-world/>

Smith, J Wesley. "Obamacare Driving Doctors Out of Medicine." 16 March 2010. *FirstThings.com*. Web. 26 May 2010. <http://www.firstthings.com/blogs/secondhandsmoke/2010/03/16/obamacare-driving-doctors-out-of-medicine/>

"Obamacare and the Nursing Shortage." 7 January 2010. *Slublog.com*. Web. 26 May 2010. <http://www.slublog.com/archives/2010/01/obamacare_and_t.html>

Examiner Editorial. "Obamacare Won't Survive Coming Doctor Shortage." 28 June 2009. *Washington Examiner*. Web. 26 May 2010. <http://www.washingtonexaminer.com/opinion/Obamacare-won_t-survive-coming-doctor-shortage-7886872-49202437.html>

REFERENCES

Oliner, Henry. "Distractions Used to Hide Obamacare's Failures." 5 April 2010. *Myyesnetwork.com.* Web. 26 May 2010. <http://www.myyesnetwork.com/go/thread/view/82290/23082773/Distractions_used_to_hide_Obamacares_failures?pg=last>

"A Doctor's Perspective on Obamacare – Healthcare Delivery Bankruptcy." 20 March 2010. *Freerepublic.com.* Web. 26 May 2010. <http://www.freerepublic.com/focus/news/2475223/posts>

Morrissey, Ed. "Exclusive: Study Shows Obamacare Will Destroy As Many As 700,000 Jobs by 2019" 17 March 2010. *Hotair.com.* Web. 26 May 2010. <http://hotair.com/archives/2010/03/17/exclusive-study-shows-obamacare-will-destroy-as-many-as-700000-jobs-by-2019/>

Reed, John. "Obama's 'You've Had a Good Life Now Drop Dead' Plan: Preventative Medicine." *JohnReed.com* Web. 28 May 2010. <http://www.johntreed.com/Obamapreventive.html>

Conn, Carroll. "Obamacare Does Cut Your Medicare Benefits" 29 July 2009. *Heritage.org.* Web. 28 May 2010. <http://blog.heritage.org/2009/07/29/obamacare-does-cut-your-medicare-benefits/>

Cheplick, Thomas. "President's Plan Limits Flexible Spending Accounts." 24 March 2010. *The Heartland Institute.* Web. 28 May 2010. <http://www.heartland.org/healthpolicy-news.org/article/27326/Presidents_Plan_Limits_Flexible_Spending_Accounts.html>

Feldstein, Martin. "Obamacare is All About Rationing." 18 August 2009. *Wall Street Journal.* Web. 28 May 2010. <http://online.wsj.com/article/SB10001424052970204683204574358233780260914.html>

"Obamacare Rationing Confirmed." 5 May 2010. *Timesfreepress.* Web. 28 May 2010. <http://www.timesfreepress.com/news/2010/may/05/fp3-obamacare-rationing-confirmed/>

Crane, Edward. "Obamacare: Medical Malpractice." June 2009. *The Cato Institute.* Web. 29 May 2010. <http://www.cato.org/pubs/policy_report/v31n3/cpr31n3-2.html>

Atlas, Scott. "Obamacare: Kiss Your Access Goodbye." 23 June 2009. *Realclearpolitics. Web. 29 May 2010.* <http://www.realclearpolitics.com/articles/2009/06/23/obamacare_kiss_your_access_goodbye_97122.html>

"Will Obamacare Force U.S. to Take Medications?" 20 May 2010. *Lubbockonline.* Web. 29 May 2010. <http://lubbockonline.com/interact/blog-post/may/2010-05-20/will-obamacare-force-us-take-medications>

Klein, Joseph. "The True Agenda of Obamacare Progressives Exposed." 25 March 2010. *Newsrealblog.* Web. 29 May 2010. <http://www.newsrealblog.com/2010/03/25/the-true-agenda-of-obamacare-progressives-exposed/>

"Reconciliation Act H.R.4872 Brings Microchipping to America. 30 March 2010. *Infowars.com.* Web. 29 May 2010. <http://current.com/1gipg4c Reconciliation Act H.R.4872 Brings Microchipping to America>

"Barack Obama Finally Has Jobs Bill, 16,000 New IRS Workers Will Be Needed For Obamacare." 21 March 2010. *Scaredmonkeys.com.* Web. 29 May 2010. <http://scaredmonkeys.com/2010/03/21/barack-obama-finally-has-jobs-bill-16000-new-irs-workers-will-be-needed-for-obamacare/>

Quinn, Jim. "Commentary: Analysis Obamacare Leads to Big Brother." 12 April 2010. *Dailyestimate.com.* Web. 29 May 2010. <http://www.dailyestimate.com/article.asp?id=30695>

Fred. "Some Unexpected Effects of Obamacare, Part 2: Gaming the System." 19 April 2010. *Guarino.typepad.com.* Web. 29 May 2010. <http://guarino.typepad.com/guarino/2010/04/some-unexpected-effects-of-obamacare-part-2-gaming-the-system.html>

"Obamacare's Folly: More Unemployment for Low-Skilled Workers." 10 May 2010. *Under The Hill.* Web. 29 May 2010. <http://underthehill.wordpress.com/2010/05/10/obamacares-folly-more-unemployment/>

REFERENCES

Gardner, Amanda. "6 Million Americans Travel Abroad Each Year for Surgeries, Medical Treatments." 8 April 2009. *Healthday*. Web. 30 May 2010. <http://news.health.com/2009/04/08/traveling-treatment/>

Woodman, Josef. "What Exactly is Medical Tourism?" *Patients Beyond Borders Second Edition*. USA and Hong Kong. Healthy Travel Media, 2008. 7-8. Print.

Smith, S.E. "What is Elective Surgery?" *Wisegeek.com*. Web. 30 May 2010. <http://www.wisegeek.com/what-is-elective-surgery.htm>

"McGraw-Hill Concise Dictionary of Modern Medicine: Emergency Surgery." 2002. *The McGraw-Hill Companies Inc*. Web. 30 May 2010. <http://medical-dictionary.thefreedictionary.com/emergency+surgery>

"Definition of Chronic Disease." 22 June 2004. *Medterms.com*. Web. 30 May 2010. <http://www.medterms.com/script/main/art.asp?articlekey=33490>

Wessel, Charles B. "The Alternative Medicine Homepage." July 2008. *Pitt.edu*. Web. 30 May 2010. <http://www.pitt.edu/~cbw/altm.html the alternative medicine homepage>

Ford-Martin, Paula. "Elective Surgery." *SurgeryEncyclopedia*. Web. 30 May 2010. <http://www.surgeryencyclopedia.com/Ce-Fi/Elective-Surgery.html>

American Society for Aesthetic Plastic Surgery. "Cosmetic Plastic Surgery Research, Statistics and Trends for 2001-2008." *Cosmeticplasticsurgerystatistics.com. Web. 30 May 2010*. <http://www.cosmeticplasticsurgerystatistics.com/statistics.html Cosmetic Plastic>

"Costs of Dental Implants and Price Ranges." 22 August 2006. *Dental-Resouces.com*. Web. 31 May 2010. <http://www.dental-resources.com/dental-implants-cost.html>

Brandt, Dr. Carl J. "Biopsy." 15 December 2009. *Netdoctor*. Web. 31 May 2010. <http://www.netdoctor.co.uk/health_advice/examinations/biopsy.htm>

Heisler, Jennifer. "What to Expect From Emergency Surgery." 4 January 2009. *About.com.* Web. 31 May 2010. <http://surgery.about.com/od/proceduresaz/ss/EmergencySurger_2.htm>

"Chronic Diseases and Health Promotion." 17 December 2009. *National Center for Chronic Disease Prevention and Health Promotion.* Web. 31 May 2010. <http://www.cdc.gov/chronicdisease/overview/index.htm>

"Health Affairs." 2006. *Project Hope.* Web. 31 May 2010. <http://content.healthaffairs.org/cgi/content/abstract/25/6/1712>

Wong, Cathy. "12 Common Questions About Insurance and Complementary/Alternative Medicine." 11 August 2006. *About.com.* Web. 31 May 2010. <http://altmedicine.about.com/od/alternativemedicinebasics/a/Insurance.htm>

"Alternative Medicine in Panama–Pt 1." 9 April 2007. *Panama Expertos.* Web. 31 May 2010. <http://www.panamaexpertos.com/alternative-medicine-in-panama-pt-1>

"Alternative Medicine Cont." 1996-2010. M*edicineNet* Inc. Web. 31 May 2010. <http://www.medicinenet.com/alternative_medicine/page2.htm#tocd>

"Disadvantages of Medical Tourism." *Healism.com.* Web 31 May 2010. <http://www.healism.com/medical_tourism/overview/disadvantages_of_medical_tourism/>

"Medical Tourism Benefits and Advantages." 3 June 2010. *Health-Tourism.* Web. 1 June 2010. <http://www.health-tourism.com/medical-tourism/benefits/>

"Advantages and Disadvantages of Medical Tourism." *Scumdoctor.* Web. 1 June 2-010. <http://www.scumdoctor.com/medical-tourism/Advantages-And-Disadvantages-Of-Medical-Tourism.html>

"Joint Commission Resources." 2002-2009. *JCR, Inc.* Web. 1 June 2010. <http://www.jointcommissioninternational.org/>

REFERENCES

Marsek, Patrick and Frances Sharpe. "Chapter Ten: Hospital Hints." *The Complete Idiot's Guide to Medical Tourism*. New York. The Penguin Group, 2009. 121-122. Print.

"Questions to Ask Your Doctor Before Having Surgery." *The Health Pages*. Web. 2 June 2010. <http://www.the-health-pages.com/topics/education/surgery_questions.html>

"Questions to Ask Before Surgery." *The University of Chicago Medical Center*. Web. 2 June 2010. <http://www.uchospitals.edu/online-library/content=P01409>

"Definition of Breast Augmentation." 27 September 2007. *MedTerms*. Web. 2 June 2010. <http://www.medterms.com/script/main/art.asp?articlekey=2525>

"Breast Augmentation Benefits." 2008. *DocShop*. Web. 2 June 2010. <http://www.docshop.com/education/cosmetic/breast/augmentation/benefits/>

"Risks of Breast Augmentation." 2001-2010. *A Board Certified Plastic Surgeon Resource*. Web. 2 June 2010. <http://www.aboardcertifiedplasticsurgeonresource.com/breast_augmentation/risk.html>

"Cost of Plastic Surgery." *Infoplasticsurgery*. Web. 2 June 2010. <http://www.infoplasticsurgery.com/cost-plastic-surgery/cost>

"Breast Augmentation Surgery – A Complete Consumer Guide." 26 April 2010. *Ceatus Media Group LLC*. Web. 2 June 2010. <http://www.yourplasticsurgeryguide.com/breast-augmentation/>

Marsek, Patrick and Frances Sharpe. "Chapter Four: Cosmetic Procedures and Popular Destinations. Breast Augmentation." *The Complete Idiot's Guide to Medical Tourism*. New York. The Penguin Group, 2009. 46-47. Print.

"Breast Augmentation (Breast Enlargement) Panama Medical Tourism" 20 December 2007. *PRLog*. Web 2 June 2010. <http://www.prlog.org/10042958-breast-augmentation-breast-enlargement-panama-medical-tourism.html>

"Breast Augmentation in Mexico – It Changed My Life (For The Better)" *Realself.com. Web 2 June 2010.* <http://www.realself.com/review/breast-augmentation-mexico>

"Breast Augmentation Information, Pictures, Photos Before/After Dr. Pichet." 2008. *Aesthetic Plastic Surgery Center.* Web. 2 June 2010. <http://www.bangkokplasticsurgery.com/breast-augmentation-surgery.html>

Lickstein, David. "Facelift." *Medlineplus.com*. Web. 2 June 2010. <http://www.nlm.nih.gov/medlineplus/ency/article/002989.htm>

"Benefits of Face Lift Surgery." 2008. *DocShop.* Web. 2 June 2010. <http://www.docshop.com/education/cosmetic/face/face-lift/benefits/>

Fallon Jr., Dr. L. Fleming. "Facelift." 2010. *Encyclopedia of Surgery.* Web. 2 June 2010. <http://www.surgeryencyclopedia.com/Ce-Fi/Face-Lift.html>

"Facelift Information – Face Lift Photos." 2000-2010. *iEnhance.com.* Web. 2 June 2010. <http://www.ienhance.com/procedure/description.asp?ProcID=5&BodyID=&specialtyid=1#5>

Marsek, Patrick and Frances Sharpe. "Chapter Four: Cosmetic Procedures and Popular Destinations. Face Lift." *The Complete Idiot's Guide to Medical Tourism*. New York. The Penguin Group, 2009. 41-42. Print.

"How Much is Facelift Surgery?" 2005-2010. *Ceatus Media Group LLC*. Web 2 June 2010. <http://www.yourplasticsurgeryguide.com/face-lift/cost.htm>

REFERENCES

"Cheap Cosmetic Surgery in India." *Indiaprofile.com*. Web. 3 June 2010. <http://www.indiaprofile.com/medical-tourism/surgeries/cheap-cosmetic-surgery.html>

Lotter, Karen. "Affordable Cosmetic Surgery Makes Scalpel Safaris Popular." 12 October 2007. *Suite101.com*. Web. 3 June 2010. <http://south-africa-travel.suite101.com/article.cfm/medical_tourism_to_south_africa>

"Cosmetic Surgery in Mexico." *Kwintessential*. Web. 3 June 2010. <http://www.kwintessential.co.uk/articles/article/Mexico/Cosmetic-Surgery-in-Mexico/1088>

"Definition of Liposuction." 16 December 1998. *MedTerms*. Web. 3 June 2010. <http://www.medterms.com/script/main/art.asp?articlekey=7855>

Olvera, Christina. "Liposuction: the Benefits Versus the Dangers and Risks." 13 June 2006. *AssociatedContent*. Web. 3 June 2010. <http://www.associatedcontent.com/article/37171/liposuction_the_benefits_versus_the.html?cat=69>

"10 Frequently Asked Questions About Liposuction." 2002-2010. *Looking Your Best*. Web. 4 June 2010. <http://www.lookingyourbest.com/bodycontouring/articles/Liposuction/liposuctionfaq#10 Frequently Asked Questions About Liposuction>

"Cost of Liposuction Surgery." April 2010. *Ceatus Media Group LLC*. Web. 4 June 2010. <http://www.yourplasticsurgeryguide.com/liposuction/cost.htm>

"Cost of Liposuction?" *Realself, Inc*. Web. 4 June 2010. <http://www.realself.com/Liposuction/cost Cost of Liposuction?>

"You are Comparing Liposuction Traveling from the USA." *AllMedical Tourism*. Web. 4 June 2010. <http://www.allmedicaltourism.com/usa/cosmetic/liposuction/>

"Definition of Rhinoplasty." 26 March 1998. *MedTerms.* Web. 4 June 2010. <http://www.medterms.com/script/main/art.asp?articlekey=5363>

"Rhinoplasty FAQ." *A Board Certified Plastic Surgeon Resource.* Web. 4 June 2010. <http://www.aboardcertifiedplasticsurgeonresource.com/rhinoplasty/rhinoplasty-faq.html>

"Rhinoplasty–Nose Surgery." *iEnhance.com.* Web. 4 June 2010. <http://www.ienhance.com/procedure/description.asp?procid=21&subbodyid=5#6>

"Rhinoplasty (Nose Surgery)" *Plastic Surgery Portal.* Web. 4 June 2010. <http://www.plasticsurgeryportal.com/rhinoplasty/2001061503560122225606>

"Panama Health: Price Guide for Cosmetic and Surgical Procedures in Panama." *Panama-Health.* Web. 4 June 2010. <http://www.panama-health.com/Surgery_Prices.htm>

"Cost of Revision Rhinoplasty?" Realself, Inc. Web. 4 June 2010. <http://www.realself.com/Revision-rhinoplasty/cost>

"Blepharoplasty." *Mayo Foundation for Medical Education and Research.* Web. 4 June 2010. <http://www.mayoclinic.com/health/blepharoplasty/my00298>

"Eyelid Surgery Tips." *Indobase.com.* Web. 4 June 2010. <http://beauty.indobase.com/cosmetic-surgery/eyelid-surgery.html>

"Eyelid Surgery (Blepharoplasty) Benefits." *DocShop.* Web. 4 June 2010. <http://www.docshop.com/education/cosmetic/face/eyelid-surgery/benefits/>

Schrieber, Trudi. "Eyelid Surgery Risks and Side Effects." *Plastic Surgery Portal.* Web. 4 June 2010. <http://www.plasticsurgeryportal.com/articles/blepharoplasty-risks/159>

"Eyelid Surgery (Blepharoplasty)" *iEnhance.com.* Web. 4 June 2010. <http://www.ienhance.com/procedure/description.asp?ProcID=137&bodyid=1&specialtyid=1#6>

REFERENCES

Loftus, Dr. "Cost of Plastic Surgery." *Infoplasticsurgery.com*. Web. 4 June 2010. <http://www.infoplasticsurgery.com/cost-plastic-surgery/cost>

"Dental Implant Surgery." 27 June 2008. *Mayo Foundation for Medical Education and Research*. Web. 4 June 2010. <http://www.mayoclinic.com/health/dental-implant-surgery/my00084>

"Dental Implants." *Dental Related Internet Resources*. Web. 4 June 2010. <http://www.dental-resources.com/dental-implants.html>

"Implant Dentistry Risks." *DocShop*. Web. 4 June 2010. <http://www.docshop.com/education/dental/general-dentistry/dental-implants/risks/>

"Dental Implants." *iEnhance.com*. Web. 4 June 2010. <http://www.ienhance.com/procedure/description.asp?ProcID=90&BodyID=&specialtyid=3#5>

"Implant Dentistry – A Solution for Missing Teeth." *DocShop*. Web. 4 June 2010. <http://www.docshop.com/education/dental/general-dentistry/dental-implants/>

"Bone Grafting for Dental Implants." *Medic8*. Web. 4 June 2010. <http://www.medic8.com/cosmetic-dentistry/bone-grafting.htm>

"Bone Grafting Materials Their Uses, Advantages and Disadvantages." American Dental Association. Web. 4 June 2010. <http://jada.ada.org/cgi/content/full/133/8/1125>

"You are Comparing Dental Bone Graft Traveling from the USA." *AllMedicalTourism*. Web. 4 June 2010. <http://www.allmedicaltourism.com/usa/dental/dental-bone-graft/>

"Endodontic Surgery." *American Association of Endodontists*. Web. 4 June 2010. <http://www.aae.org/patients/patientinfo/faqs/endosurgery.htm>

Fallon Jr., Dr. L. Fleming. "Tooth Extraction." *Surgery Encyclopedia*. Web. 4 June 2010. <http://www.surgeryencyclopedia.com/St-Wr/Tooth-Extraction.html>

Johnstone, Greg. "Bridging the Gap with a Dental Bridge." May 2009. *Your Dentistry Guide*. Web. 4 June 2010. <http://www.yourdentistryguide.com/bridges/>

Soni, Dr. Mukesh and Dr. Kailesh Solanki. "Porcelain Veneers for Smile Makeovers." *CosmeticDentistryGuide*. Web. 4 June 2010. <http://www.cosmeticdentistryguide.co.uk/veneers.html>

"Porcelain Veneers Benefits." *DocShop*. Web. 4 June 2010. <http://www.docshop.com/education/dental/cosmetic-dentistry/porcelain-veneers/benefits/>

"Dental Health and Veneers." *WebMD Medical Reference*. Web. 4 June 2010. <http://www.webmd.com/oral-health/veneers>

Ducasse, Dr. Don. "Dental Fillings. Which Type is Best for You?" *TheBestKeptSecret*. Web. 4 June 2010. <http://www.thebestkeptsecret.ca/Articles.aspx?ArtID=335>

"Benefits of Dentures." *Medic8*. Web. 4 June 2010. <http://www.medic8.com/cosmetic-dentistry/dentures/benefits-dentures.html>

Peterson, Dr. Dan. "Family Gentle Dental Care." 27 February 2007. *Dental Gentle Care*. Web. 4 June 2010. <http://www.dentalgentlecare.com/scaling__root_planning.htm>

"Laser Gum Treatment." *Futuredontics, Inc*. Web. 4 June 2010. <http://www.1800dentist.com/dental-encyclopedia/laser-gum-treatment>

Erstad, Shannon. "Hip Replacement Surgery." 17 April 2009. *WebMD*. Web. 4 June 2010. <http://arthritis.webmd.com/hip-replacement-surgery>

Cluett, Dr. Jonathan. "What Are the Risks of Hip and Knee Replacement?" 6 May 2009. *Orthopedics Guide*. Web. 4 June 2010. <http://orthopedics.about.com/od/hipkneereplacement/f/risks.htm>

"What to Expect During Pacemaker Surgery." *Nhlbi.nih.gov*. Web. 4 June 2010. <http://www.nhlbi.nih.gov/health/dci/Diseases/pace/pace_duringsurgery.html>

REFERENCES

Heisler, Jennifer. "Pacemaker Surgery: All About Pacemakers." 5 June 2010. *About.com*. Web. 5 June 2010. <http://surgery.about.com/od/proceduresaz/ss/Pacemaker_3.htm>

"Definition of a Hysterectomy." 13 February 2002. *MedTerms*. Web. 5 June 2010. <http://www.medterms.com/script/main/art.asp?articlekey=3876>

"What You Need to Know About Hysterectomy." *The Cleveland Clinic Foundation*. Web. 5 June 2010. <http://my.clevelandclinic.org/services/hysterectomy/hic_what_you_need_to_know_about_hysterectomy.aspx>

"How Much Does a Biopsy Cost?" August 2009. *CostHelper.com*. Web. 5 June 2010. <http://www.costhelper.com/cost/health/biopsy.html>

"Definition of In Vitro Fertilization." 12 May 2002. *MedTerms*. Web. 5 June 2010. <http://www.medterms.com/script/main/art.asp?articlekey=7298>

"Advantages of In Vitro Fertilization." *eHow*. Web. 5 June 2010. <http://www.ehow.com/about_4760556_advantages-vitro-fertilization.html>

Best-Boss, Angie. "Frozen Embryo Transfer." *Conceiving Concepts*. Web. 5 June 2010. <http://www.conceivingconcepts.com/infertility-treatment/assisted-reproduction/ivf/fet-frozen-embryo-transfer>

"Definition of Intracytoplasmic Sperm Injection (ICSI)" 2 July 2001. *MedTerms*. Web. 5 June 2010. <http://www.medterms.com/script/main/art.asp?articlekey=7299>

"Intracytoplasmic Sperm Injection: ICSI" May 2007. *American Pregnancy Association*. Web. 5 June 2010. <http://www.americanpregnancy.org/infertility/icsi.html>

"Definition of Gamete Intrafallopian Transfer (GIFT)" 12 January 2000. *MedTerms*. Web. 5 June 2010. <http://www.medterms.com/script/main/art.asp?articlekey=12288>

"A First: Ovary Transplant and 2 Births." 24 February 2010. *MSNBC*. Web. 5 June 2010. <http://www.msnbc.msn.com/id/35559268/ns/health-kids_and_parenting/>

"LASIK" *DocShop.* Web. 5 June 2010. <http://www.docshop.com/education/vision/refractive/lasik/>

Segre, Liz. "The LASIK Procedure: A Complete Guide." April 2010. *AllAboutVision.com. Web. 5 June 2010.* <http://www.allaboutvision.com/visionsurgery/lasik.htm>

"LASIK Eye Surgery Definition." 12 December 2008. *Mayo Foundation for Medical Education and Research.* Web. 5 June 2010. <http://www.mayoclinic.com/health/lasik-eye-surgery/MY00376>

"Health Issues." 9 October 2000. *National Center for Policy Analysis.* Web. 5 June 2010. <http://www.ncpa.org/sub/dpd/index.php?Article_ID=9413>

"At a Glance." *Kosmix Corporation.* Web. 5 June 2010. <http://www.righthealth.com/topic/After_Surgery/overview/rh_uniquecontent?fdid=rhuniquecontent_e97a9365609d38ac6d06ed431408859b>

Vansickle, Carol. "How Much Does an Air Ambulance Cost?" *eHow.* Web. 5 June 2010. <http://www.ehow.com/about_4674530_much-does-air-ambulance-cost.html>

"Free and Low Cost Medical Transport Services." *Bridges4Kids.* Web. 5 June 2010. <http://www.bridges4kids.org/Disabilities/Transport.html>

"Definition of Peptic Ulcer." 26 March 1998. *MedTerms.* Web. 5 June 2010. <http://www.medterms.com/script/main/art.asp?articlekey=4829>

Bingham, JR. "The Evaluation of Emergency Gastrectomy for Hæmorrhage from the Upper Gastrointestinal Tract." *Department of Medicine, the Toronto Western Hospital and the University of Toronto.* Web. 6 June 2010. <http://www.ncbi.nlm.nih.gov/pmc/articles/PMC1830841/?page=1>

Timpone, Dr. P.J. and Dr. Ludwig Gross. " Emergency Gastrectomy in the Surgical Treatment of Perforated Peptic Ulcer." *Interscience.* Web. 6 June 2010. <http://www3.interscience.wiley.com/journal/120171195/abstract?CRETRY=1&SRETRY=0>

REFERENCES

Mahnke, Dr. Daus. "Gastrectomy (Total Gastrectomy, Partial Gastrectomy, Subtotal Gastrectomy, Stomach Removal)" 22 June 2008. *Thirdage*. Web. 6 June 2010. <http://www.thirdage.com/encyclopedia/gastrectomy-total-gastrectomy-partial-gastrectomy-subtotal-gastrectomy-stomach-remov>

Hussain, Dr. Nasir and Dr. Bernard Karnath. "GI Consult: Perforated Peptic Ulcer."*Emedmag.com*. Web. 6 June 2010. <http://www.emedmag.com/html/pre/gic/consults/071503.asp>

"Apollo Hospital Chennai." 7 March 2010. *Health-Tourism*. Web. 6 June 2010. <http://www.health-tourism.com/medical-centers/apollo-hospital-chennai/>

"Distance from India to USA." *True Knowledge LTD*. Web. 6 June 2010. <http://www.trueknowledge.com/q/distance_from_india_to_usa>

"Chapter 5: The Surgery of the Stomach." *Meb.uni-bonn.de*. Web. 6 June 2010. <http://www.meb.uni-bonn.de/dtc/primsurg/docbook/html/x3617.html>

"Gallbladder Removal: Laparoscopic Method." September 2000. *American Academy of Family Physicians*. Web. 6 June 2010. <http://familydoctor.org/online/famdocen/home/articles/114.html>

Gulli, Dr. Laith. "Gallstone Removal." *Surgeryencyclopedia*. Web. 6 June 2010. <http://www.surgeryencyclopedia.com/Fi-La/Gallstone-Removal.html>

"Affordable Gallbladder Surgery Package in Mexico Center Profile: Laparoscopic Solutions" *Placidway.com*. Web. 6 June 2010. <http://www.placidway.com/package/155/Affordable-Gallbladder-Surgery-Package-in-Mexico Center Profile: Laparoscopic Solutions>

"Appendectomy – Open Surgery." *Doctorsofusc.com*. Web. 6 June 2010. <http://www.doctorsofusc.com/condition/document/2>

Cowles, Dr. R.A. "Appendectomy." 2 May 2009. *Medlineplus*. Web. 6 June 2010. <http://www.nlm.nih.gov/medlineplus/ency/article/002921.htm>

"Patient Information for Laparoscopic Appendectomy." March 2004. *Society of American Gastrointestinal Endoscopic Surgeons.* Web. 6 June 2010. <http://www.sages.org/publication/id/PI08/>

"Bangkok Hospital Pattaya." *Bangkokpattayahospital.com.* Web. 6 June 2010. <http://www.bangkokpattayahospital.com/index.html>

Heisler, Jennifer. "Hernia Defined." 4 January 2009. *About.com.* Web. 6 June 2010. <http://surgery.about.com/od/glossaryofsurgicalterms/g/HerniaDefined.htm>

Nicks, Dr. Bret. "Hernias." 25 January 2010. *Emedicine.* Web. 6 June 2010. <http://emedicine.medscape.com/article/775630-overview Hernias>

"Inguinal Hernia – What Happens." 29 April 2009. *WebMD.* Web. 6 June 2010. <http://www.webmd.com/digestive-disorders/tc/inguinal-hernia-what-happens>

"Inguinal Hernia – Treatment Overview." 29 April 2009. *WebMD.* Web. 6 June 2010. <http://www.webmd.com/digestive-disorders/tc/inguinal-hernia-treatment-overview>

"Patient Information for Laparoscopic Inguinal Hernia Repair from SAGES." 2004. *The Society of American Gastrointestinal and Endoscopic Surgeons (SAGES).* Web. 6 June 2010. <http://www.sages.org/publication/id/PI06/>

"Mastectomy" 2010. *MedlinePlus.* Web. 6 June 2010. <http://www.nlm.nih.gov/medlineplus/mastectomy.html>

"Types of Mastectomy to Treat Breast Cancer." 2010. *WebMD.* Web. 6 June 2010. <http://www.webmd.com/breast-cancer/mastectomy>

"What You Can Expect." 17 October 2009. *MayoClinic.* Web. 7 June 2010. <http://www.mayoclinic.com/health/mastectomy/MY00943/DSECTION=what-you-can-expect>

REFERENCES

"Low Cost Mastectomy Surgery Abroad." *Medicaltourismco.com*. Web 7 June 2010. <http://www.medicaltourismco.com/oncology/mastectomy-surgery-abroad.php>

Longstreth, George F. "Spleen Removal." *MedlinePlus*. Web. 7 June 2010. <http://www.nlm.nih.gov/medlineplus/ency/article/002944.htm>

"Spleen Removal Surgery (Splenectomy)." *Health Grades Inc*. Web. 7 June 2010. <http://www.healthgrades.com/procedures/profile/Spleen_Removal_Surgery_(Splenectomy)>

"Why It's Done Splenectomy." 21 May 2010. *MayoClinic*. Web. 7 June 2010. <http://www.mayoclinic.com/health/splenectomy/MY01271/DSECTION=why-its-done Splenectomy>

"Splenectomy." 2010. *WebMD*. Web. 7 June 2010. <http://www.webmd.com/digestive-disorders/splenectomy Splenectomy>

"BNH Hospital." 24 February 2010. *Health Tourism*. Web. 7 June 2010. <http://www.health-tourism.com/medical-centers/bnh-hospital/ BNH Hospital>

"Lung Transplantation." 12 April 2010. *MedlinePlus*. Web. 7 June 2010. <http://www.nlm.nih.gov/medlineplus/lungtransplantation.html>

Moffatt-Bruce, Dr. Susan D. "Lung Transplantation." 13 May 2009. *Emedicine*. Web. 7 June 2010. <http://emedicine.medscape.com/article/429499-overview Lung Transplantation>

"What You Can Expect Lung Transplant." 26 September 2008. *MayoClinic*. Web. 7 June 2010. <http://www.mayoclinic.com/health/lung-transplant/MY00106/DSECTION=what-you-can-expect>

"Transplantation Surgery in Turkey." 20 April 2010. *Your Surgery Abroad*. Web. 7 June 2010. <http://www.yoursurgeryabroad.com/transplantation-surgery/turkey/#pid=828>

"Definition of Hemorrhoid." 8 February 2004. *MedTerms*. Web. 7 June 2010. <http://www.medterms.com/script/main/art.asp?articlekey=3702 Definition of Hemorrhoid>

"Hemorrhoids Surgery." 29 September 2008. *WebMD*. Web. 7 June 2010. <http://www.webmd.com/a-to-z-guides/hemorrhoids-surgery>

"Surgery Hemorrhoids Cont." 2010. *WebMD*. Web. 7 June 2010. <http://www.emedicinehealth.com/hemorrhoids/page7_em.htm#Surgery Hemorrhoids (cont.)>

Mohan, Dr. Venkat. "Hemorrhoid Surgery." 21 September 2009. *WebMD*. Web. 7 June 2010. <http://www.webmd.com/a-to-z-guides/surgery-treat-hemorrhoids?page=2>

"SINTEZA Health Centre." *Global Health Consulting*. Web. 7 June 2010. <http://www.mydoctor.com.hr/default.aspx?page=229&article=3880>

Heisler, Jennifer. "Neurosurgery Definition." 7 January 2009. *About.com*. Web. 7 June 2010. <http://surgery.about.com/od/glossaryofsurgicalterms/g/NeuroSurgery.htm>

Gulli, Dr. Laith Farid, Dr. Miguel A. Melgar and Nicole Mallory. "Neurosurgery." *Surgeryencyclopedia*. Web. 7 June 2010. <http://www.surgeryencyclopedia.com/La-Pa/Neurosurgery.html>

Jasmin, Dr. Luc. "Brain Tumor – Primary –Adults." 14 October 2009. *MedlinePlus*. Web. 7 June 2010. <http://www.nlm.nih.gov/medlineplus/ency/article/007222.htm>

"Brain Tumor Cont." 2010. *MedicineNet, Inc*. Web. 7 June 2010. <http://www.medicinenet.com/brain_tumor/page7.htm>

"University Medical Center Freiburg." 2010. *Health Tourism*. Web. 7 June 2010. <http://www.health-tourism.com/medical-centers/university-medical-center-freiburg/>

"Orthopedic Surgery." *Surgeryencyclopedia*. Web. 7 June 2010. <http://www.surgeryencyclopedia.com/La-Pa/Orthopedic-Surgery.html>

"Orthopedic Surgery." *Gale Encyclopedia of Medicine*. Web. 7 June 2010. <http://medical-dictionary.thefreedictionary.com/orthopedic+surgery>

REFERENCES

Benjamin, Dr. C. "Spinal Stenosis." 10 July 2009. *MedlinePlus*. Web. 7 June 2010. <http://www.nlm.nih.gov/medlineplus/ency/article/000441.htm>

Benjamin, Dr. C. "Spinal Fusion." 4 March 2009. *MedlinePlus*. Web. 7 June 2010. <http://www.nlm.nih.gov/medlineplus/ency/article/002968.htm>

Eck, Jason C. "Minimally Invasive Lumbar Spinal Fusion." *MedicineNet.com*. Web. 7 June 2010. <http://www.medicinenet.com/minimally_invasive_lumbar_spinal_fusion/article.htm>

"Mahkota Medical Centre." 4 May 2010. *Health Tourism*. Web. 7 June 2010. <http://www.health-tourism.com/medical-centers/mahkota-medical-centre/>

Vega, Dr. Jose. "Vascular Surgery." 30 April 2008. *About.com*. Web. 7 June 2010. <http://stroke.about.com/od/glossary/g/vascularsgy.htm>

Lee, Dr. James. "Abdominal Aortic Aneurysm." 21 August 2009. *Medline Plus*. Web. 7 June 2010. <http://www.nlm.nih.gov/medlineplus/ency/article/000162.htm>

"Aortic Aneurysm Surgery." 7 March 2008. WebMD. Web. 7 June 2010. <http://www.webmd.com/heart-disease/tc/aortic-aneurysm-surgery>

"Sahel General Hospital." 18 March 2009. *Health Tourism*. Web. 7 June 2010. <http://www.health-tourism.com/medical-centers/sahel-general-hospital/>

"Definition of Aortic Valve." 5 April 2000. *MedTerms*. Web. 7 June 2010. <http://www.medterms.com/script/main/art.asp?articlekey=2298>

"Aortic Valve Replacement." *Surgeryencyclopedia*. Web. 7 June 2010. <http://www.surgeryencyclopedia.com/A-Ce/Aortic-Valve-Replacement.html>

"Krishna Heart and Super Specialty Institute." 16 November 2009. *Health Tourism*. Web. 7 June 2010. <http://www.health-tourism.com/medical-centers/krishna-heart-and-super-specialty-institute/>

Gulli, Dr. Laith Farid. "Pediatric Surgery." *Surgeryencyclopedia*. Web. 7

June 2010. <http://www.surgeryencyclopedia.com/Pa-St/Pediatric-Surgery.html>

Reid, Dr. Janet. "Hypertrophic Pyloric Stenosis." 3 August 2009. *EMedicine*. Web. 7 June 2010. <http://emedicine.medscape.com/article/409621-overview>

"Pyloromyotomy: Surgery for Pyloric Stenosis." *Aboutkidshealth.com*. Web. 7 June 2010. <http://www.aboutkidshealth.ca/HealthAZ/Pyloromyotomy-Surgery-for-Pyloric-Stenosis.aspx?articleID=8543&categoryID=AZ1d>

"Pyloromyotomy – Open Technique (Fredet-Ramstedt Operation)." 27 May 2009. *InsideSurgery.com*. Web. 7 June 2010. <http://insidesurgery.com/2007/05/pyloromyotomy-open-technique-fredet-ramstedt-operation/>

"KK Women's and Children's Hospital." 29 March 2010. *Health Tourism*. Web. 7 June 2010. <http://www.health-tourism.com/medical-centers/kk-womens-and-childrens-hospital/>

Marks, Dr. James. "Tackling Chronic Diseases." CDCFoundation. Web. 8 June 2010. <http://www.cdcfoundation.org/frontline/2003/tackling_chronic_diseases.aspx>

"About Half of Americans Have Chronic Conditions, CDC Report Finds." 28 April 2010. *Californiahealthline.com*. Web. 8 June 2010. <http://www.californiahealthline.org/articles/2010/4/28/about-half-of-americans-have-chronic-condition-cdc-report-finds.aspx>

"About the Crisis." *Fightchronicdisease.com*. Web. 8 June 2010. <http://www.fightchronicdisease.org/issues/about.cfm>

Brownstein, Joseph. "Millions of Families Struggle to Pay for Care, Even Those With Health Insurance." 5 February 2009. *ABC News Medical Unit*. Web. 8 June 2010. <http://abcnews.go.com/Health/OnCall/story?id=6811555&page=1 Cancer Care Costs Squeeze Millions of Americans>

Stuckey, Mick. "When Staying Alive Means Going Bankrupt." 15 August 2007. *MSNBC.com*. Web. 8 June 2010. <http://www.msnbc.msn.com/id/20201807/ When staying alive means going bankrupt>

REFERENCES

"Moving Clinical Trials Overseas Tests the System's Safety, Efficacy." 19 February 2009. *Medicalnewstoday.com*. Web. 8 June 2010. <http://www.medicalnewstoday.com/articles/139528.php>

"Medical Records – Frequently Asked Questions." *State of California*. Web. 8 June 2010. <http://www.medbd.ca.gov/consumer/complaint_info_questions_records.html>

"SEER Cancer Statistics Review." 2010. *SEER website*. Web. 8 June 2010. <http://seer.cancer.gov/csr/1975_2007/>

"How Many People Die From Cancer Each Year." 1 February 2010. *Nano Medicine Center*. Web. 8 June 2010. <http://www.nanomedicinecenter.com/article/how-many-people-die-from-cancer-each-year/>

"Cancer Data and Statistics." 18 May 2010. Division of Cancer Prevention and Control, National Center for Chronic Disease Prevention and Health Promotion. Web. 8 June 2010. <http://www.cdc.gov/cancer/dcpc/data/Cancer Prevention and Control>

"What Causes Cancer?" 24 February 2009. *Cancer.org*. Web. 8 June 2010. <http://www.cancer.org/docroot/CRI/content/CRI_2_4_2x_Do_we_know_what_causes_cancer.asp>

Stephen, Pam. "What is Breast Cancer?" 30 January 2009. *About.com*. Web. 8 June 2010. <http://breastcancer.about.com/od/definition/a/bc_definition.htm>

"Dictionary of Cancer Terms Hematological Cancer." *Cancer.gov*. Web. 8 June 2010. <http://www.cancer.gov/dictionary/?CdrID=45708>

"Statistics on Leukemia: 2006 Estimates." 5 March 2009. *EmedTV.com*. Web. 8 June 2010. <http://leukemia.emedtv.com/leukemia/leukemia-statistics.html>

"Dictionary of Cancer Terms Lung Cancer." *Cancer.gov*. Web. 8 June 2010. <http://www.cancer.gov/dictionary/?CdrID=445043>

"Lung Cancer Statistics." 11 March 2010. Division of Cancer Prevention and Control, National Center for Chronic Disease Prevention and Health Promotion. Web. 8 June 2010. <http://www.cdc.gov/cancer/lung/statistics/ Lung Cancer Statistics>

"Definition of Prostate Cancer." 26 March 1998. *MedTerms*. Web. 8 June 2010. <http://www.medterms.com/script/main/art.asp?articlekey=5072>

"What are the Key Statistics about Prostate Cancer?" 29 April 2010. *Cancer.org*. Web. 8 June 2010. <http://www.cancer.org/docroot/cri/content/cri_2_4_1x_what_are_the_key_statistics_for_prostate_cancer_36.asp>

"Dictionary of Cancer Terms Skin Cancer." *Cancer.gov*. Web. 8 June 2010. <http://www.cancer.gov/dictionary/?CdrID=445084>

Polsky, Dr. David and Dr. Steven Wang. "Skin Cancer Facts." *Skincancer.org*. Web. 8 June 2010. <http://www.skincancer.org/Skin-Cancer-Facts/>

"Definition of Endometrial Cancer." 17 February 2009. *MedTerms*. Web. 8 June 2010. <http://www.medterms.com/script/main/art.asp?articlekey=31740>

"What are the Key Statistics about Endometrial Cancer?" 22 October 2010. *Cancer.org*. Web. 8 June 2010. <http://www.cancer.org/docroot/cri/content/cri_2_4_1x_what_are_the_key_statistics_for_endometrial_cancer.asp>

"Definition of Colon Cancer." 3 February 2002. *MedTerms*. Web. 8 June 2010. <http://www.medterms.com/script/main/art.asp?articlekey=2788>

"What are the Key Statistics for Colorectal Cancer?" 16 February 2010. *Cancer.org*. Web. 8 June 2010. <http://www.cancer.org/docroot/cri/content/cri_2_4_1x_what_are_the_key_statistics_for_colon_and_rectum_cancer.asp>

"Definition of Pancreatic Cancer." 10 October 2010. *MedTerms*. Web. 8 June 2010. <http://www.medterms.com/script/main/art.asp?articlekey=4746>

REFERENCES

"What are the Key Statistics about Cancer of the Pancreas?" 13 October 2009. *Cancer.org*. Web. 9 June 2010. <http://www.cancer.org/docroot/cri/content/cri_2_4_1x_what_are_the_key_statistics_for_pancreatic_cancer_34.asp>

"Surgery." 19 June 2009. *Cancer.org*. Web. 9 June 2010. <http://www.cancer.org/docroot/ETO/content/ETO_1_2X_Surgery.asp>

"How Does Radiation Work to Treat Cancer?" 17 July 2009. *Cancer.org*. Web. 9 June 2010. <http://www.cancer.org/docroot/ETO/content/ETO_1_4X_How_does_radiation_work_to_treat_cancer.asp?sitearea=ETO>

"Goals of Radiation Therapy." 17 July 2009. *Cancer.org*. Web. 9 June 2010. <http://www.cancer.org/docroot/ETO/content/ETO_1_4X_Goals_of_radiation_therapy.asp?sitearea=ETO>

"Chemo: What it is, How it Helps." 28 April 2009. *Cancer.org*. Web. 9 June 2010. <http://www.cancer.org/docroot/ETO/content/ETO_1_2X_Chemotherapy_What_It_Is_How_It_Helps.asp>

"What is Targeted Therapy?" 16 March 2009. *Cancer.org*. Web. 9 June 2010. <http://www.cancer.org/docroot/ETO/content/ETO_1_2x_Targeted_Therapy.asp>

"Medical Tourism and Cancer Treatments." 7 June 2010. *Alanahu.org*. Web. 9 June 2010. <http://www.alanahu.org/medical-tourism-and-cancer-treatments/>

"Bumrungrad International Hospital Horizon Regional Cancer Centre." 2010. *Bumrungrad.com*. Web. 9 June 2010. <http://www.bumrungrad.com/overseas-medical-care/medical-services/clinics-and-centers/horizon-regional-cancer-center.aspx>

"Type 2." American Diabetes Association. Web. 9 June 2010. <http://www.diabetes.org/diabetes-basics/type-2/ Type 2>

"Type 2 Diabetes Definition." 13 June 2009. *MayoClinic*. Web. 9 June 2010. <http://www.mayoclinic.com/health/type-2-diabetes/ds00585>

"Type 2 Diabetes Overview." *WebMD Medical Reference*. Web. 9 June 2010. <http://diabetes.webmd.com/guide/type-2-diabetes Type 2 Diabetes Overview>

Zieve, Dr. David and Dr. Deborah Wexler. "Type 2 Diabetes." 20 May 2009. *MedlinePlus*. Web. 9 June 2010. <http://www.nlm.nih.gov/medlineplus/ency/article/000313.htm>

"Diabetes Statistics." *Diabetes.org*. Web. 9 June 2010. <http://www.diabetes.org/diabetes-basics/diabetes-statistics/>

"Heart Disease Definition." 8 April 2010. *MayoClinic*. Web. 9 June 2010. <http://www.mayoclinic.com/health/heart-disease/ds01120>

"Definition of Heart Disease." 2 March 2003. *MedTerms*. Web. 9 June 2010. <http://www.medterms.com/script/main/art.asp?articlekey=31193>

"Heart Disease Overview." *WebMD Medical Reference*. Web. 9 June 2010. <http://www.webmd.com/heart-disease/default.htm>

"Heart Disease Statistics." *Mamashealth, Inc.* Web. 9 June 2010. <http://www.mamashealth.com/Heart_stat.asp>

"Cardiovascular Disease Statistics." *American Heart Association*. Web. 9 June 2010. <http://www.americanheart.org/presenter.jhtml?identifier=4478>

"Kidney and Urologic Disease Statistics for the United States." February 2009. NIH Publication. Web. 9 June 2010. <http://kidney.niddk.nih.gov/kudiseases/pubs/kustats/index.htm>

Patel, Dr. Parul. "Kidney Disease." 27 August 2009. *MedlinePlus*. Web. 9 June 2010. <http://www.nlm.nih.gov/medlineplus/ency/article/000457.htm>

REFERENCES

"Understanding Kidney Disease – Basic Information." *WebMD Medical Reference*. Web. 9 June 2010. <http://www.webmd.com/a-to-z-guides/understanding-kidney-disease-basic-information>

"Chronic Kidney Disease." *Emedicinehealth.com*. Web. 9 June 2010. <http://www.emedicinehealth.com/chronic_kidney_disease/article_em.htm>

"Chronic Obstructive Pulmonary Disease (COPD)" 18 January 2010. *CDC/National Center for Health Statistics*. Web. 9 June 2010. <http://www.cdc.gov/nchs/fastats/copd.htm>

"Definition of Chronic Obstructive Pulmonary Disease." 21 February 2004. *MedTerms*. Web. 9 June 2010. <http://www.medterms.com/script/main/art.asp?articlekey=7784>

"COPD (Chronic Obstructive Pulmonary Disease) – Overview." 8 May 2008. *WebMD Medical Reference*. Web. 9 June 2010. <http://www.webmd.com/lung/copd/tc/chronic-obstructive-pulmonary-disease-copd-overview>

"Chronic Respiratory Diseases." *World Health Organization*. Web. 9 June 2010. <http://www.who.int/respiratory/en/ Chronic respiratory diseases>

"Definition of Obesity." 2 February 2002. *MedTerms*. Web. 9 June 2010. <http://www.medterms.com/script/main/art.asp?articlekey=4607 Definition of Obesity>

"Obesity." *WebMD Medical Reference*. Web. 9 June 2010. <http://www.webmd.com/diet/guide/what-is-obesity>

"Obesity" *World Health Organization*. Web. 9 June 2010. <http://www.who.int/topics/obesity/en/>

Balentine, Jerry and Dr. Ruchi Mathur. "Obesity Weight Loss." *MedicineNet.com*. Web. 9 June 2010. <http://www.medicinenet.com/obesity_weight_loss/article.htm>

"Understanding Adult Obesity." November 2008. *NIH Publication*. Web. 9 June 2010. <http://win.niddk.nih.gov/publications/understanding.htm>

"Definition of Stem Cell." 12 September 2001. *MedTerms.* Web. 9 June 2010. <http://www.medterms.com/script/main/art.asp?articlekey=10597>

"Stem Cell Basics." 28 April 2009. *National Institute of Health.* Web. 9 June 2010. <http://stemcells.nih.gov/info/basics/basics1>

"Fetal Stem Cell Treatment." *Medra Inc.* Web. 9 June 2010. <http://www.medra.com/ Fetal Stem Cell Treatment>

"Stem Cell Therapies Today." *NIH Publication.* Web. 9 June 2010. <http://learn.genetics.utah.edu/content/tech/stemcells/sctoday/ STEM CELL>

"Statistics." 6 August 2009. *NIH Publication.* Web. 9 June 2010. <http://www.nimh.nih.gov/health/topics/statistics/index.shtml>

"Mental Illness Definition." 4 September 2008. *MayoClinic.* Web. 9 June 2010. <http://www.mayoclinic.com/health/mental-illness/ds01104>

"Mental Health Overview." *WebMD Medical Reference.* Web. 10 June 2010. <http://www.webmd.com/mental-health/default.htm>

"What is Mental Illness: Mental Illness Facts." *Nami.org.* Web. 10 June 2010. <http://www.nami.org/Content/NavigationMenu/Inform_Yourself/About_Mental_Illness/About_Mental_Illness.htm>

"Depression Glossary." *WebMD Medical Reference.* Web. 10 June 2010. <http://www.webmd.com/depression/depression-glossary Depression: Depression Glossary>

"Definition of Addiction." *MedTerms.* Web. 10 June 2010. <http://www.medterms.com/script/main/art.asp?articlekey=10177>

"The Definition of Addiction." 20 March 2010. *Addictions and Recovery.* Web. 10 June 2010. <http://www.addictionsandrecovery.org/definition-of-addiction.htm>

"Addiction Statistics." *U.S. Substance Abuse and Mental Health Services Administration.* Web. 10 June 2010. <http://www.coachinginternational.com/stats.html Addiction Statistics>

REFERENCES

Hicks, Jennifer. "What Kind of Diabetes Do I Have?" 15 August 2009. *About.com*. Web. 10 June 2010. <http://diabetes.about.com/od/symptoms diagnosis/a/typesofdiabetes.htm>

"What are The Different Types of Diabetes?" *Allaboutlifechallenges.org*. Web. 10 June 2010. <http://www.allaboutlifechallenges.org/types-of-diabetes-faq.htm>

"Types of Diabetes." *Eastern Virginia Medical School*. Web. 10 June 2010. <http://www.mfm-evms.org/dm2diabetestypes.html>

Pilkington, Nicky. "The Different Types of Diabetes." *Healthguidence.org*. Web. 10 June 2010. <http://www.healthguidance.org/entry/4942/1/The-Different-Types-of-Diabetes.html>

Barby, Ernest. "The Different Types of Heart Disease." *Selfgrowth.com*. Web. 10 June 2010. <http://www.selfgrowth.com/articles/The_Different_Types_of_Heart_Disease_27542.html>

"Symptoms and Types." *WebMD Medical Reference*. Web. 10 June 2010. <http://www.webmd.com/heart-disease/guide/heart-disease-symptoms-types>

"Common Cardiovascular Diseases." *American Heart Association*. Web. 10 June 2010. <http://www.americanheart.org/presenter.jhtml?identifier=2873>

"Definition of Heart Attack." 17 July 2004. MedTerms. Web. 10 June 2010. <http://www.medterms.com/script/main/art.asp?articlekey=3669>

"Definition of Coronary Artery Disease." 19 September 2003. *MedTerms*. Web. 10 June 2010. <http://www.medterms.com/script/main/art.asp?articlekey=10267>

"Definition of Cardiomyopathy." 6 September 2003. MedTerms. Web. 10 June 2010. <http://www.medterms.com/script/main/art.asp?articlekey=13590>

Bryg, Robert J. "Heart Disease and Cardiomyopathy." 7 March 2009. *WebMD Medical Reference*. Web. 10 June 2010. <http://www.webmd.com/heart-disease/guide/muscle-cardiomyopathy>

"What is Cardiomyopathy?" June 2010. *Health Grades Inc.* Web. 10 June 2010. <http://www.wrongdiagnosis.com/c/cardiomyopathy/basics.htm>

"Definition of Atrial Fibrillation." 26 March 1998. *MedTerms*. Web. 10 June 2010. <http://www.medterms.com/script/main/art.asp?articlekey =2384>

"Atrial Fibrillation – The Common Arrhythmia." *Heart Rhythm Society*. Web. 10 June 2010. <http://www.hrsonline.org/education/afib360/afibss/>

"Statistics About Atrial Fibrillation." June 2010. *Health Grades Inc.* Web. 10 June 2010. <http://www.wrongdiagnosis.com/a/atrial_fibrillation/stats.htm>

"Heart Valve Disease." *WebMD Medical Reference*. Web. 10 June 2010. <http://www.webmd.com/heart-disease/guide/heart-valve-disease>

Bryg, Robert J. "Heart Disease and Pericarditis." 7 March 2009. *WebMD Medical Reference*. Web. 10 June 2010. <http://www.webmd.com/heart-disease/guide/heart-disease-pericardial-disease-percarditis>

"Different Types of Kidney Disease." 1 April 2004. *Netwellness.org*. Web. 10 June 2010. <http://www.netwellness.org/healthtopics/kidney/kidneydisease.cfm>

"Types of Kidney Disease." June 2010. *Health Grades Inc.* Web. 10 June 2010. <http://www.wrongdiagnosis.com/k/kidney_disease/subtypes.htm#typeslist>

"Renal Tubular Acidosis." October 2008. *NIH Publication*. Web. 10 June 2010. <http://kidney.niddk.nih.gov/kudiseases/pubs/tubularacidosis/>

"Definition of Polycystic Kidney Disease." 3 September 2003. *MedTerms*. Web. 10 June 2010. <http://www.medterms.com/script/main/art.asp?articlekey=4980>

REFERENCES

"Definition of Alport Syndrome." 21 June 2004. *MedTerms*. Web. 10 June 2010. <http://www.medterms.com/script/main/art.asp?articlekey=10745>

"Statistics About Alport Syndrome." *Health Grades Inc.* Web. 10 June 2010. <http://www.wrongdiagnosis.com/a/alport_syndrome/stats.htm>

Patel, Dr. Parul. "Reflux Nephropathy – Overview." 18 September 2009. *Umm.Edu.* Web. 10 June 2010. <http://www.umm.edu/ency/article/000459.htm>

"Chronic Renal Insufficiency." June 2010. *Health Grades Inc*. Web. 10 June 2010. <http://www.wrongdiagnosis.com/c/chronic_renal_insufficiency/intro.htm>

"Definition of Asthma." 8 April 2004. *MedTerms*. Web. 10 June 2010. <http://www.medterms.com/script/main/art.asp?articlekey=2373>

"Definition of Pulmonary Hypertension." 22 October 2004. *MedTerms*. Web. 10 June 2010. <http://www.medterms.com/script/main/art.asp?articlekey=5126>

"Statistics About Pulmonary Hypertension." June 2010. *Health Grades Inc*. Web. 10 June 2010. <http://www.wrongdiagnosis.com/p/primary_pulmonary_hypertension/stats.htm>

"Definition of Emphysema." 26 March 1998. *MedTerms*. Web. 10 June 2010. <http://www.medterms.com/script/main/art.asp?articlekey=3228>

"Statistics About Emphysema." June 2010. *Health Grades Inc*. Web. 10 June 2010. <http://www.wrongdiagnosis.com/e/emphysema/stats.htm>

"Definition of Chronic Bronchitis." 13 December 1998. *MedTerms*. Web. 10 June 2010. <http://www.medterms.com/script/main/art.asp?articlekey=7792>

"Statistics About Chronic Bronchitis." June 2010. *Health Grades Inc*. Web. 10 June 2010. <http://www.wrongdiagnosis.com/c/chronic_bronchitis/stats.htm>

"Definition of Stroke." 4 July 1999. *MedTerms*. Web. 10 June 2010. <http://www.medterms.com/script/main/art.asp?articlekey=9791>

"High Blood Pressure (Hypertension)." *MedicineNet.com*. Web. 10 June 2010. <http://www.medicinenet.com/high_blood_pressure/article.htm>

Marks, Dr. Jay. "Gallstones." *MedicineNet.com*. Web. 10 June 2010. <http://www.medicinenet.com/gallstones/article.htm>

"Definition of Sleep Apnea." 9 March 2004. *MedTerms*. Web. 10 June 2010. <http://www.medterms.com/script/main/art.asp?articlekey=5510>

"Definition of Heart Failure." 18 June 2002. *MedTerms*. Web. 10 June 2010. <http://www.medterms.com/script/main/art.asp?articlekey=3672>

"Pickwickian Syndrome." *The HealthScout Network*. Web. 10 June 2010. <http://www.healthscout.com/ency/68/745/main.html>

"Hodgkin's Lymphoma (Hodgkin's Disease) Definition." 11 July 2009. *MayoClinic*. Web. 10 June 2010. <http://www.mayoclinic.com/health/hodgkins-disease/ds00186>

"Definition of Parkinson's Disease." 31 October 2003. *MedTerms*. Web. 10 June 2010. <http://www.medterms.com/script/main/art.asp?articlekey=4783>

"Definition of Multiple Sclerosis." 20 December 2003. *MedTerms*. Web. 10 June 2010. <http://www.medterms.com/script/main/art.asp?articlekey=4457>

"Types of Mental Illness." *WebMD Medical Reference*. Web. 10 June 2010. <http://www.webmd.com/mental-health/mental-health-types-illness>

"Gambling Addiction Statistics." *Clearleadinc.com*. Web. 10 June 2010. <http://www.clearleadinc.com/site/gambling-addiction.html>

"Statistics About Schizophrenia." June 2010. *Health Grades Inc*. Web. 10 June 2010. <http://www.wrongdiagnosis.com/s/schizophrenia/stats.htm>

REFERENCES

"Bipolar Disorder Statistics." 4 May 2006. *Dbsalliance.org*. Web. 10 June 2010. <http://www.dbsalliance.org/site/PageServer?pagename=about_statistics_bipolar>

"Statistics About Borderline Personality Disorder." June 2010. Health Grades Inc. Web. 10 June 2010. <http://www.wrongdiagnosis.com/b/borderline_personality_disorder/stats.htm>

"Anorexia Statistics." *Mirror-mirror.org*. Web. 10 June 2010. <http://www.mirror-mirror.org/anorexia-statistics.htm>

"Statistics About Drug Abuse." June 2010. *Health Grades Inc*. Web. 10 June 2010. <http://www.wrongdiagnosis.com/d/drug_abuse/stats.htm>

Herkov, Dr. Michael. "What is Sexual Addiction?" 10 December 2006. *PsychCentral.com*. Web. 10 June 2010. <http://psychcentral.com/lib/2006/what-is-sexual-addiction/>

"Sex Addiction Statistics and Facts." *MyAddiction.com*. Web. 10 June 2010. <http://www.myaddiction.com/education/articles/sex_statistics.html>

"Type 2 Diabetes." 13 June 2009. *MayoClinic*. Web. 10 June 2010. <http://www.mayoclinic.com/health/type-2-diabetes/ds00585/dsection=treatments-and-drugs>

"Coronary Artery Disease." April 2005. *Surgical Associates of Texas*. Web. 10 June 2010. <http://www.texheartsurgeons.com/cad.htm>

"About Medi-Clinic Heart Hospital." *Mediclinic.co.za*. Web. 10 June 2010. <http://www.mediclinic.co.za/hospitals/Pages/about.aspx?h=45>

"Kidney Failure: Choosing a Treatment That's Right for You." November 2007. *NIH Publications*. Web. 10 June 2010. <http://kidney.niddk.nih.gov/kudiseases/pubs/choosingtreatment/>

Simon, Dr. Harvey. "Chronic Obstructive Pulmonary Disease Medications." 20 April 2009. *New York Times*. Web. 10 June 2010. <http://health.nytimes.com/health/guides/disease/chronic-obstructive-pulmonary-disease/medications.html>

"Surgical Treatments Chronic Obstructive Pulmonary Disease (COPD)" *Columbia University Medical Center.* Web. 10 June 2010. <http://www.columbiasurgery.org/thoracic/copd_treatment.html>

"Beijing Anzhen Hospital." *Anzhen.com.* Web. 10 June 2010. <http://www.anzhen.org/english/rd.html>

"Gastric Bypass Surgery Definition." 2 October 2009. *MayoClinic.* Web. 10 June 2010. <http://www.mayoclinic.com/health/gastric-bypass/my00825>

"Obesity Treatments and Drugs." 9 May 2009. *MayoClinic.* Web. 10 June 2010. <http://www.mayoclinic.com/health/obesity/ds00314/dsection=treatments-and-drugs>

"Cancer *Treatment:* Stem Cell Transplantation." *Cancercompass.com.* Web. 10 June 2010. <http://www.cancercompass.com/cancer-treatment/stem-cell-transplantation.htm>

"About EmCell." *EmCell.com.* Web. 10 June 2010. <http://www.emcell.com/en/about_emcell.htm>

"Mental Illness Treatment and Drugs." *MayoClinic.* Web. 10 June 2010. <http://www.mayoclinic.com/health/mental-illness/ds01104/dsection=treatments-and-drugs>

"Mental Health Care Treatment in South Africa." *Life Path Group.* Web. 10 June 2010. <http://www.lifepathgroup.co.za/>

Grayson, Charlotte. "New Prescriptions for Addiction Treatment." *MedicineNet.com.* Web. 10 June 2010. <http://www.medicinenet.com/script/main/art.asp?articlekey=50394>

"Nova Vida Recovery Centre." 28 May 2010. *Health Tourism.* Web. 10 June 2010. <http://www.health-tourism.com/medical-centers/nova-vida-reccovery-centre/>

"Alternative Medicine Cont." 26 July 2006. *MedicineNet.com.* Web. 11 June 2010. <http://www.medicinenet.com/alternative_medicine/page3.htm>

REFERENCES

"Alternative Medicine: Evaluate Claims of Treatment Success." 8 April 2010. *MayoClinic*. Web. 11 June 2010. <http://www.mayoclinic.com/health/alternative-medicine/sa00078>

"Alternative Medicine – Avenue for Medical Tourism." 11 February 2010. *Aardf Health*. Web. 11 June 2010. <http://www.aardf.org/2010/02/alternative-medicine-avenue-for-medical-tourism/>

"What is Immunotherapy?" 25 August 2009. *American Cancer Society*. Web. 11 June 2010. <http://www.cancer.org/docroot/eto/content/eto_1_4x_what_is_immunotherapy.asp>

Guthrie, Michael. "Alternative Cancer Treatments." 7 May 2006. *Alternative-cancer-treamtents.com*. Web. 11 June 2010. <http://www.alternative-cancer-treatments.com/>

"Immuno-Augmentative Therapy" 1 November 2008. *American Cancer Society*. Web. 11 June 2010. http://www.cancer.org/docroot/eto/content/eto_5_3x_immuno-augmentative_therapy.asp

"Unconventional Cancer Treatments." *Quackwatch.com*. Web. 11 June 2010. <http://www.quackwatch.org/01QuackeryRelatedTopics/OTA/ota06.html>

"Issels Treatment Summary." June 2010. Issels.com. Web. 11 June 2010. <http://www.issels.com/TreatmentSummary.aspx>

"Issels Foundations Inc." *Whale.to*. Web. 11 June 2010. <http://www.whale.to/cancer/issels.html>

"Dictionary of Cancer Terms Nutrition Therapy." *Cancer.gov*. Web. 11 June 2010. <http://www.cancer.gov/dictionary/?CdrID=463725>

"Definition of Macrobiotic Diet." 2 June 2006. *MedTerms*. Web. 11 June 2010. <http://www.medterms.com/script/main/art.asp?articlekey=11616>

Wigmore, Ann. "Wheatgrass Treatment for Cancer." *Cancertutor.com*. Web. 11 June 2010. <http://www.cancertutor.com/Cancer/Wheatgrass.html>

"Hyperthermia." 17 July 2009. *American Cancer Society.* Web. 11 June 2010. <http://www.cancer.org/docroot/ETO/content/ETO_1_2x_Hyperthermia.asp>

"DMSO – The Magic Bullet for Cancer." *Cancertutor.com.* Web. 11 June 2010. <http://cancertutor.com/Cancer/DMSO.html>

"What is Biological Therapy?" *Cancer.gov.* Web. 11 June 2010. <http://www.cancer.gov/cancertopics/biologicaltherapy>

"Revici's Guided Chemotherapy." 1 November 2008. *Cancer.org.* Web. 11 June 2010. <http://www.cancer.org/docroot/ETO/content/ETO_5_3X_Revicis_Guided_Chemotherapy.asp>

"The Budwig Center: Private Cancer Treatment in Spain." *Treatment Abroad.* Web. 11 June 2010. <http://www.treatmentabroad.com/cancer-treatment-abroad/cancer-spain/ta-the-budwig-center/>

"Homeopathy – Topic Overview." 30 June 2009. *WebMD Medical Reference.* Web. 11 June 2010. <http://www.webmd.com/balance/tc/homeopathy-topic-overview>

Schmukler, Alan V. "What is Homeopathy? Definition and Details." 25 November 2009. *Hpathy.com.* Web. 11 June 2010. <http://hpathy.com/abc-homeopathy/what-is-homeopathy-definition-and-details/>

"Types of Homeopathic Medicines, Practitioners." 14 June 2007. *Pharmpress.com.* Web. 11 June 2010. <http://www.pharmpress.com/shop/samples/HPPC_sample.pdf>

"Homeopathic Medicine FAQ." 16 May 2010. *Rite Care Pharmacy Inc.* Web. 11 June 2010. <http://www.ritecare.com/homeopathic/guide_general.asp>

"Natural Healthcare for the Whole Family." *The Fountain Centre.* Web. 11 June 2010. <http://www.fountaincentre.com.au/>

REFERENCES

Vann, Madeline. "Can Chelation Therapy Help Heart Disease?" 26 August 2009. *Everydayhealth.com*. Web. 11 June 2010. <http://www.everydayhealth.com/alternative-health/chelation-therapy-and-heart-disease.aspx>

"Definition of Naturopathy." 6 June 2004. *MedTerms*. Web. 11 June 2010. <http://www.medterms.com/script/main/art.asp?articlekey=11735>

"Naturopathic Medicine." *Naturopathic Medicine Network*. Web. 11 June 2010. <http://www.pandamedicine.com/naturopathic_medicine.html>

"Naturopathy." *Uniklinik-freiburg.de*. Web. 11 June 2010. <http://www.uniklinik-freiburg.de/ims/live/hospital/naturopathy_en.html>

"Definition of Ayurveda." 23 June 2004. *MedTerms*. Web. 11 June 2010. <http://www.medterms.com/script/main/art.asp?articlekey=10787>

Lad, Dr. Vasant. "An Introduction to Ayurveda." *The Ayurveda Institute*. Web. 11 June 2010. <http://www.healthy.net/scr/article.aspx?Id=373>

"Ayurvedic Medicine: An Introduction." July 2009. *NCCAM Publication*. Web. 11 June 2010. <http://nccam.nih.gov/health/ayurveda/introduction.htm>

"Definition of Acupuncture." 23 June 2004. *MedTerms*. Web. 11 June 2010. <http://www.medterms.com/script/main/art.asp?articlekey=2132>

"Acupuncture." 11 December 2009. *MayoClinic*. Web. 12 June 2010. <http://www.mayoclinic.com/health/acupuncture/my00946>

Stuart, Annie. "Hyperbaric Oxygen Therapy." November 2009. *NYU Langone Medical Center*. Web. 12 June 2010. <http://www.med.nyu.edu/patientcare/library/article.html?ChunkIID=101004>

Medoff, Dr. Benjamin. "Hyperbaric Oxygen Therapy." 24 September 2008. *MedlinePlus*. Web. 12 June 2010. <http://www.nlm.nih.gov/medlineplus/ency/article/002375.htm>

"Definition of Biofeedback" 6 April 2002. MedTerms. Web. 12 June 2010. <http://www.medterms.com/script/main/art.asp?articlekey=10810>

Brown, Anitra. "What is a Spa?" *About.com*. Web. 12 June 2010. <http://spas.about.com/cs/spa101/a/whatisaspa.htm>

Brown, Anitra. "What is a Destination Spa?" *About.com*. Web. 12 June 2010. <http://spas.about.com/od/destinationspas/p/destinationspa.htm>

Brown, Anitra. "What is a Resort Spa? *About.com*. Web. 12 June 2010. <http://spas.about.com/od/resortspas/a/resortspa.htm>

Brown, Anitra. "Day Spas." *About.com*. Web. 12 June 2010. <http://spas.about.com/od/dayspas/a/dayspa.htm>

Brown, Anitra. "What is a Mineral Springs Spa?" *About.com*. Web. 12 June 2010. <http://spas.about.com/od/choosingaspabasics/a/mineralsprings.htm>

Brown, Anitra. "What is a Medical Spa." *About.com*. Web. 12 June 2010. <http://spas.about.com/od/medispas/a/medicalspa.htm>

"Electromyographic Biofeedback" *Medical Dictionary*. Web. 12 June 2010. <http://medical-dictionary.thefreedictionary.com/electromyographic+biofeedback>

"Thermal Biofeedback." *Medical Dictionary*. Web. 12 June 2010. <http://medical-dictionary.thefreedictionary.com/thermal+biofeedback>

"Neurofeedback and EEG Biofeedback Dictionary." *Eeginfo.com*. Web. 12 June 2010. <http://www.eeginfo.com/glossary-definition.html>

"Types of Biofeedback Devices Used." *Nwhealth.edu*. Web. 12 June 2010. <http://www.nwhealth.edu/healthyU/chillOut/biofb1.html>

"Oxygen Concentrator." *Vitalitymedical.com*. Web. 12 June 2010. <http://www.vitalitymedical.com/Catalog/What-is-an-oxygen-concentrator-75.html>

Latham, Dr. Emi. "Hyperbaric Oxygen Therapy." 19 May 2010. *Emedicine*. Web. 12 June 2010. <http://emedicine.medscape.com/article/1464149-overview>

REFERENCES

"St. Augustine's Hyperbaric Medicine Centre." *Sahmc.com*. Web. 12 June 2010. <http://www.sahmc.co.za/>

"Types of Acupuncture." *Psychology Today*. Web. 12 June 2010. <http://healthprofs.com/cam/content/acupuncture_types.html>

"Types of Acupuncture." 4 July 2008. *The Health Guide*. Web. 13 June 2010. <http://www.thehealthguide.org/acupuncture/types-of-acupuncture/>

"ACURA Acupuncture Clinic Tokyo Japan." *Acuraclinic.com*. Web. 13 June 2010. <http://www.acuraclinic.com/en/Overview_Home.aspx>

"Ayurvedic Medicine: An Introduction." July 2009. *NCCAM Publication*. Web. 13 June 2010. <http://nccam.nih.gov/health/ayurveda/introduction.htm>

"The Retreat." Ayurveda.*org*. Web. 13 June 2010. <http://www.ayurveda.org/retreat.html>

"Chelation Therapy By Advanced Medical Group." *Placidway.net*. Web. 13 June 2010. <http://placidway.net/package/195/>

"Crime Statistics Murder per Capita By Country."*NationMaster.com*. Web. 14 June 2010. <http://www.nationmaster.com/graph/cri_mur_percap-crime-murders-per-capita>

"Joint Commission International Accreditation." *Joint Commission International*. Web. 14 June 2010. <http://www.jointcommissioninternational.org/Accreditation-and-Certification-Process/>

Marsek, Patrick and Frances Sharpe. "The Complete Idiot's Guide to Medical Tourism." New York. The Penguin Group, 2009. Parts 2-4. 91-281 Print.

Woodman, Josef. "Patients Beyond Borders." Chapel Hill, NC. Healthy Travel Media, 2008. Chapter 2,3,4,5,6. 35-161. Print.

Gahlinger, Dr. Paul. "The Medical Tourism Travel Guide." North Branch, MN. Sunrise River Press, 2008. Chapter 3. 59-75. Print.

"Orthopedic Surgery in Panama – Hospitals Guide." *Health Tourism*. Web. 17 June 2010. <http://www.health-tourism.com/orthopedic-surgery/panama/>

"Strategic Location." *Dubai Smile Dental Center*. Web. 17 June 2010. <http://www.dubaismile.com/overseas.htm>

"Health Care in Dubai." 8 August 2009. *Expatforum.com*. Web. 17 June 2010. <http://www.expatforum.com/articles/health/health-care-in-dubai.html>

"Health Care in South Africa." 10 August 2009. *Expatforum.com*. Web. 17 June 2010. <http://www.expatforum.com/articles/health/health-care-in-south-africa.html>

"Healthcare in Singapore." *Singapore Expats*. Web. 17 June 2010. <http://www.singaporeexpats.com/guides-for-expats/healthcare-in-singapore.htm>

"Spike in Diabetes in Saudi Arabia." 10 March 2009. *Diabetes.co.uk*. Web. 17 June 2010. <http://www.diabetes.co.uk/news/2009/Mar/spike-in-diabetes-in-saudi-arabia.html>

"Health Care in New Zealand." 8 August 2009. *Expatforum.com*. Web. 17 June 2010.<http://www.expatforum.com/articles/health/health-care-in-new-zealand.html>

"Panama Language." *Mapsofworld.com*. Web. 17 June 2010. <http://www.mapsofworld.com/panama/society-and-culture/language.html>

"Language in Dubai." *Mapsofworld.com*. Web. 17 June 2010. <http://www.mapsofworld.com/dubai/language-in-dubai.html>

"The Languages of South Africa." *Southafrica.info*. Web. 17 June 2010. <http://www.southafrica.info/about/people/language.htm>

"Saudi Arabia Language." *Mapsofworld.com*. Web. 17 June 2010. <http://www.mapsofworld.com/saudi-arabia/society-and-culture/language.html>

REFERENCES

"New Zealand Language." *Tourism.net*. Web. 17 June 2010. <http://www.tourism.net.nz/new-zealand/about-new-zealand/language.html>

"India – Language, Culture, Customs and Etiquette." *Kwintessential*. Web. 17 June 2010. <http://www.kwintessential.co.uk/resources/global-etiquette/india-country-profile.html>

"Medical Tourism in Panama." *Health Tourism*. Web. 17 June 2010. <http://www.health-tourism.com/panama-medical-tourism/>

McBrewster, John, Frederik P. Miller and Agnes F. Vandome, eds. "Medical Tourism." USA. Alphascript Publishing, 2009. Print.

Index

A

Abdominal Aortic Aneurysm
   Repair *204, 214*
ACHSI Accreditation (Australian Council for Healthcare Standards International) *291*
Acupuncture *273, 274, 275, 276, 286, 362, 399, 403, 446, 448*
Addiction – treatments *246*
   Counseling or
      Group Therapy *246*
   Prescribed Medication *246*
   Rehabilitation *185, 246, 247*
Addiction – variants
   Drug and Alcohol Abuse
      246, 368
   Gambling Addiction *246, 441*
   Sexual Addiction *246, 442*
Adjunctive Therapies *263*
Adult Stem Cell Treatment
   254, 362
Advanced Medical Group
   268, 448
Air Ambulance *118, 186, 398, 425*
Alfano, Madelyn *42*
Alliance *402*

Alport Syndrome *231, 362, 440*
American Air Ambulance *186*
American Cancer Society *217, 221, 403, 444, 445*
American Hospital, Dubai
   227, 339
AmeriMed American Hospital *332*
Anadolu Medical Center *358*
Angel Flight *186*
Antineoplaston Therapy *264*
Aortic Valve Replacement *206, 214, 363, 430*
Apollo Gleneagles Hospital *195*
Apollo Hospital in Chennai *189*
Appendectomy *101, 191, 212, 363, 401, 426, 427*
Argentina *147, 157, 166, 167, 168, 169, 174, 176, 178, 207, 214, 265*
Ars Medica Laser Clinic *358*
ART Fertility Clinic *351*
ASAN Medical Center
   International Clinic *355*
Asthma *234, 363, 440*
Atrial Fibrillation *228, 364, 439*
Australian Homeopathic
   Society *267*

REFERENCES

Ayurvedic Medicine *272, 284, 285, 364, 446, 448*

B

Bali *101, 128*
Bangkok Hospital *192, 427*
Barbados *166, 167, 168, 169, 178*
Beijing Anzhen Hospital *236, 443*
Beijing Institute of Heart, Lung and Blood Vessel Diseases *236*
Belhoul Specialty Hospital *339*
Belize *101, 114, 200, 285, 317, 324, 328, 329, 330*
Belize Medical Associates *330*
Big Pharma *47, 48, 49, 59, 64, 65, 75, 88, 390, 393, 410*
Biofeedback Therapy *278, 364*
    Electromyography (EMG) *279, 368*
    Finger Pulse Measurements *280*
    Respiration Biofeedback *280*
    Thermal Biofeedback *279, 379, 447*
Biological Therapies *263, 364*
Biopsy *164, 177, 364, 416, 424*
Blepharoplasty *148, 149, 171, 175, 364, 421*
BNH Hospital, Thailand *197*
Brain Tumor Surgery *201, 213, 263*

Brazil *147, 164, 170, 174, 177, 179, 190, 212, 247*
Breast Augmentation *144, 174, 365, 399, 418, 419*
Budwig Center, Spain *264*
Bumrungrad International Hospital *224, 434*
Burnham, Andy *63*

C

Cancer *88, 217, 218, 221, 222, 238, 241, 251, 261, 343, 358, 365, 366, 369, 370, 373, 375, 377, 402, 403, 427, 431, 432, 433, 434, 443, 444, 445*
Cape Town Medi-Clinic *340*
Cardiac Surgery *206, 342*
Cardiomyopathy *228, 365, 438, 439*
Cardiovascular Surgery *163*
CDC *216, 304, 431, 436*
Centro Medico Paitilla *327, 328*
Changi General Hospital *343*
Charles Krauthammer *43, 408*
Chelation Therapy *267, 285, 366, 403, 446, 448*
Chemotherapy *223, 251, 366, 434, 445*
Childhood Obesity Task Force Report *30*

Chinese Medicine *258*
Cholecystectomy *210, 366*
Christiaan Barnard Memorial Hospital *341, 342*
Chronic Bronchitis *235, 366, 440*
Chronic Obstructive Pulmonary Disease (COPD) *436, 443*
Chronic Renal Insufficiency *231, 366, 440*
CIMA Hospital *335*
City Hospital *338*
Clinica Biblica Hospital *173, 336*
Clinical Trials *432*
Coahuila, Mexico *190*
Commerce Clause *54*
Constitutional Medicine *265*
Coronary Artery Disease *228, 367, 438, 442*
Cosmetic Surgery *71, 113, 143, 293, 321, 325, 331, 340, 359, 367, 393, 397, 398, 412, 420*
Cosmetic Surgery Loan Company *293*
Costa Rica *145, 149, 152, 153, 154, 155, 158, 159, 160, 161, 170, 174, 175, 176, 177, 179, 193, 199, 202, 205, 212, 213, 214, 251, 252, 253, 285, 324, 325, 333, 334, 335, 336*

Council for Health Services Accreditation of Southern Africa *291*
Croatia *148, 152, 174, 175, 199, 200, 213*
Cyfeed Biofeedback Center *280*

D

Denmark *169, 178*
Dental Care Dubai *321*
Dentistry *344, 400, 422, 423*
   Dental Bridge *154, 176, 367, 423*
   Dental Fillings *158, 176, 423*
   Dental Implants *150, 416, 422*
   Dental Surgery *150, 175, 331, 334*
   Dental Veneers *157, 176*
   Dentures *159, 176, 368, 423*
   Gum Treatment *160, 177, 423*
Diabetes – treatment
   Blood Sugar Levels *226*
   Diet *225, 229, 444*
   Insulin and Medication *226*
   Surgery *226, 380*
Diabetes – types
   Gestational Diabetes *225*
   Prediabetes *377*
   Pregestational Diabetes *225, 377*

Type 1 *225, 377*
Type 2 *224, 368, 434,*
435, 442
Diagnostic Surgery *164, 368*
Dialysis *232, 368, 376, 402*
Dingell, John *92*
DMSO Therapy *285*
DRK Kliniken Berlin *357*
Dubai *148, 174, 227, 251, 321,*
336, 337, 338, 339, 449

E

Egyptian Health Care Accreditation Organization *291*
Emcell Clinic *242*
Emphysema *234, 369, 440*
Endodontic Surgery *152, 175, 369, 400, 422*
Europe *22, 110, 290, 304, 323, 356, 357, 399*
Extraction *153, 154, 175, 400, 422*

F

Face and Neck Lift *145*
Fair Labor and Standards Act *72*
Fertility Treatment *165*
Financing *135, 293*
Fortis Kidney Institute *233*
Fountain Center *267*

Frozen Embryo Transfer *166, 178, 369, 400, 424*

G

Gall Bladder Removal *189, 210*
Gamete Intrafallopian Transfer (GIFT) *369, 424*
Gastrectomy *188, 212, 251, 370, 401, 425, 426*
General Surgery *186, 342, 346, 401*
Gleneagles Medical Center *361*
Guatemala *157, 176*
Gynecology *370*

H

HA Accreditation – The Thailand Hospital Accreditation *291*
Harvard Medical International Hospital *233*
Healthcare Bill *32*
Heart Attack *228, 370, 438*
Heart Disease *227, 228, 366, 370, 403, 435, 438, 439, 446*
Heart Valve Disease *228, 370, 439*
Hemorrhoidectomy *371*
Himalayas *172, 284, 301*
Homeopathy *264, 265, 267, 270, 371, 403, 445*
　Allergodes, Nosodes and Sarcodes *266*

Classical Medicine *265*
Complex Medicine *266*
Constitutional Medicine *265*
Polychrests *266*
House of Representatives *27, 39*
Hungary *151, 152, 153, 155, 158, 159, 175, 176, 290, 323, 357, 358*
Hyperbaric Oxygen Therapy *276, 371, 446, 447*
   Compressed Oxygen Cylinders *277*
   Liquid Oxygen Systems *277, 373*
   Multiplace Chamber *278, 374*
   Oxygen Concentrators *277, 375*
Hyperthermia *263, 371, 403, 445*
Hypertrophic Pyloric Stenosis *208, 371, 431*
Hysterectomy *164, 177, 211, 371, 400, 424*

I

Immuno-Augmentative Therapy *261, 262, 371, 444*
Immunotherapy *223, 261, 444*
India *110, 125, 146, 153, 162, 164, 165, 171, 172, 174, 175, 177, 188, 189, 192, 195, 198, 200, 204, 205, 207, 208, 209, 212, 213, 214, 220, 233, 249, 250, 251, 252, 253, 254, 265, 272, 273, 284, 285, 286, 290, 301, 303, 305, 322, 348, 349, 381, 420, 426, 450*
Inguinal Hernia Repair *192, 212, 372, 427*
Internal Revenue Service *68, 93, 94, 396, 411, 415*
Intracytoplasmic Sperm Injection *167, 178, 372, 424*
In Vitro Fertilization *166, 178, 372, 424*
Irish Health Services Accreditation Board *291*
ISQua Accreditation – The International Society for Quality in Healthcare *291*
Israel *164, 177*
Issels Whole Body Immunotherapy *261, 372*

J

Japan *124, 274, 276, 286, 291, 308, 354, 448*
Japan Council for Quality in Healthcare *291*
Jaw Bone Grafting *151, 175, 372*
Johns Hopkins International *194, 326*

Joint Commission International
(JCI) *129, 132, 134, 189,
190, 192, 197, 198, 209, 291,
325, 326, 328, 331, 332, 334,
335, 336, 339, 340, 342, 343,
344, 345, 346, 348, 349, 350,
351, 352, 353, 354, 356, 358,
359, 360, 384*

K

Karl Heusner Memorial
Hospital *329*
Kidney Disease *231, 372, 377,
435, 436, 439*
Kidney Medication *232*
Kidney Reflux *231, 372*
King Faisal Specialist Hospital
and Research Center *345*
KK Women's and Children's
Hospital *209, 431*
Krishna Heart and Super Specialty
Institute *208, 349, 430*

L

La Catolica Hospital Hotel *335*
Laser Eye Surgery (LASIK) *169,
170, 179, 324, 398, 400, 425*
Lebanon *206*
Lifeline Pilots *186*
Life Path Health Group,
South Africa *245*

Lifetime Coverage
Insurance Plans *96*
Liposuction *146, 171, 174, 373,
400, 420*
Lung Disease *253, 402*
Lung Transplant *197, 213,
373, 428*

M

Macrobiotic Nutrition *262, 374*
Mahkota Medical Centre *204, 430*
Malaysia *196, 204, 213, 214,
290, 323, 324, 350, 359,
360, 361*
Maria's Italian Kitchen *42*
Marks, Dr. James *216, 430, 431*
Marriage penalty *69, 411*
Massachusetts *97*
Mastectomy *194, 213, 374, 401,
427, 428*
Mayo Clinic *148, 169, 381*
Medevac *119*
Medical Bills *72, 397*
Medical Malpractice *89, 415*
Medical Tourism Agencies *19*
Medicare or Medicaid *38, 40, 41,
44, 45, 48, 53, 66, 67, 76, 77,
83, 86, 388, 395, 414*
Medication *226, 229, 230, 232,
233, 235, 243, 244, 246,
310, 313*

Medi-Clinic Heart Hospital
230, 442
Memorial Health Group *198*
Mental Illness – treatment
   Electroconvulsive
      Therapy *244*
   Medication and Behavioral
      Therapy *243*
   Psychotherapist *244*
Mental Illness – types
   Anxiety Disorders *243, 363*
   Eating Disorders *243*
   Impulse Control Disorders
      243, 372
   Mood Disorders *243*
   Personality Disorders *243, 376*
   Psychotic Disorders *243, 377*
Metropolitan Medical Center *353*
Mexico *101, 102, 105, 108, 109, 114, 119, 125, 145, 146, 151, 152, 154, 155, 157, 160, 161, 164, 170, 173, 174, 175, 176, 177, 179, 184, 188, 190, 195, 199, 200, 203, 204, 205, 209, 210, 211, 212, 213, 214, 218, 251, 252, 253, 254, 268, 285, 286, 322, 324, 328, 329, 331, 332, 333, 397, 401, 419, 420, 426*

MSQH Accreditation – Malaysian Society for Quality in Health *291*
Myth *32, 33, 34, 35, 36, 37, 38*

N

National Cancer Center
   Singapore *343*
National Sales Tax *43, 408*
Naturopathic Medicine *269, 446*
   Botanical Medicine *270, 365*
   Light Surgery *270*
   Naturopathic Obstetrics
      271, 374
   Nutrition *262, 270, 374, 444*
   Physical Medicine *269, 376*
   Psychological Medicine *269*
Netcare Olivedale Hospital *341*
Neurosurgery *201, 321, 342, 348, 375, 429*
New England Journal
   of Medicine *78*
New River Cove *330, 331*
New Zealand *23, 162, 177, 200, 207, 214, 290, 322, 346, 347, 449, 450*
Non-Surgical Dental
   Procedures *156*
Nova Vida Recovery Center *247*
Nutritional Therapies *262*

REFERENCES

O

Obamacare *26, 27, 28, 29, 30, 31, 35, 36, 39, 40, 42, 46, 49, 50, 51, 54, 61, 62, 63, 66, 71, 72, 73, 74, 75, 76, 77, 78, 79, 82, 83, 87, 88, 91, 93, 95, 97, 98, 99, 100, 101, 104, 108, 109, 114, 116, 120, 121, 162, 184, 187, 216, 385, 386, 387, 388, 389, 390, 391, 392, 393, 394, 395, 396, 397, 398, 405, 406, 407, 408, 409, 410, 411, 412, 413, 414, 415*

Obama, President Barack *27, 28, 29, 30, 31, 32, 33, 36, 38, 39, 43, 45, 46, 47, 48, 49, 50, 51, 59, 60, 61, 62, 63, 65, 66, 69, 71, 72, 73, 74, 75, 76, 78, 79, 82, 83, 85, 86, 87, 90, 92, 93, 94, 95, 97, 98, 99, 104, 117, 130, 241, 385, 387, 390, 393, 394, 395, 396, 405, 407, 410, 411, 414, 415*

Obesity Clinic 365MC *239*

Obesity – diseases linked with
   Cancer *88, 217, 218, 221, 222, 238, 241, 251, 261, 343, 358, 365, 366, 369, 370, 373, 375, 377, 402, 403, 427, 431, 432, 433, 434, 443, 444, 445*
   Gallstones *189, 237, 369, 441*
   Heart Failure *238, 370, 441*
   High Blood Pressure *237, 371, 441*
   Pickwickian Syndrome *238, 376, 441*
   Sleep Apnea *237, 378, 441*
   Stroke *237, 379, 441*

Obesity – treatment
   Gastric Bypass Surgery *104, 238, 370, 397, 443*
   Lifestyle Change *238*
   Medication *226, 229, 230, 232, 233, 235, 243, 244, 246, 310*

Oophorectomy *375*

Orthodontic Surgery *153*

Orthopedic Surgery *162, 202, 429, 449*

Ovary Transplant *169, 178, 375, 424*

P

Pacemaker Implant *163, 177, 252*

Panama *21, 22, 23, 101, 108, 114, 125, 134, 145, 148, 165, 174, 177, 190, 193, 194, 200, 212, 251, 253, 285, 286, 317, 321, 324, 325, 326, 327, 328, 329, 333, 417, 419, 421, 449, 450*

Patient Protection and Affordable Care Act *27, 31, 53, 385, 405*
Patriot Act *28, 95, 396*
Paul, Ron *51, 60, 391, 410*
Payment Plans *293*
Pediatric Surgery *208, 430*
Penalties *37, 41, 43, 44, 53, 63, 68, 82, 99*
Pericarditis *229, 376, 439*
Peru *151, 175*
Pharmaceutical Companies *409*
Philippines *323, 352, 353, 354*
Polycystic Kidney Disease *231, 377, 439*
Poverty *43*
Prince Court Medical Center *360*
Pulmonary Arterial Hypertension *234, 377*
Punta Pacifica Hospital *19, 21, 22, 23, 24, 134, 194, 326, 328*
Pyloromyotomy *208, 377, 431*

Q
QHA Accreditation – Trent *291*

R
Radiation Therapy *222, 378, 434*
Rationing *45, 85, 385, 391, 395, 408, 409, 414*
Rehabilitation *185, 246, 247*

Renal Acidosis *378*
Reserve Force Army *69*
Revici Therapy *264, 378*
Rhinoplasty *147, 172, 174, 378, 400, 421*

S
Safety Abroad *128, 140, 290, 301, 303, 313, 314, 357, 383*
Sahel General Hospital *206, 430*
Saudi Arabia *322, 344, 345, 449*
Seoul St. Mary's Hospital *356*
SHA Wellness Clinic *283*
Sime Darby Medical Centre *361*
Singapore *196, 198, 209, 213, 214, 321, 342, 343, 344, 449*
Sinteza Health Centre *200*
Socialized Medicine *30, 406, 407*
South Africa *19, 101, 108, 112, 125, 146, 149, 173, 174, 175, 200, 230, 245, 252, 254, 278, 286, 321, 340, 341, 383, 443, 449*
South America *23, 110, 324, 325*
South Korea *149, 154, 158, 159, 166, 175, 176, 178, 188, 202, 212, 213, 252, 253, 285, 290, 323, 354, 355, 356*
Spain *167, 168, 169, 178, 264, 283, 328, 357, 445*

Spa Retreats *281*
   Day Spa *282*
   Health Spa *281, 284*
   Medical Spa *283, 399, 447*
   Mineral Springs Spa *283, 447*
   Resort Spa *282, 447*
Specialists *88, 200, 386, 389*
Specialist Surgery *200*
Spinal Fusion *202, 378, 401, 430*
Spleen Removal *195, 213, 428*
Starship Children's Health Service *347*
St. Augustine's Hyperbaric Medicine Centre *278, 448*
Stem Cell Treatment *240, 241, 254, 323, 356, 362, 437*
Stimulus Plan *28*
St. Luke's Medical Center *353*

T
Targeted Therapy *223, 434*
Taxes *43, 68, 388, 394, 397, 407, 408*
Teeth Whitening *176, 400*
Thailand *110, 125, 145, 147, 164, 165, 174, 177, 192, 193, 196, 197, 200, 212, 213, 224, 251, 252, 274, 291, 323, 350, 351*
Travel Insurance *100, 304*

U
Unemployment *41, 98, 389, 415*
Universal Healthcare *28*
University Medical Center Freiburg *429*

V
Vascular Surgery *204, 352, 430*

W
Wall Street *48, 49, 385, 389, 391, 392, 409, 414*
Welcare Hospital *337*
Wheatgrass Therapy *262, 379*

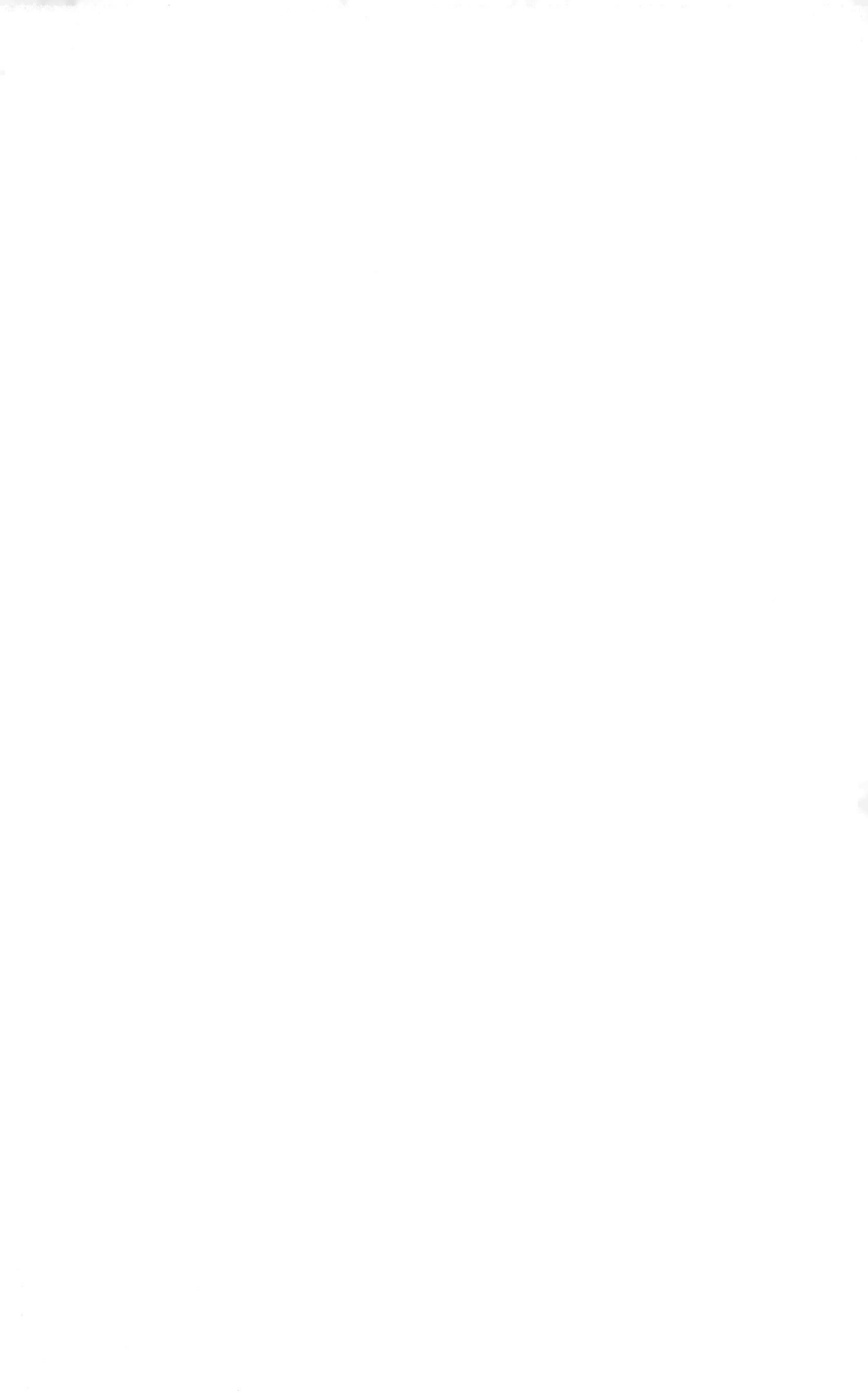